Transesophageal Echocardiography in Pediatric Congenital Cardiac Surgery and Catheter Intervention

Shen-Kou Tsai • Jou-Kou Wang
Shyh-Jye Chen

Transesophageal Echocardiography in Pediatric Congenital Cardiac Surgery and Catheter Intervention

Springer

Shen-Kou Tsai, MD, PhD
Professor, Anesthesiologist
Cheng Hsin General Hospital
Professor of Anesthesiology
School of Medicine
National Taiwan University, and Hospital
Taipei, Taiwan

Shyh-Jye Chen, MD, PhD
Professor and Chairman
Department of Medical Imaging/Center of Radiation Protection
National Taiwan University Hospital
Director, Department of Radiology
School of Medicine
National Taiwan University
Taipei, Taiwan

Jou-Kou Wang, MD, PhD
Professor of Pediatrics, School of Medicine
National Taiwan University
Pediatric Cardiologist
National Taiwan University Hospital
Taipei, Taiwan

ISBN 978-981-99-6584-7 ISBN 978-981-99-6582-3 (eBook)
https://doi.org/10.1007/978-981-99-6582-3

This Springer imprint is published by the registered company Springer Nature Singapore Pte Ltd.
The registered company address is: 152 Beach Road, #21-01/04 Gateway East, Singapore 189721, Singapore

Paper in this product is recyclable

Preface

Over the past 25 years, we have successfully carried out over 3000 surgeries for congenital heart diseases (CHD), over 5000 pediatric catheter interventions and over 10,000 computed tomography (CT) or magnetic resonance imaging (MRI). This book provides a review of our experience using intraoperative transesophageal echocardiography (TEE) in various pediatric surgeries including congenital heart surgeries, catheter interventions, and hybrid surgeries.

TEE monitoring plays a crucial role in providing essential information for the surgeon throughout each procedure. From pre-operative planning to real-time assistance during the surgery, TEE helps confirm intended results and identify any residual lesions that may require additional surgical intervention. Intraoperative TEE can significantly reduce the risk of unintended surgical events (Part I).

Catheter-based interventions and hybrid surgeries are alternative treatments for CHD. By combining TEE with fluoroscopy, the risk of radiation exposure for children can be reduced. TEE images provide important information for preoperative patient selection, guide the entire procedure, and confirm the correct deployment of devices. This book also explores the growing complexity and diversity of CHD catheter interventions (Part II).

To effectively use intraoperative TEE images for monitoring and guidance during a procedure, it is important for the provider to be familiar with current surgical methods and catheter-based procedures. This book presents various CHD surgical methods using actual intraoperative photographs to enhance understanding of how to use TEE images to assess the completeness of the procedure. We also provide pre- and postoperative images, such as cardiac CT, MRI, or 3D reconstructions, to complement TEE images.

This book is both comprehensive and practical, providing well-documented figures that clearly illustrate the complex anatomy of various CHD. This makes it a valuable resource for perioperative management. Transesophageal echocardiography plays a crucial role in providing essential information for perioperative decision-making and fosters effective teamwork among pediatric cardiologists, surgeons, anesthesiologists, radiologists and intensivists by employing a common language.

We would like to express our sincere gratitude to our team of pediatric cardiologists (Hung-Chi Lue, Mei-Hwan Wu), surgeons (Chung-I Chang, Ing-Sh Chiu, Yieh-Sharng Chen Shu Chien Huang), anesthesiologists (Ming-Jiuh Wang, Chi-Hsiang Huang, Su-Man Lin, Ching Huei Ou), and illustrators (Yea-Wen Lee, Yung

Wei Huang). Additionally, we extend our thanks to Dr. Jui-Yu Hsu, a pediatric cardiologist and Dr. Ching Huei Ou, who not only contributed significantly to the preparation of most of the manuscripts but also provided numerous special requests for the production of this book. Their invaluable knowledge, extensive experience, and expertise have been generously shared in this book with the aim of improving healthcare delivery and clinical outcomes

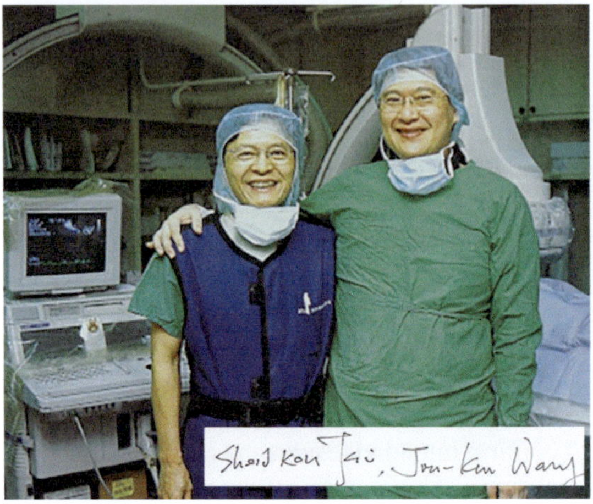

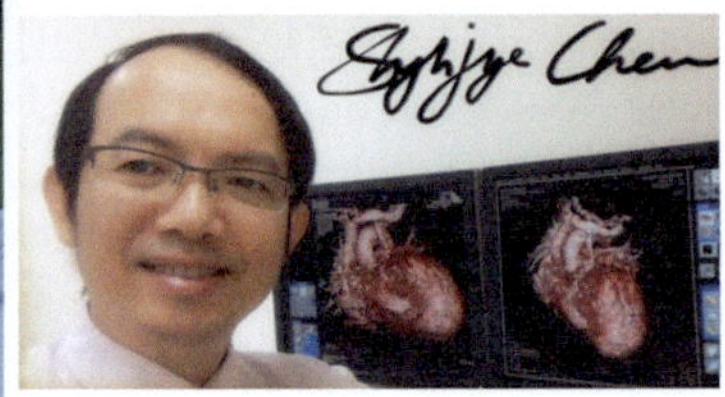

Shen-Kou Tsai
Jou-Kou Wang
Shyh-Jye Chen

Contents

Abbreviations

AAo/AAO	Ascending aorta
ADO II	Amplatzer Duct Occluder II
ADO	Amplatzer Duct Occluder
ALVT	Aorta to left ventricular tunnel
Ao/AO	Aorta
AR	Aortic regurgitation
ASD	Atrial septal defect
ASO	Aterial swith operation
AV	Aortic valve
BAS	Balloon atrial septostomy
C	Catheter
CA	Common atrium
CAVC	Complete atrioventricular canal
ccTGA	Congenitally Corrected TGA
CHD	Congenital heart diseases
CoA	Coractation of aorta
CPB	Cardiopulmonary bypass
CSO	Coronary sinus ostium
CT	Computed tomography
DAo/DAO	Descending aorta
DCRV	Double chambered right ventricle
DILV	Double inlet left ventricle
DIRV	Double inlet right ventricle
DORV	Double outlet right ventricle
ECMO	Extracorporeal Membrane Oxygeneation
HLHS	Hypoplastic left heart syndrome
IA rim	Anterior inferior rim
IAA	Interrupted aortic arch
IAS	Interatrial septum
IP rim	Posterior inferior rim
IVS	Interventricular septum
LA	Left atrium
LAA	Left atrial appendage

LAI	Left atrial isomerism
LAX	Long-axis view
LB	Left bronchus
LCC	Left coronary cusp
LD	Left Disc
LPA	Left pulmonary artery
LV	Left ventricle
LVOT	Left ventricular outflow tract
ME LAX	Mid-esophageal long axis view
ME SAX	Mid-esophageal short axis view
MPR	Multiplanar reformatting
MV	Mitral valve
NCC	Noncoronary cusp
O	Occulder
PA	Pulmonary artery
PAPVC	Partial anomalous pulmonary venous connection
PDA	Patent ductus arteriosus
pmVSD	Perimembranous ventricular septal defect
PV	Pulmonary valve
RA	Right atrium
RAA	Right atrial appendage
RAI	Right atrial isomerism
RB	Right bronchus
RCA	Right coronary artery
RCAA	Right coronary artery aneurysm
RCC	Right coronary cusp
RD	Right Disc
RPA	Right pulmonary artery
RSVA	Ruptured sinus of Valsalva Aneurysm
RUPV	Right upper pulmonary vein
RV	Right ventricle
RVOT	Right ventricular outflow tract
SA rim	Anterior superior rim
SAX	Short-axis view
SP rim	Superior posterior rim
SVASD	Sinus Venous ASD
TA	Tricuspid atresia
TAPVC	Total anomalous pulmonary venous connection
TEE	Transesophageal echocardiography
TG	Transgastric view
TGA	Transposition of the great arteries
TOF	Tetralogy of Fallot
TPV	Transcatheter pulmonary valve

T	Trachea
TrA	Truncus arteriosus
TV	Tricuspid valve
UE LAX	Upper-esophageal long axis view
UE SAX	Upper-esophageal short axis view
VSD	Ventricular septal defect

Part I

Introduction of Transesophageal Echocardiography (TEE) for Pediatric Congenital Heart Diseases

1 Overview of Pediatric Echocardiography

Echocardiography is an imaging method that uses ultrasound waves to visualize the heart's structures and functions. Pediatric echocardiography [1–4] has a history that dates back to the 1950s, when ultrasound imaging was first developed for medical applications. However, it was not until the 1970s that two-dimensional (2D) echocardiography became a widely available diagnostic tool for pediatric use. Dr. Helen Taussig, a renowned pediatric cardiologist known for developing the Blalock-Taussig shunt, recognized the potential of echocardiography as a diagnostic tool and worked with engineers and scientists to create the first pediatric echocardiography machine. Over time, technological advancements led to the development of more sophisticated imaging techniques. Nowadays, pediatric echocardiography [5, 6] is widely used in diagnosing and managing congenital and acquired heart disease in infants and children (as shown in Fig. 1.1).

Transthoracic echocardiography (TTE) is one of the techniques that involves placing a transducer on the chest to create images of the heart from outside the body. The choice of transducer used in pediatric TTE echocardiography depends on the child's age and size. Smaller transducers with higher frequencies are typically used for newborns and young infants to obtain clear images, while larger transducers with low frequency may be required for deeper structures as children grow and their chest size increases.

M-mode echocardiography [7, 8] which is a common mode in TTE was first developed in the 1950s as a diagnostic tool for cardiology. This technique is allowed for the production of high-frequency sound waves that could be focused and directed to produce detailed images of internal structures. Initially, M-mode echocardiography was used to measure the thickness of heart walls and assess cardiac function in adults with heart disease (as shown in Fig. 1.2). Today, M-mode echocardiography is often used in pediatric cardiology to monitor heart function, and assess response to therapy.

S.-K. Tsai et al., *Transesophageal Echocardiography in Pediatric Congenital Cardiac Surgery and Catheter Intervention*, https://doi.org/10.1007/978-981-99-6582-3_1

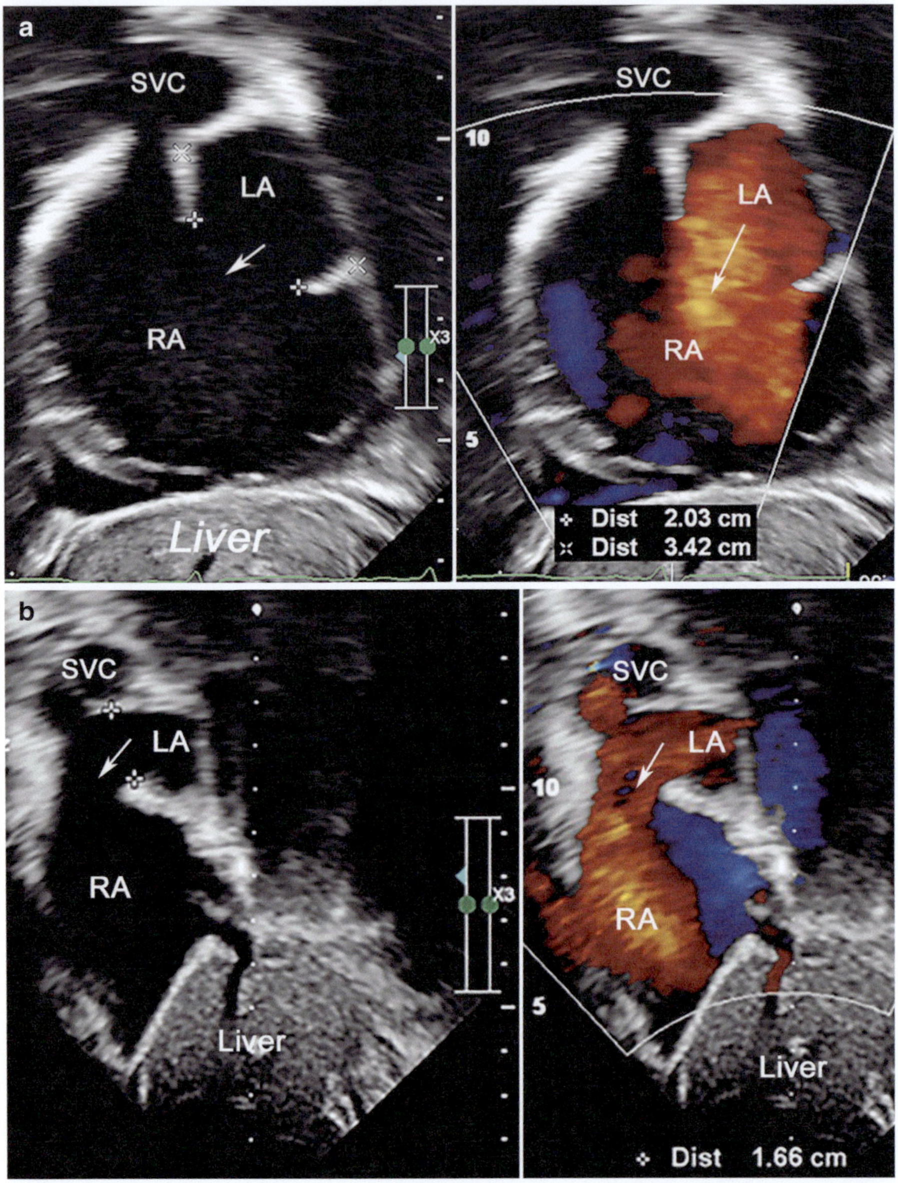

Fig. 1.1 Transthoracic echocardiography (TTE) depicts a secundum atrial septal defect (ASD) and a superior sinus venous ASD in a child. (**a**) A TTE taken from the subxiphoid short-axis view displays a large secundum atrial septal defect (ASD) measuring 2.03 cm in diameter. The right diagram, using color Doppler, demonstrates a left-to-right shunt. (**b**) A TTE taken from the subxiphoid short-axis view reveals that blood flow drains from the superior vena cava (SVC) into the left atrium (LA), indicating a superior sinus venous atrial septal defect (ASD) measuring 1.66 cm in diameter. The right diagram, using color Doppler, demonstrates a left-to-right shunt

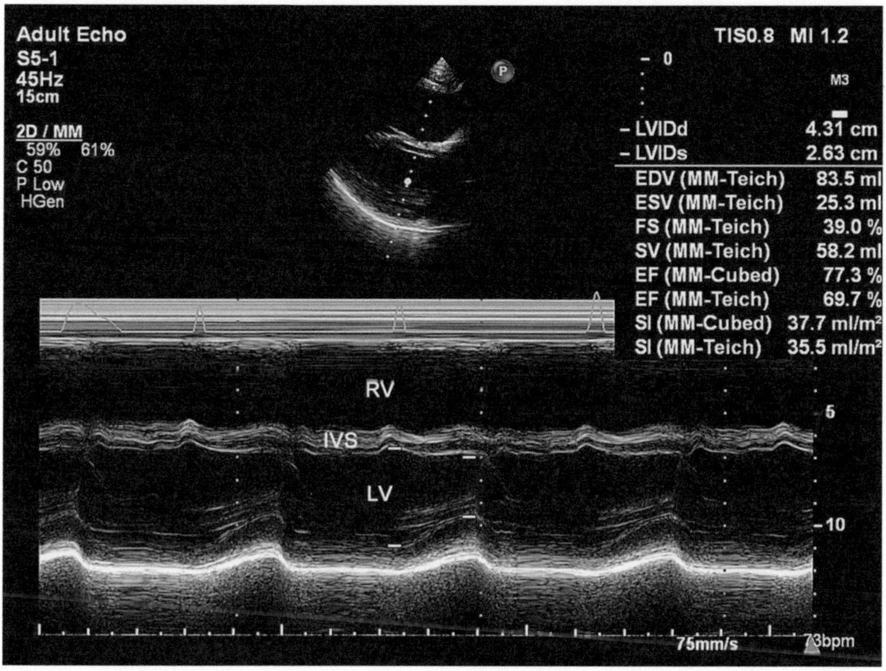

Fig. 1.2 Depicts an M-mode echocardiogram image that illustrates right ventricular volume overload in a child who has undergone surgery for tetralogy of Fallot, with severe pulmonary regurgitation. The image demonstrates paradoxical motion, which indicates dilation of the right ventricle

Color Doppler echocardiography [9, 10], which utilizes Doppler technology to generate a color-coded image of blood flow and velocities, was initially introduced in the mid-1980s. This technology enabled a more in-depth assessment of blood flow patterns and velocities in the heart and surrounding vessels (as shown in Fig. 1.1 right diagram). Nowadays, it is a fundamental component of most echocardiography systems.

The development of intracardiac echocardiography (ICE) technology began in the 1980s, and the first clinical applications of ICE were reported in the early 1990s. This technology involves the insertion of a small ultrasound probe into the heart through a catheter sheath, typically introduced from the femoral vein into the right atrium. Once the probe is inside the heart, it provides high-resolution real-time images of the heart structures (as depicted in Fig. 1.3). ICE [11, 12] has emerged as a crucial tool in the diagnosis and management of various cardiac conditions, including arrhythmias, valvular heart disease, and congenital heart defects (as shown in Fig. 1.3).

Transesophageal echocardiography (TEE) is another kind of echocardiography that is performed by passing a flexible probe (transducer) through the mouth and into the esophagus, which is located behind the heart. The transducer emits

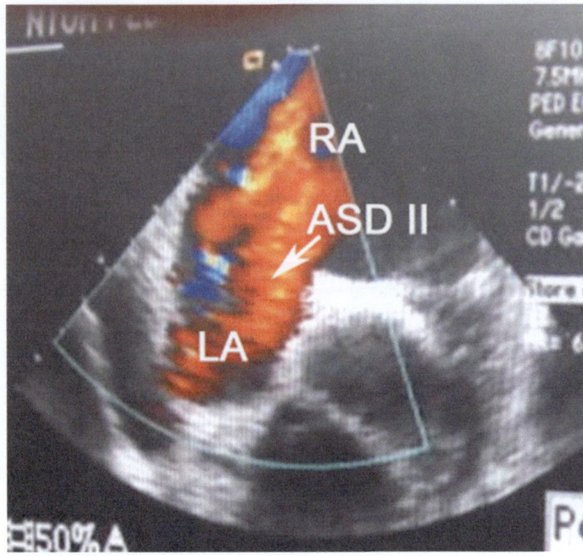

Fig. 1.3 Demonstrates the use of intracardiac echocardiography (ICE) for detecting a secundum atrial septal defect (ASD II). The color Doppler image shows a left-to-right shunt during the transcatheter closure of the ASD

ultrasound waves that bounce back from the heart and are then converted into images that can be viewed on a monitor. TEE may provide a more detailed view of the heart than TTE and will be further discussed in Chap. 2.

The inception of 3D echocardiography [13–15] dates back to the 1970s, with its first clinical application in adults reported in 1974. Nevertheless, it was not until the 1990s that 3D echocardiography became commercially available and commonly used in clinical practice (as shown in Fig. 1.4).

4D echocardiography [16, 17], which includes the time dimension in 3D images, was developed in the 2000s. These advanced imaging techniques offer more intricate information on the structures and functions of the heart than conventional 2D echocardiography, and they are especially helpful in visualizing complex cardiac structures (as shown in Figs. 8.34b1 and 9.4).

Advancements in pediatric cardiac imaging have posed significant challenges due to the intricate nature of pediatric heart disease and its growth-related impact. However, the use of artificial intelligence [18, 19] (AI) in pediatric echocardiography has the potential to enhance the quality, interpretation, and clinical application of echocardiographic data for sonographers, echocardiographers, and clinicians. The echocardiogram is the primary imaging modality utilized by cardiologists. With AI in medical imaging, we can expand the usefulness of cardiac ultrasounds beyond their immediate observations, uncovering previously undetected patterns and enabling more accurate and efficient diagnoses.

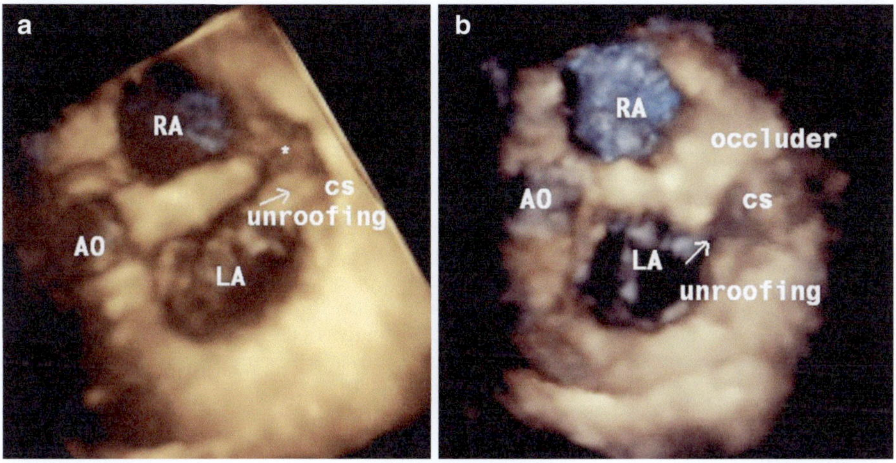

Fig. 1.4 Shows a three-dimensional (3D) echocardiogram of an unroofed coronary sinus (CS) atrial septal defect (ASD) in a 5-year-old child who underwent transcatheter closure using an occluder. (**a**) En face views of the atrium and aorta were obtained using 3D full volume cropping with Philips QLab. The images clearly show a defect between the coronary sinus (CS) and the left atrium (LA). A star indicated the ostium of the CS. (**b**) Successful transcatheter closure of the ostium of CS using an occluder was demonstrated

References

1. Kulkarni SS, Griffin BP. Pediatric echocardiography: a historical perspective. Echocardiography. 2017;34(12):1808–16.
2. Schilling WH, Nield LS. History of echocardiography in children. J Card Fail. 2016;22:544–6.
3. Garg VK, Saxena S. Pediatric echocardiography: a journey through time. Indian Pediatr. 2018;55(4):295–301.
4. Lu L, Penny DJ, Mahle WT. Pediatric echocardiography: historical perspectives and future directions. J Am Soc Echocardiogr. 2016;29(11):1021–9.
5. Lai WW, Geva T, Shirali GS, et al. Guidelines and standards for performance of a pediatric echocardiogram: a report from the Task Force of the Pediatric Council of the American Society of Echocardiography. J Am Soc Echocardiogr. 2006;19(12):1413–30.
6. Lopez L, Colan SD, Frommelt PC, et al. Recommendations for quantification methods during the performance of a pediatric echocardiogram: a report from the Pediatric Measurements Writing Group of the American Society of Echocardiography Pediatric and Congenital Heart Disease Council. J Am Soc Echocardiogr. 2010;23(5):465–95.
7. Nagueh SF, Kopelen HA, Zoghbi WA. Relation of mean right atrial pressure to echocardiographic and Doppler parameters of right atrial and right ventricular function. Circulation. 1996;93(8):1160–9.
8. Lopez L, Colan SD, Frommelt PC, Ensing GJ, Kendall K, Younoszai AK, Lai WW, Geva T. Recommendations for quantification methods during the performance of a pediatric echocardiogram: a report from the Pediatric Measurements Writing Group of the American Society of Echocardiography Pediatric and Congenital Heart Disease Council. J Am Soc Echocardiogr. 2010;23(5):465–95.

9. Huhta JC. Color Doppler in pediatric echocardiography. Pediatr Cardiol. 2019;11(4):199–203.
10. Reller MD, Thornburg KL. Color Doppler echocardiography in infants and children. Am J Cardiol. 1990;66(16):1249–54.
11. Sacher F, Scherr D. Intracardiac echocardiography in electrophysiology: a review of current applications and future directions. J Interv Card Electrophysiol. 2017;49(2):157–67.
12. Hung J, Lang RM. Intracardiac echocardiography: state of the art. J Am Soc Echocardiogr. 2019;32(3):340–55.
13. Friedberg MK, Silverman NH. Three-dimensional echocardiography in congenital heart disease: an expert consensus document from the European Association of Cardiovascular Imaging and the American Society of Echocardiography. J Am Soc Echocardiogr. 2016;29(8):1–26.
14. Lang RM, Badano LP, Tsang W, et al. EAE/ASE recommendations for image acquisition and display using three-dimensional echocardiography. J Am Soc Echocardiogr. 2012;25(1):3–46.
15. Haeck ML, Scherptong RW, Marsan NA, et al. Usefulness of three-dimensional speckle tracking echocardiography for the evaluation of right ventricular function in patients with pulmonary hypertension. Am J Cardiol. 2012;109(8):1144–50.
16. Liang HY, Cui H, Li QL, Li Z, Li L. Four-dimensional echocardiography in the diagnosis and evaluation of congenital heart disease: a systematic review. Echocardiography. 2017;34(4):557–64.
17. Yared K, Noseworthy P, Weyman AE, et al. Four-dimensional echocardiography: the future or already a reality? J Am Soc Echocardiogr. 2019;32(7):844–56.
18. Nguyen MB, Villemain O, Friedberg MK, et al. Artificial intelligence in the pediatric echocardiography laboratory: automation, physiology, and outcomes. Front Radiol. 2022;2:1–13.
19. Quer G, Arnaout R, Henne M, Arnaout R. Machine learning and the future of cardiovascular care: JACC state-of-the-art review. J Am Coll Cardiol. 2021;77:300–13.

Transesophageal Echocardiography (TEE) for Pediatric Congenital Cardiac Surgery and Catheter Intervention

2

2.1 The History and Development of Pediatric TEE

Pediatric transesophageal echocardiography (TEE) has been developed since the 1990s [1, 2] (Fig. 2.1) and was initially used for critical care in adults. As technology of TEE advanced and its benefits became more apparent, it was extended to use in pediatric patients. Its usefulness in improving outcomes in cardiac surgery has been extensively documented [3, 4] (Fig. 2.2), and it is now also used as a navigation tool during interventional procedures for CHDs [5, 6] (Fig. 2.3). This has made TEE an important tool in the diagnosis and treatment of CHDs. However, it is important to understand the anatomy, techniques, indications, contraindications, and risks associated with TEE usage in pediatric patients, since it is a semi-invasive diagnostic modality. In children, the insertion and manipulation of the ultrasound probe during TEE may result in esophageal or gastric trauma, respiratory impairment, or vascular compression. Therefore, comprehensive multiplane TEE examinations should be performed following guidelines and standards set from the American Society of Echocardiography and the Society of Cardiovascular Anesthesiologists [7, 8].

2.1.1 The Evolutionary Development of Pediatric TEE Transducers

The development of TEE probes for children has been a gradual process that has taken place over several decades. The first TEE probe was reported in 1976 by Frazin [9], but it was primitive and consisted of a single M-mode crystal probe attached to a rigid endoscope. As TEE became more commonly used in pediatric

S.-K. Tsai et al., *Transesophageal Echocardiography in Pediatric Congenital Cardiac Surgery and Catheter Intervention*, https://doi.org/10.1007/978-981-99-6582-3_2

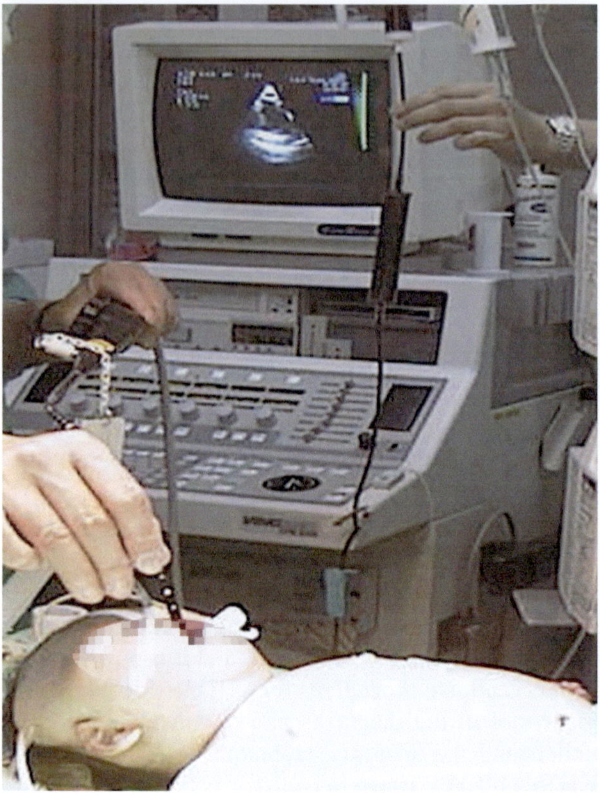

Fig. 2.1 Depicts a baby undergoing transesophageal echocardiography (TEE) monitoring for congenital heart disease (CHD) surgery. During this procedure, a pediatric TEE probe is inserted into the baby's esophagus and connected to an ultrasound machine (GE Vingmed CFM 800 ultrasound, Norway) under nasal endotracheal anesthesia. To facilitate probe insertion and minimize interference with TEE imaging, the baby's head is positioned in the midline and slightly flexed. Before the procedure, nasogastric or feeding tubes are removed, and lubricating jelly can be used, although excessive force should be avoided. To minimize the risk of complications, hemodynamic changes such as blood pressure, pulse rate, and oxygenation are closely monitored. Following the procedure, the TEE probe should be properly cleaned with glutaraldehyde to reduce the risk of infection

patients, there was a growing need for smaller and more flexible probes. In 1988, Omoto [10] improved TEE technology by creating a single-plane phased array with 24 elements, which was more suitable for pediatric use, with a frequency of 5 Hz and a diameter of 6.8 mm. Over the years, transducers have been miniaturized, and advancements in phased array ultrasound technology have led to the development of smaller and more flexible probes that offer higher resolution imaging. These probes

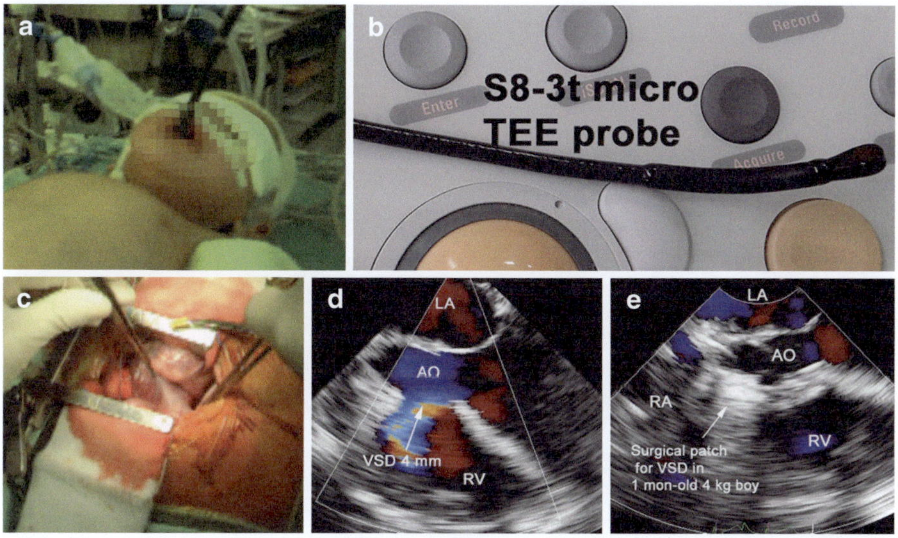

Fig. 2.2 Intraoperative TEE in an infant undergoing VSD Repair. (**a**) An operative photograph shows the insertion of a TEE probe into the esophagus of the infant. (**b**) A diagram of the TEE probe used during the procedure, the S8-3t Philips microTEE transducer. (**c**) An intraoperative photograph showing the infant undergoing heart surgery. (**d**) Preoperative TEE imaging in color displays a 4 mm diameter ventricular septal defect (VSD) with left-to-right shunting, as seen in the five-chamber view. (**e**) Postoperative TEE imaging in the five-chamber view shows complete closure of the VSD using a patch

are now available in a range of sizes and shapes, including miniaturized probes for use in neonates and infants (Figs. 2.4 and 2.5b). Furthermore, with advancements in phased array ultrasound technology and miniaturized crystals, TEE technology has rapidly evolved. Consequently, it now offers 3D real-time imaging [11] (Fig. 2.4), enabling more accurate visualization of cardiac structures.

2.1.2 The Current TEE Transducer for Infants in Pediatrics

The diameter of the esophagus in neonates, children, and adolescents varies as a function of weight. In a 3 kg child, the diameter of the esophagus ranges from 4.8 to 8.48 mm, with a variation range of 1.5 to 2 mm [12]. The recommended mean maximal diameter of the esophagus based on age [13] and weight [14] is displayed in Fig. 2.5a, and the corresponding size of TEE probes is shown in Fig. 2.5b. The GE Vingmed multiplane and Philips mini-multilane transducer can be used in newborns weighing 3.5 kg, while the Philips microTEE probe can be used in premature infants weighing 2.5 kg.

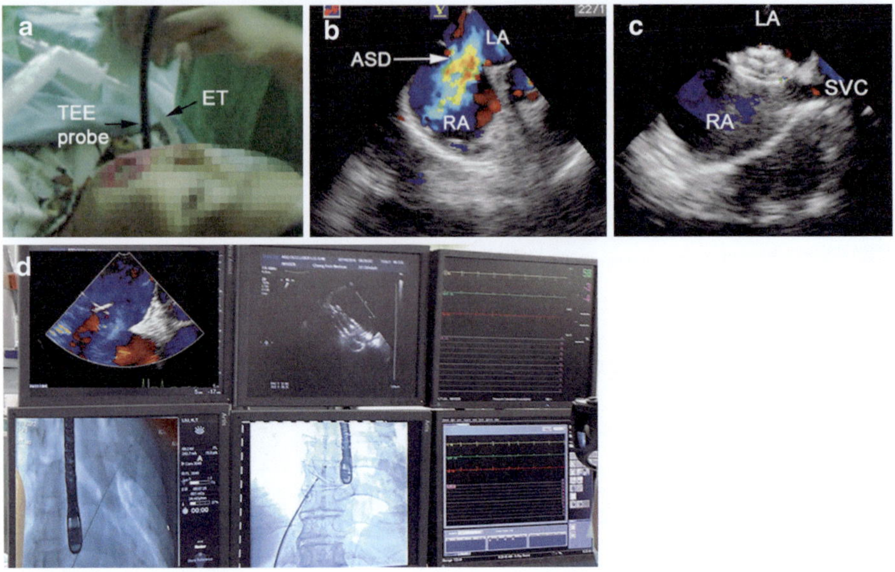

Fig. 2.3 TEE during pediatric interventional procedure (detailed discussion to follow in Part II). (**a**) During transcatheter closure under an endotracheal general anesthesia, a TEE probe, with a bite guard in place, is inserted into the esophagus of a child with an atrial septal defect (ASD). (**b**) Preprocedural color TEE imaging shows a large ASD between the left and right atria with a left-to-right shunting. (**c**) "Postprocedural color TEE imaging displays successful deployment of the Amplatzer Septal Occluder device, without residual shunting, as seen in the bicaval view. (**d**) A photograph captures the multichannel monitoring during the interventional procedure, including TEE imaging, fluoroscopy imaging, and hemodynamic data"

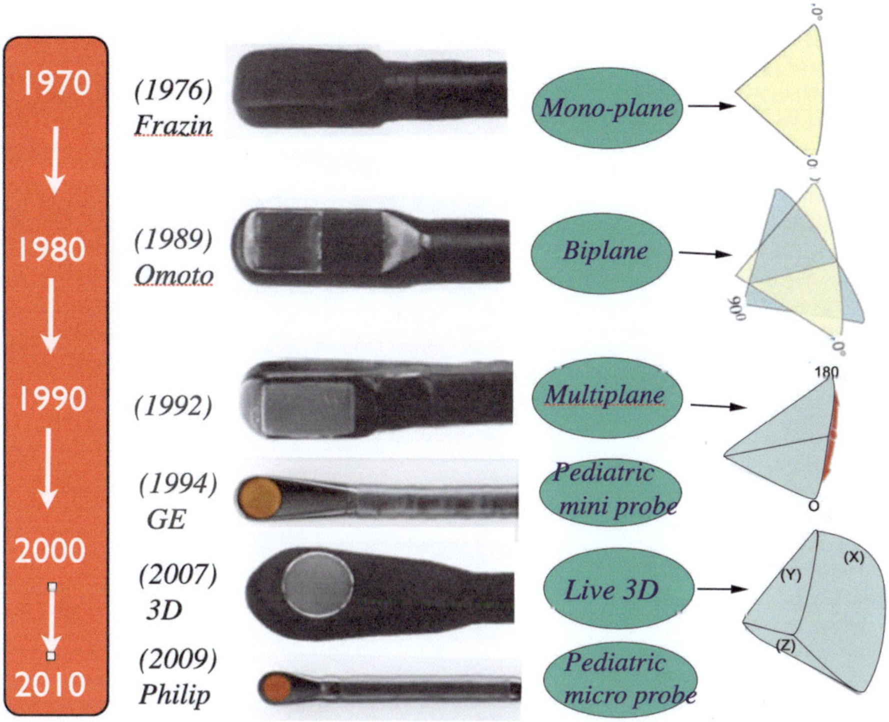

Fig. 2.4 Displays the various commercially available transesophageal echocardiography (TEE) probes that have been developed over time. The probes include: (1) Monoplane (single plane) TEE probe with a linear array transducer, which provides a single image of the heart (2). Biplane TEE probe with separate transducer arrays, which combines transverse and longitudinal axis images to provide a more comprehensive view of the heart. (3) Multiplane TEE probe, which comprises a linear phased array of 64–128 piezoelectric crystals arranged in a circular pattern to provide continuous visualization of the cardiac anatomy. This probe can be electronically or manually steered to produce images from various angles. (4) Live 3D TEE probe (matrix array probe), which consists of 2500 piezoelectric crystals that allow for volume scanning and acquisition of raw 3D data for processing and image display. The 3D TEE probe provides accurate evaluation of the cardiac anatomy and ventricular function. (5) Until recently, the smallest pediatric TEE probe with multiplane imaging was 7.5–10.8 mm in diameter, making it suitable for use in small babies

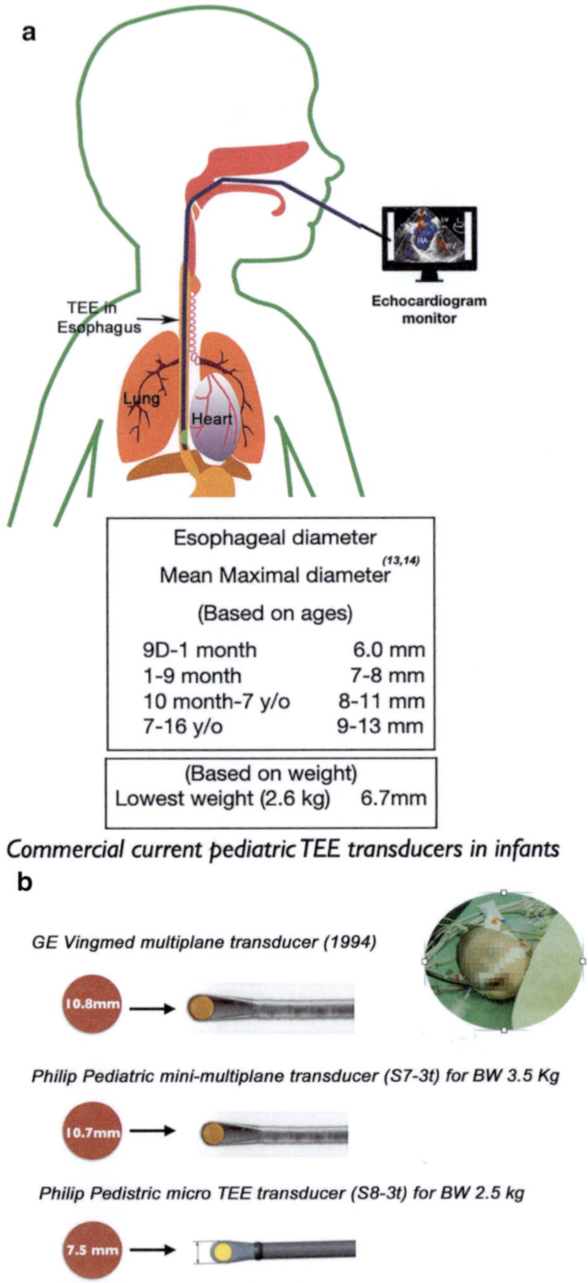

Fig. 2.5 (**a**) The upper diagram shows the basic principle of pediatric transesophageal echocardiography (TEE). This technique uses ultrasound waves to scan the heart, creating images that are displayed on a monitoring screen for children. The lower diagram displays the mean diameter of the esophagus at the cranial point of measurement, based on age and weight, respectively [13, 14]. (**b**) The safety and efficacy of using pediatric transesophageal echocardiography (TEE) probes, with a diameter ranging from 7.5 to 10.8 mm, have been extensively studied and proven for use in infants, including premature babies weighing as little as 2.5 kg. Clinical utilization of these probes, as shown in the upper right diagram, provides a valuable tool for evaluating various congenital heart conditions

2.2 Indication of TEE

TEE is considered as the most sensitive method for evaluating cardiac structures and function. The most common indications for TEE include the evaluation of cardiac emboli or masses, endocarditis, valvular dysfunction, and aortic aneurysms. Furthermore, TEE is not only used as a diagnostic tool, but also as a monitoring tool during cardiac surgery or percutaneous procedures. In this chapter, our focus is specifically on the use of intraoperative TEE for monitoring congenital heart disease surgeries and guiding intervention procedures.

2.2.1 Indication of the Pediatric TEE Monitoring of Congenital Heart Surgery

The use of Intraoperative TEE helps confirm the preoperative diagnosis and can alter the surgical plan if hidden or additional findings are uncovered during the procedures. These changes may occur inside the operating room. Intraoperative TEE is used to ensure that the heart is de-aired before separation from cardiopulmonary bypass (CPB) and to identify any new or residual surgical lesions after CPB, which may require a second run or early surgical revision (Fig. 2.2).

2.2.2 Pediatric TEE Guidance of Cardiac Catheter Intervention

Up to 40% of congenital heart diseases (CHD) can be treated with transcatheter procedures. TEE can facilitate these procedures by combining with fluoroscopy and reduce radiation exposure for both patients and personnel in the catheter room. The use of TEE in CHD interventions is aimed at enhancing the safety and efficacy of the treatment. TEE serves several important functions, including:

1. Patient Selection by Providing Imaging Information to Determine Suitability for the Procedure
2. Assessment of the Morphology and Characteristics of the Defects, Including the Size, Number, and Relationship to Valves and Surrounding Vessels
3. Guiding Device Positioning, Deployment, and Successful Anchoring to Tissue
4. Monitoring Residual Effects and Assessing the Impact on Valvular Function and Surrounding Vessels
5. Early Detection of Complications Related to Catheter Procedures (Fig. 2.3)

2.3 Fundamental Aspect of Pediatric TEE

The fundamentals of pediatric TEE involve inserting a probe with a transducer into the esophagus to create a computerized image of the heart in motion. This is achieved by using ultrasound or high-frequency sound waves, which reflect off the heart to produce real-time images on the monitoring screen. The TEE also provides a means of monitoring the heart's function. TEE provides a clearer image of the heart compared to a transthoracic echocardiogram (TTE) as it avoids interference from the chest wall, ribs, and lungs, allowing for more accurate imaging (Figs. 2.5a and 2.6). According to the ACE Guidelines and standards [7, 8, 15], pediatric TEE probes are limited to anteflexion and retroflexion, without the ability to flex right or left.

2.3.1 Key Views in Pediatric TEE Imaging

The basic TEE imaging examination can be performed at three key perspectives: the mid-esophageal (ME) view (Fig. 2.7), the upper-esophageal (UE) view (Fig. 2.8), and the transgastric view (Fig. 2.9).

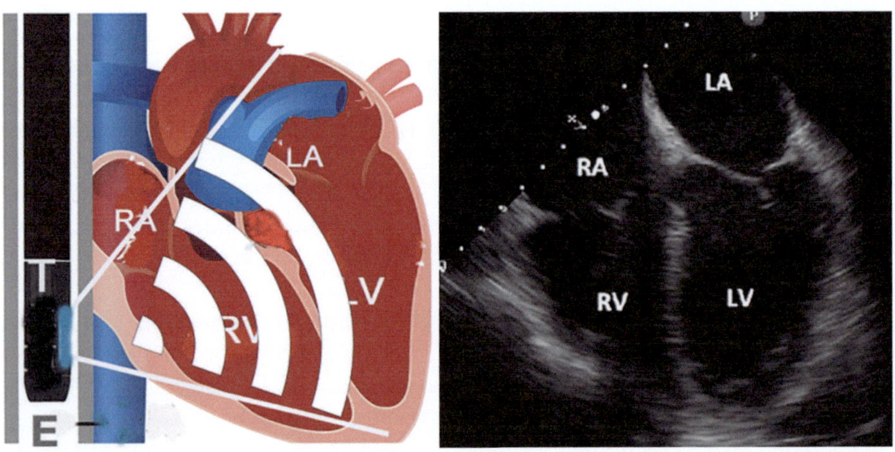

Fig. 2.6 Illustrates the application of transesophageal echocardiography (TEE). The TEE probe (T) is inserted into the esophagus (E) (left diagram) and sends ultrasound waves that reflect off the heart. These waves produce real-time images of the cardiac structure and provide a clear and detailed image of the heart's anatomy and function, which can be viewed on the monitor (right diagram). Therefore, variations in the images of cardiac structures are anticipated when the TEE probe is positioned in different regions of the esophagus

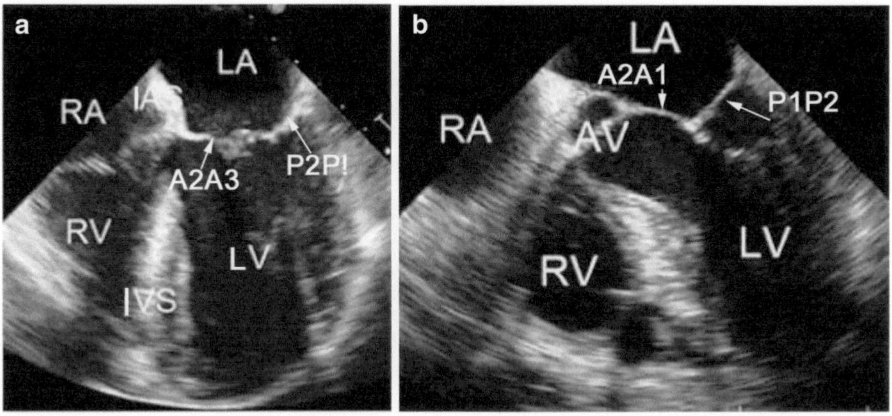

Fig. 2.7 The middle-esophageal (ME) transesophageal echocardiography (TEE) view is obtained by positioning the TEE probe in the middle part of the esophagus, which is located just behind the heart and aorta. The ME view is used to obtain detailed images of the aorta and its surrounding structures, including the atria, ventricles, and great vessels. The ME TEE view is often used to diagnose and monitor a variety of cardiac conditions, including valvular heart disease, endocarditis, and congenital heart diseases. (**a**) TEE examination in the mid-esophageal (ME) four-chamber view, with the transducer angled at 0° degrees, provides a clear visualization of the following structures: the right atrium (RA), left atrium (LA), right ventricle (RV), left ventricle (LV), interatrial septum (IAS), interventricular septum (IVS), and mitral valve (MV) scallops (A2 and A3, P2 and P1). The function of this view is to provide a detailed and accurate evaluation of the heart's four chambers, enabling the detection and assessment of any abnormalities or issues that may affect their function. (**b**) The five-chamber view with the transducer angled at 0° degrees provides a clear visualization of the following structures: the aortic valve (AV), left ventricular outflow tract (LVOT), RA, LA, RV, LV, interatrial septum (IAS), IVS, and MV scallops (A2 and A1, P1 and P2). (**c**) The aortic valve short-axis (AV SAX) view, with the transducer angled between 0° and 45° degrees, provides a clear visualization of the following structures: the aortic valve (right coronary cusp (RCC), left coronary cusp (LCC), noncoronary cusp (NCC)), right ventricular outflow tract (RVOT), pulmonary artery (PA), RA, LA, RV, IAS, and IVS. The MEAV SAX view provides a clear and detailed view of the AV, enabling the evaluation of its structure and function, including the presence and severity of aortic stenosis, aortic regurgitation, atrial and ventricular septal defects, or other abnormalities. (**d**) The two-chamber view, also known as the bicommissural view, with the transducer angled between 80° and 90° degrees, provides a clear visualization of the following structures: the LA, LV, left atrial appendage (LAA), and MV scallops (P3, A2, and P1). This view is particularly important in guiding procedures related to the MV. (A indicates anterior, B indicates posterior). (**e**) The aortic valve long-axis (AV LAX) view, with the transducer angled between 90° and 120° degrees, provides a clear visualization of the following structures: the LA, left ventricular outflow tract (LVOT), AV, proximal ascending aorta (AAo), RV, and MV scallops (P2 and A2). This view is useful for evaluating the anatomy and function of the aortic valve, mitral valve, and the left side of the heart. (**f**) The bicaval view, with the transducer angled between 90° and 120° degrees, provides a clear visualization of the following structures: the RA, LA, superior vena cava (SVC), inferior vena cava (IVC), and IAS. This view is useful for evaluating the anatomy and function of the right-side heart chambers and the major veins that drain blood into the RA. (For the abbreviations, please refer to Part IV Appendix)

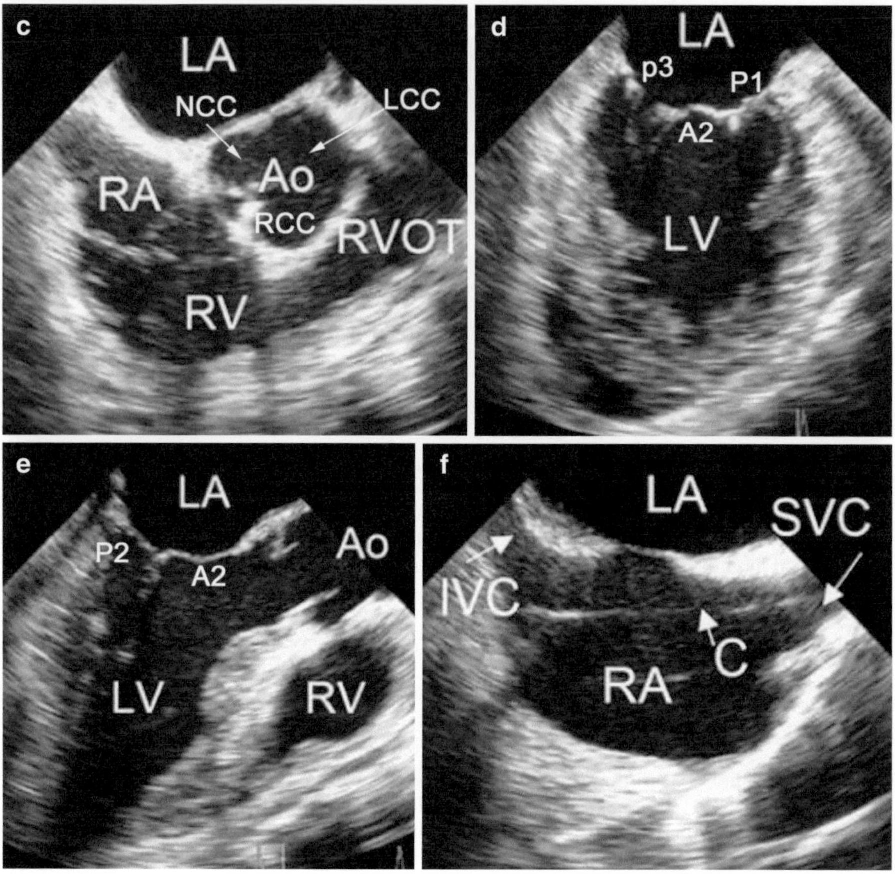

Fig. 2.7 (continued)

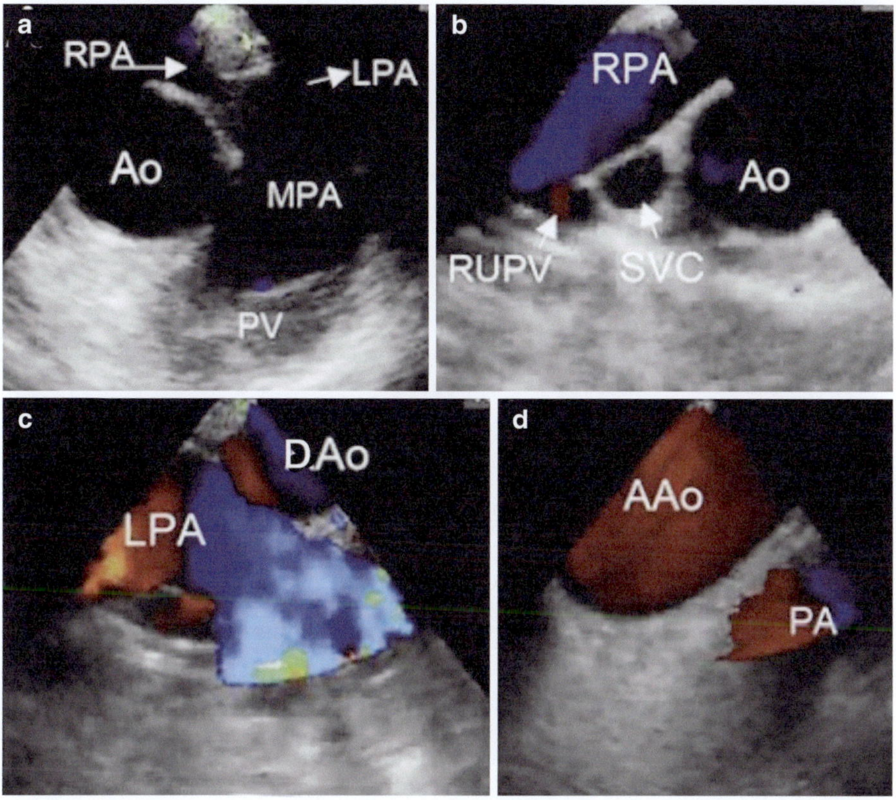

Fig. 2.8 The upper-esophageal (UE) transesophageal echocardiography (TEE) view is used to visualize the structures above the heart, such as the great vessels, the aortic arch, and the superior vena cava. The UE TEE view can help diagnose conditions such as aortic stenosis, aortic dissection, and pulmonary embolism, pulmonary stenosis, among others. (**a**) The PA view (with a transducer angle of 20°) displays the main pulmonary artery (PA), right PA, left PA, and mid-ascending aorta (AAo). (**b**) The RPA view (with a transducer angle of 20°) displays the descending aorta (DAo), superior vena cava (SVC), right upper pulmonary vein (RUPV), and RPA. (**c**) The DAo view (with a transducer angle of 20°) displays the DAo and LPA. (**d**) The AAo view (with a transducer angle of 20°) displays the AAo and PA

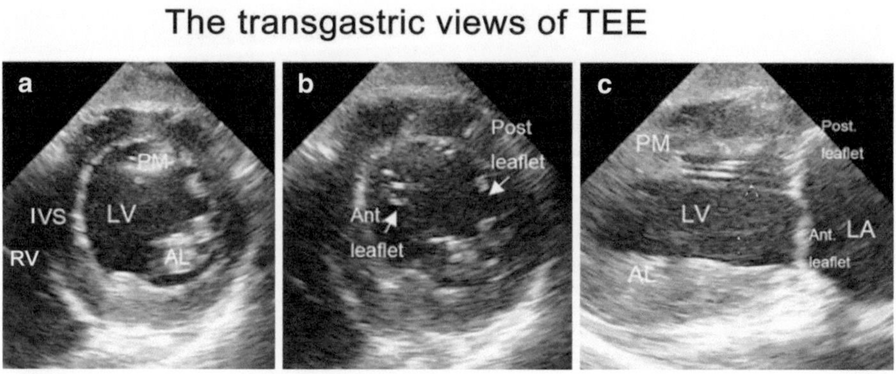

Fig. 2.9 TEE examination of transgastric (TG) view. (**a**) The TG mid SAX view displays the middle left ventricle (LV), middle right ventricle (RV), interventricular septum (IVS), posterior medial papillary muscle (PM), and anterior lateral papillary muscle (AL). (**b**) The basal SAX view illustrates the scallops of mitral valve (MV) (anterior/posterior leaflets). (**c**) The TG LAX view (with the transducer angle set at 120°) shows the left atrium (LA), LV, MV, and PM and AL

2.3.1.1 Additional Left Paracarinal View for Visualizing Left Pulmonary Artery (LPA)

Furthermore, the TEE imaging of the proximal left pulmonary artery (LPA) is hindered by a "blind spot" caused by the interposition of the left bronchus between the proximal LPA and the esophagus, resulting from air blockage (Fig. 2.10a–c). At the carinal (C) level, however, the esophagus is positioned dorsally to the left edge of the carina, between the carina and the descending aorta (Fig. 2.10d). By using the left paracarinal transverse view [16], this limitation can be overcome and the proximal LPA can be clearly seen, which is crucial for diagnostic purposes in cases of patent ductus arteriosus (PDA) or for its repair through surgery or transcatheter closure (Fig. 2.10d, e).

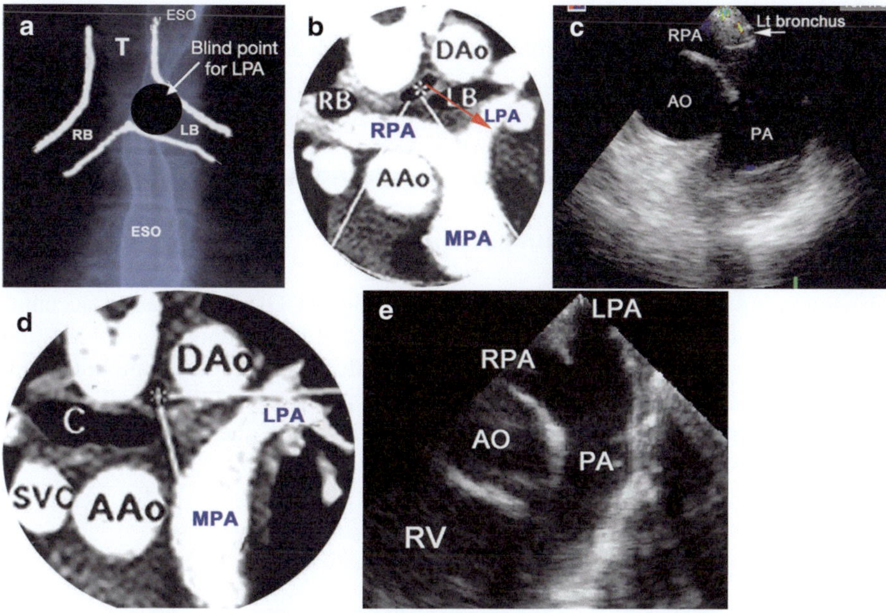

Fig. 2.10 Shows a left paracarinal view for visualizing the left pulmonary artery (LPA). The image provides a clear representation of the left pulmonary artery, allowing for accurate assessment and diagnosis. (**a**) An esophagogram reveals that the left bronchus (LB) lies in front of the esophagus (ESO) at the upper portion, causing a blind point in the ability of the TEE probe to visualize the LPA from the esophagus. (**b**) Cardiac CT image. The red arrow indicates the left bronchus (LB) which creates a blind spot between the esophagus (*) and the left pulmonary artery (LPA), hindering the visualization of the latter. On the other hand, the right pulmonary artery (RPA) can be distinguished clearly from the esophagus. (**c**) The standard view of the LPA at the upper esophagus is obstructed by the left bronchus. (**d**) Cardiac CT at the level of the carina (C) demonstrates the esophagus (*) located dorsally to the left edge of the carina and between the carina and the descending aorta (DAO). In this left paracarinal view, the LPA can be delineated from the esophagus. (**e**) TEE image of the UE AAo SAX view reveals that the left pulmonary artery (LPA) can be delineated by avoiding the left bronchus (LB) through the use of the left paracarinal transverse view

2.4 Safety and Effectiveness of Pediatric TEE

While pediatric TEE plays a significant role in CHD surgery and catheter interventions, it is considered semi-invasive, particularly in pediatric patients, nonetheless it is safer compared to other diagnostic techniques. Consequently, the insertion and handling of the ultrasound probe during the procedure can result in related injuries to the gastroesophageal system, as well as potential compromise to the cardiovascular and respiratory systems. Despite the rarity of such complications, they can be fatal if not prevented or promptly treated. To minimize the risk, it is essential to employ strategies for the prevention of these complications. Comprehensive multiplane TEE examinations are performed according to guidelines established by the American Society of Echocardiography (ASE) and the Society of Cardiovascular Anesthesiologists (SCA) [7, 8].

2.5 Potential Complications Associated with Pediatric TEE

2.5.1 Gastrointestinal Injury

TEE injury is a consistent major upper gastrointestinal (UGI) complication, accounting for 1.2% of such cases [17]. Hematoma (Fig. 2.11a), bleeding (Fig. 2.11b), and perforation [18] are possible esophageal injuries that are due to the small diameter of the esophagus in pediatric patients, particularly when using TEE. Small children, especially, may experience injury from improper insertion, inexperience, or hastily

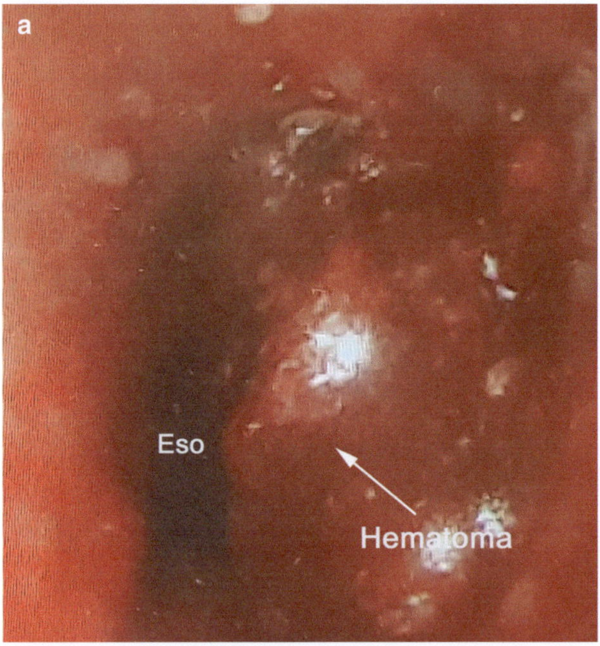

Fig. 2.11 (**a**) A patient-reported difficulty swallowing after undergoing cardiac surgery. Upon examination via panendoscopy, a large hematoma was discovered in the lower esophageal area (Eso). (**b**) Shows a 4-year-old female patient with tetralogy of Fallot who underwent surgical repair. Postsurgery, persistent esophageal bleeding was observed, and panendoscopy revealed erosion and bleeding lesions at the gastroesophageal junction (GEJ) (indicated by arrows in the two upper diagrams). Hemostasis was achieved by applying two hemoclips (H) in the two lower diagrams

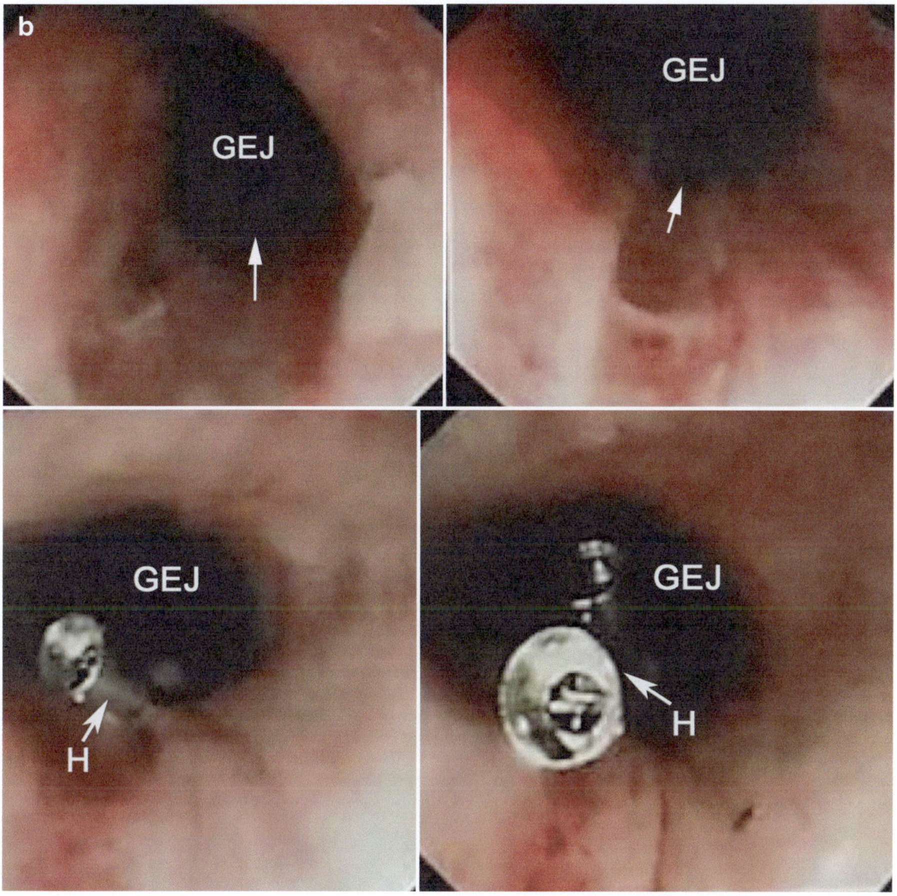

Fig. 2.11 (continued)

withdrawn TEE probe. Additionally, peptic ulcer or gastroesophageal reflux can cause inflammation or bleeding in the esophagus, particularly during heparization in cardiopulmonary bypass. The contributing factors to TEE-related esophageal injury may be due to prolonged flexion of the probe or mobilization in a locked position, particularly during prolonged cardiopulmonary bypass with nonpulsatile flow or excessive heat, which can lead to ischemic esophageal injury.

2.5.2 Airway Compression

Compression of the trachea or bronchial tree can obstruct ventilation.

1. Patients with congenital heart conditions, such as tetralogy of Fallot (TOF) or pulmonary atresia, have a high rate of tracheobronchomalacia (as shown in

Fig. 2.12), which is easily compressed by the rigid TEE probe in the esophagus, leading to airway obstruction.

2. An aneurysm in the pulmonary artery due to tetralogy of Fallot with an absent pulmonary valve can also result in tracheal and esophagus compression (as shown in Fig. 2.12a).
3. In infants with a double aortic arch or a left pulmonary sling, tracheal stenosis may occur near the carina, away from the tip of the endotracheal tube. If necessary, intubating only one lung which can relieve such atypical airway obstruction is recommended (as shown in Fig. 2.12b).
4. Children with congenital heart disease (CHD) have a higher incidence of tracheobronchial anomalies [19] (as stated in Fig. 2.12c). These anomalies, combined with extrinsic compression or an undiagnosed condition, can result in significant perioperative morbidity. Physicians should be vigilant for signs of cardiorespiratory compromise and take prompt action when necessary.

   It is important to note that if airway obstruction occurs after the insertion of a TEE probe, the probe should be immediately removed.

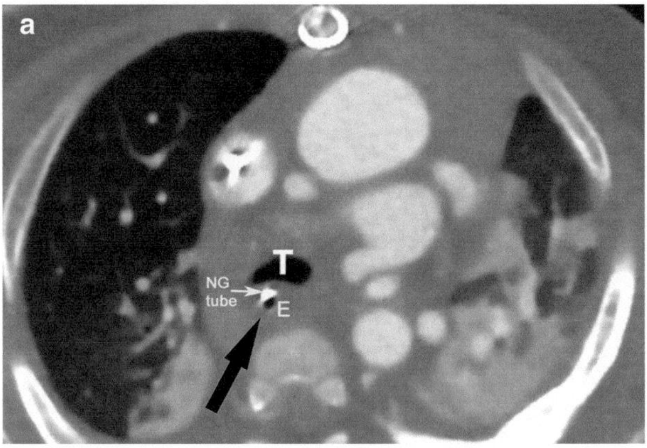

Fig. 2.12 (**a**) Contrast-enhanced cardiac CT image displayed by a lung window shows a nasogastric (NG) tube compresses on the ventral membranous portion of the trachea (T) (black arrow) in a 4-month-old male infant with diagnosed as tetralogy of Fallot (TOF) with tracheomalacia. (**b–b2**) Depicts a 7-month-old child with TOF and an absent pulmonary valve (PV) before surgical repair. The multislice CT reconstruction shows a large right pulmonary artery (RPA) aneurysm compressing the carina, right bronchus (arrows in **b** and **b1**), and esophagus, resulting in respiratory distress and potentially hindering the insertion of a transesophageal echocardiogram (TEE) probe (**b2**). The TEE probe was introduced after a sternotomy was performed. (abbreviation: T, trachea; RB, Right bronchus; C, Carina; UE, upper esophagus; LE, lower esophagus; * indicates middle esophagus). (**c–c1**) Depicts an infant experiencing respiratory distress due to a double aortic arch. The bronchogram in the left plane shows the double aortic arch forming a vascular ring and compressing the carina region. To address this, single-lung intubation was performed using an endotracheal tube with multiple handmade holes at its tip, which ensured that the tube passed through the distal stenosis at the carina and allowed gas to reach the other lung, as seen in **c1**. (**d**) Depicts an infant with a ventricular septal defect (VSD) and a 3D trachea, which shows an abnormal narrowing of the left bronchus

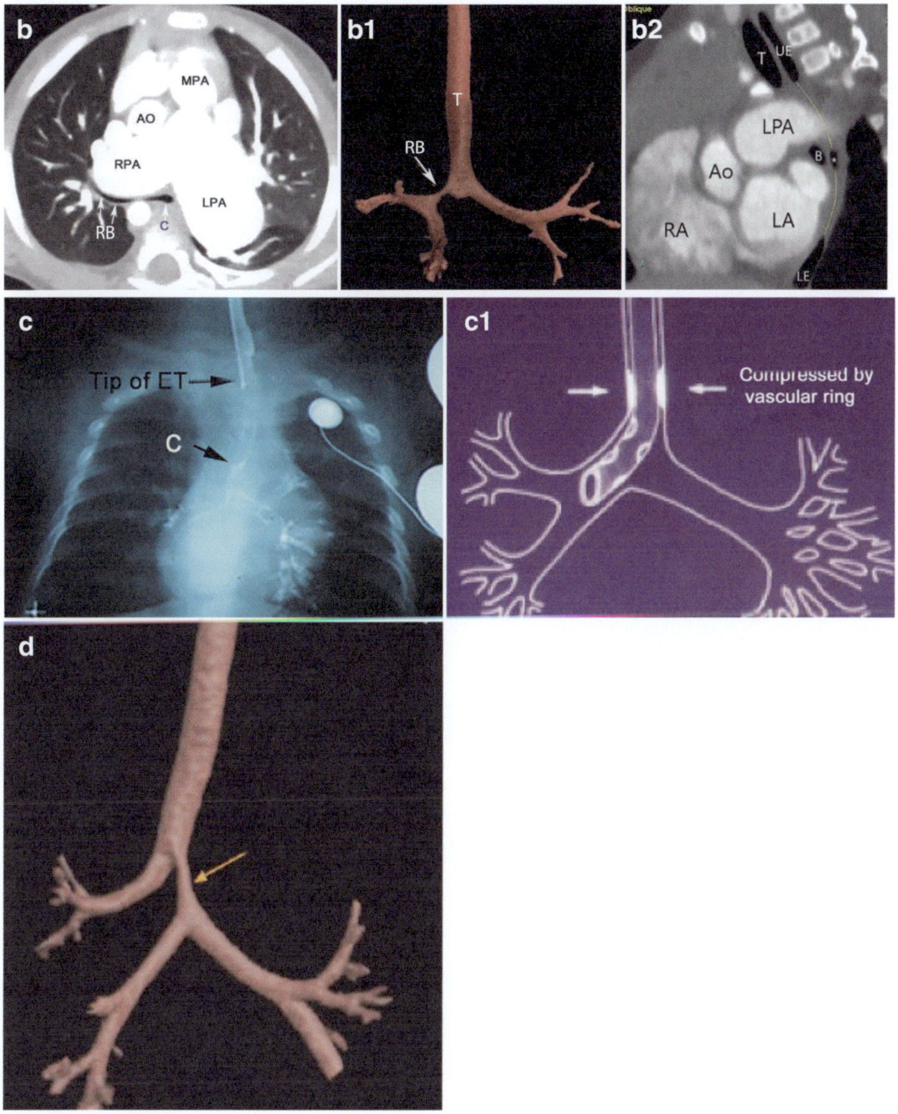

Fig. 2.12 (continued)

2.5.3 Desaturation and Systemic Hypotension

Newborns with Total Anomalous Pulmonary Venous Connection (TAPVC) have a congenital heart defect where the four pulmonary veins are not properly connected to the left atrium. Instead, they form a confluence known as the Pulmonary Venous Confluence (PVC) which is located behind the left atrium and can be easily compressed by the rigid TEE probe inserted into the esophagus. This compression can lead to hypotension or desaturation [20] (as shown in Fig. 2.13).

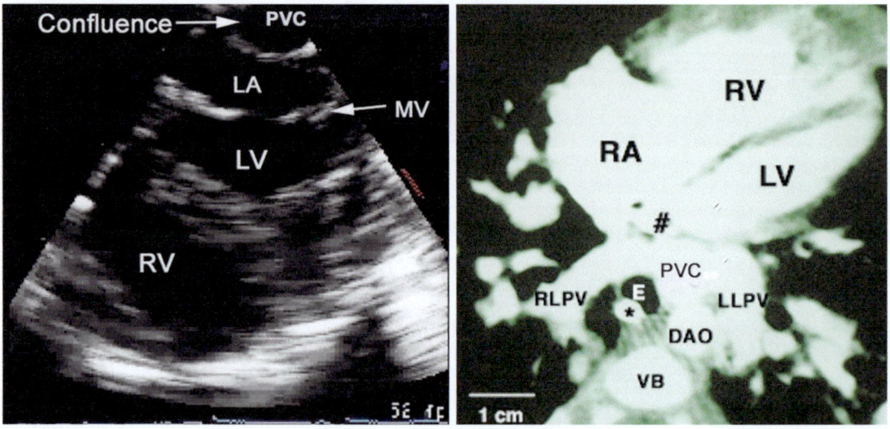

Fig. 2.13 Depicts a baby with total anomalous pulmonary venous connection (TAPVC). The transesophageal echocardiogram (TEE) image in the left diagram shows the pulmonary venous confluence (PVC) located behind the left atrium (LA), marked by a small "LA." The cardiac CT in the right diagram shows the PVC arising from both the left and right pulmonary veins, fitting closely against the back of the esophagus. Hence, placement of the TEE probe in the esophagus will compress the PVC, leading to desaturation. (Note: The "#" indicates the left atrium and the "*" indicates the nasogastric tube)

2.5.4 Systemic Hypotension

It is recommended to withdraw the TEE probe after the surgical repair of Coarctation of the aorta (CoA) due to the risk of hypotension. This is because the repaired aorta can be easily compressed by the rigid TEE probe in the esophagus. CoA is a condition in which the aorta is abnormally narrowed, but it can be treated successfully with surgery (as shown in Fig. 2.14).

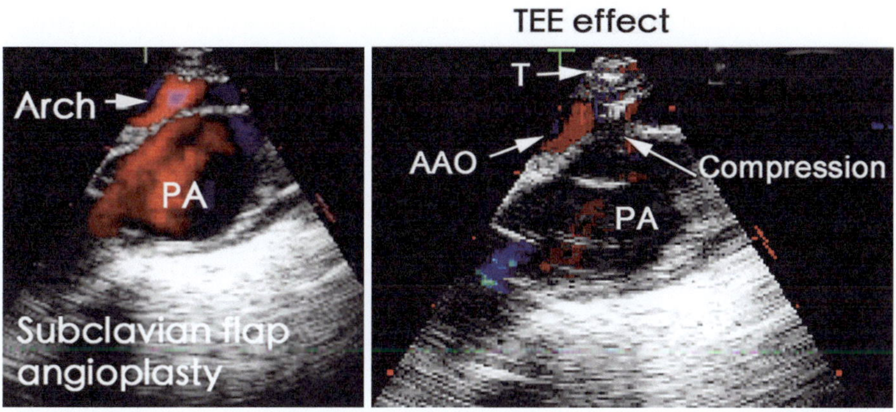

Fig. 2.14 Depicts a child with a coarctation of the aorta (CoA) who underwent angioplasty repair (as shown in left diagram). The insertion of a transesophageal echocardiogram (TEE) through the esophagus can result in systemic hypotension due to compression of the surgical flap, as depicted in the right diagram

2.6 Contraindication for Pediatric TEE (Refer to Table 2.1)

The use of TEE in cardiac surgery has been reported to result in major injury in approximately one out of every 1000 patients [21]. Although such incidents are relatively uncommon, they can occur due to problems during probe insertion or manipulation. These complications can include oropharyngeal trauma, arrhythmias, and disruptions to both respiratory and cardiac function. These contraindications are listed in Table 2.1.

Table 2.1 Contraindication in TEE used in pediatric patients

Absolute contraindications	Relative contraindications
Esophageal pathology	Specific lesions
Fistula to trachea	TAPVC[a]
Stricture	CoA[b]
Infection	Severe coagulopathy or thrombocytopenia
Bleeding	History of esophageal surgery
Trauma	
Tumor	
Diverticulum	
Poor airway control	
Respiratory distress (e.g., vascular ring)	

[a] *TAPVC* total anomalous pulmonary venous connection
[b] *CoA* coarctation of the aorta

2.7 Recommendations for Pediatric TEE (Refer to Table 2.2)

Due to the unique anatomy of infants and children, including a smaller diameter of the esophagus and a reduced safety margin, special considerations must be made when using TEE in pediatric patients. These recommendations are outlined in Table 2.2.

Table 2.2 Recommendations of TEE in pediatric patients

Required basic knowledge and skills of TEE
Monitoring of vital signs during the procedure
Avoid TEE probe-associated injury
Avoid forceful placement
Avoid the probe in locked position
Generous lubrication
Removal of nasogastric tube or feeding tube
Temporary removal of TEE probe during the long duration of CPB
Routine check the blood stains over the TEE probe when the probe was removed to ensure without trauma by TEE probe
Awareness of pathophysiology of CHD
Prevention of cardiovascular and respiratory effects during the TEE probe placement
TEE can be used safely after sternotomy in child with TAPVC (total anomalous pulmonary venous connection)

2.8 Conclusion

During surgical procedures or catheter-based treatments for CHD, accurate identification of cardiac morphological features is essential to make informed decisions and increase the likelihood of success. TEE is a useful tool for guiding decisions in pediatric cardiology, but it is a semi-invasive procedure that requires additional caution when used in children compared to adults. When performing TEE in pediatric patients, it is important to use endotracheal anesthesia and continuously monitor vital signs to ensure their safety. The procedure should involve a team of specialists, including pediatric cardiologists, cardiac surgeons, radiologists, and anesthesiologists. Figure 2.15 illustrates the importance of a teamwork in this process. If there are any difficulties with inserting the TEE probe or if the patient experiences systemic hypotension or desaturation, it is crucial to immediately stop the procedure and withdraw the probe. This step is essential to ensure the safety of the pediatric patients. In summary, TEE is a valuable tool for guiding decisions during surgical repair or interventional therapy in pediatric cardiology, but extra caution and a team approach are necessary when performing the procedure in children.

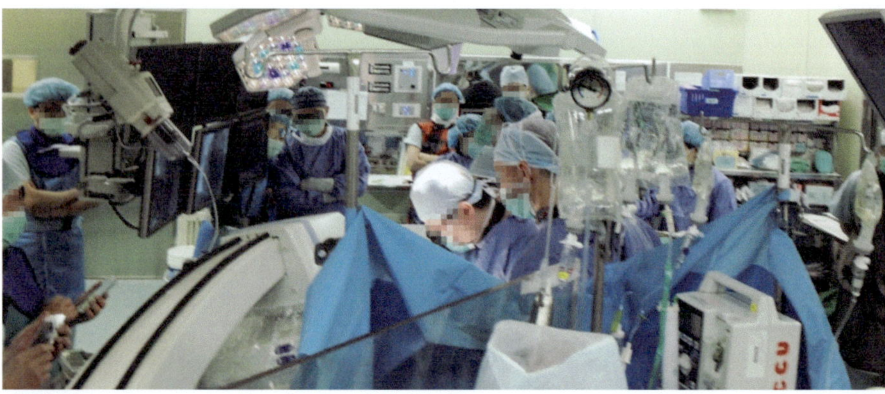

Fig. 2.15 Shows the pediatric intervention procedure that was carried out in the hybrid room. Crucial collaboration and effective communication among the staff are important in ensuring the successful completion of the operation and maintaining the safety of the patient

References

1. Cyran SE, Kimball TR, Meyer RA, et al. Efficacy of intraoperative transesophageal echocardiography in children with congenital heart disease. Am J Cardiol. 1989;63:594–8.
2. Seward JB, Khandheria BK, Oh JK, et al. Transesophageal echocardiography: technique, anatomic correlations, implementation and clinical applications. Mayo Clin Proc. 1988;63:649–80.
3. Daniel WG, Erbel R, Kasper W, Visser CA, Engberding R, Sutherland GR, et al. Safety of transesophageal echocardiography. A multicenter survey of 10,419 examinations. Circulation. 1991;83:817–21.
4. Wei J, Hsiung MC, Tsai SK, Ou CH, Chang CY, Chang YC, et al. The routine use of live three-dimensional transesophageal echocardiography in mitral valve surgery: clinical experience. Eur J Echocardiogr. 2010;11:14–8.
5. Tseng HC, Hsiao PN, Lin YH, Wang JK, Tsai SK. Transesophageal echocardiographic monitoring for transcatheter closure of atrial septal defect. J Formos Med Assoc. 2000;99:684–8.
6. Wang JK, Tsai SK, Wu MH, Lin MT, Lue HC. Short- and intermediate-term results of transcatheter closure of atrial septal defect with the Amplatzer septal occluder. Am Heart J. 2004;148:511–7.
7. Hahn RT, Saric M, Faletra FF, et al. Echocardiographic imaging and structural heart interventions: Recommended Standards for the Performance of Transesophageal Echocardiographic Screening for Structural Heart Intervention: From the American Society of Echocardiography. J Am Soc Echocardiogr. 2022;35:1–76.
8. Lai WW, Geva T, Shirali GS, Frommelt PC, Humes RA, et al. Guideline and standard for performance of a pediatric echocardiogram: a report from the Task Force of the Pediatric Council of the American Society of Echocardiography. J Am Soc Echocardiogr. 2006;19:1413–30.
9. Frazin L, Talano JV, Stephanides L, Loeb HS, Kopel L, Gunnar RM. Esophageal echocardiography. Circulation. 1976;54:102–8.
10. Omoto R, Kyo S, Matsumura M, Yamada E, Matsunaka T. Variomatrix—a newly developed transesophageal echocardiography probe with a rotating matrix biplane transducer. Technological aspects and initial clinical experience. Echocardiography. 1993;10:79–84.
11. Sugeng L, Shernan SK, Salgo IS, Weinert L, Shook D, Raman J, et al. Live 3-dimensional transesophageal echocardiography initial experience using the fully-sampled matrix array probe. J Am Coll Cardiol. 2008;52:446–9.
12. Loff S, Diez O, Ho W, Kalle TV, Hetjens S, Boettcher M. Esophageal diameter as a function of weight in neonates, children and adolescents: reference values for dilatation of esophageal stenosis. Front Pediatr. 2022;10:822271.
13. Haase FR, Brenner A. Esophageal diameter at various ages. Arch Otolaryngol. 1963;77:119–22.
14. Thomas SB, Thekla VK, Alexander S, Oliver HD. Esophageal diameter in children correlated to body weight. Eur J Pediatr Surg. 2019;29:528–32.
15. Tsai SK. The role of transesophageal echocardiography in clinical use. J Chin Med Assoc. 2013;76:661–72.
16. Tsai SK, Chang CI, Wang MJ, Chen SJ, Chiu IS, et al. The assessment of the proximal left pulmonary artery by transesophageal echocardiography and computed tomography in neonates and infants: a case series. Analgesia. 2001;93:594–7.
17. Lennon MJ, Gibbs NM, Weightman WM, Ee HC. Transesophageal echocardiography-related gastrointestinal complications in cardiac surgical patients. J Cardiothorac Vasc Anesth. 2005;19:141–5.

18. Nana AM, Stefanidis C, Chami JP, Deviere J, Barvais L, et al. Esophageal perforation during cardiac surgery: treatment by endoscopic stenting. Ann Thorac Surg. 2003;75:1955–7.
19. Foz C, Peyton J, Staffa SJ, Kovatsis P, Park R, et al. Airway abnormalities in patients with congenital heart disease: incidence and associated factors. J Cardiothorac Vasc Anesth. 2021;35:139–44.
20. Chang YY, Chang CI, Wang MJ, Lin SM, Chen YS, Tsai SK, et al. The safe use of intraoperative transesophageal echocardiography in the management of total anomalous pulmonary venous connection in newborns and infants: a case series. Pediatr Anesth. 2005;15:939–43.
21. Piercy M, McNicol L, Dinh DT, Story DA, et al. Major complications related to the use of transesophageal echocardiography in cardiac surgery. J Cardiothorac Vasc Anesth. 2009;23:62–5.

Part II

TEE Monitoring of Pediatric Congenital Cardiac Surgery

The chapters of this part focus on the use of transesophageal echocardiography (TEE) for monitoring pediatric patients undergoing surgery for congenital heart diseases.

3 Septal Defects

3.1 Atrial Septal Defect (ASD)

Atrial septal defect (ASD) is a congenital heart defect characterized by an abnormal opening in the wall (septum) between the two upper chambers (atria) of the heart.

There are several types of ASDs, including [1, 2]: (as depicted in Fig. 3.1)

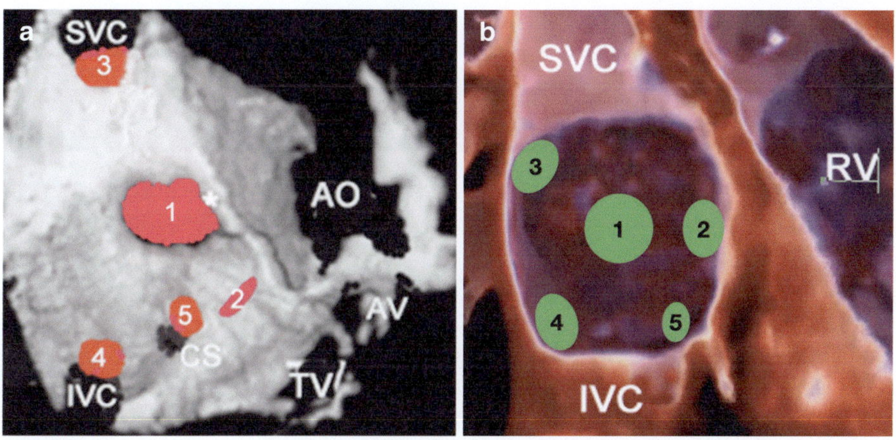

Fig. 3.1 Describes the types of atrial septal defect (ASD) based on their location as seen in a 3D TEE image (**a**) and a 3D cardiac CT image (**b**). The most common type is ostium secundum (1), located in the area of the fossa ovalis. Ostium primum (2), which affects 10–15% of cases, is located in the lower part of the atrial septum and overlies the mitral and tricuspid valves. Superior sinus venous (3) and inferior sinus venous (4), each affecting 5% of cases, are located in the upper and lower parts of the dorsal interatrial septum near the entry of the superior and inferior vena cava, respectively. The rarest type, coronary sinus septal defect (5), occurs in less than 1% of cases and is located between the coronary sinus roof and the left atrium floor

S.-K. Tsai et al., *Transesophageal Echocardiography in Pediatric Congenital Cardiac Surgery and Catheter Intervention*, https://doi.org/10.1007/978-981-99-6582-3_3

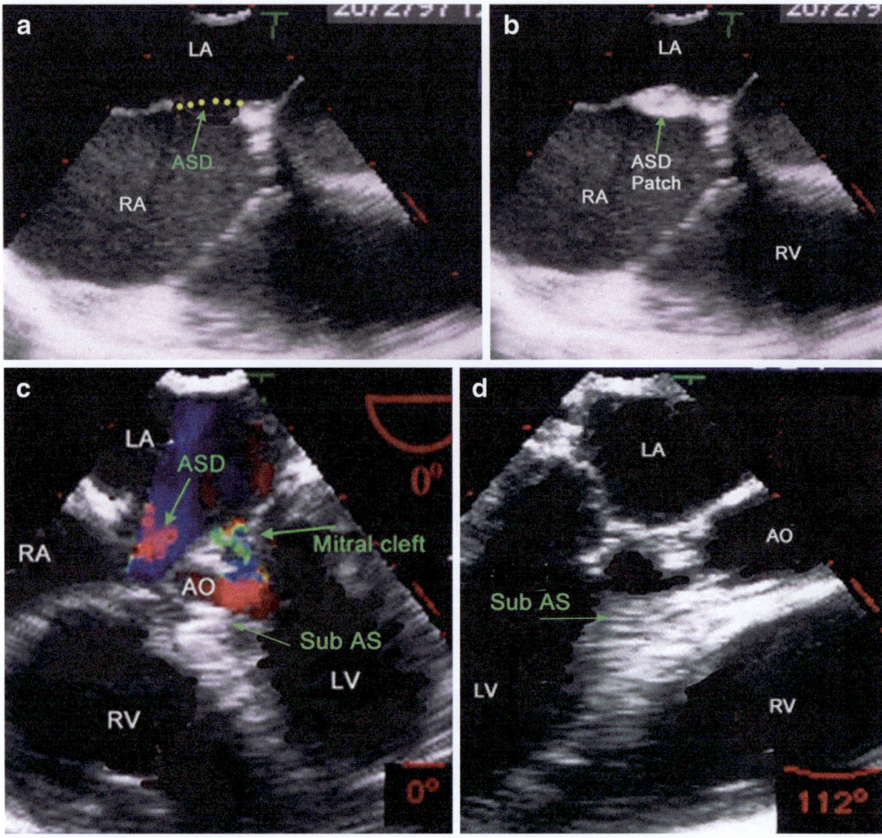

Fig. 3.2 Illustrates a surgical repair of an ostium primum atrial septal defect (ASD) in a 4-year-old boy. The preoperative TEE in ME four-chamber view (**a**) shows the defect (yellow dotted line) in the inferior part of the interatrial septum. After the repair (**b**), the postoperative TEE in ME four-chamber view shows the surgical patch without any residual shunt. Furthermore, an incompletely formed septum primum is associated with an anterior mitral leaflet cleft and mitral regurgitation, which can be observed in the four-chamber view (**c**). Additionally, subaortic stenosis can be identified in the ME AV LAX view (**d**). More details regarding this topic will be covered in Fig. 3.18

1. Primum ASD (as shown in Fig. 3.2): This type of ASD occurs at the lower part of the interatrial septum, near the tricuspid and mitral valves. It is often associated with other congenital heart defects, such as a cleft in the mitral or tricuspid valve.
2. Secundum ASD (as shown in Fig. 3.3): This is the most common type of ASD, accounting for about 70% of all cases. It occurs in the central of the interatrial septum and is often small to moderate in size.
3. Sinus venosus ASD (Figs. 3.4 and 3.5): This unusual type of ASD is located near the superior vena cava or inferior vena cava. These veins are responsible for carrying blood from the upper and lower parts of the body respectively, and this

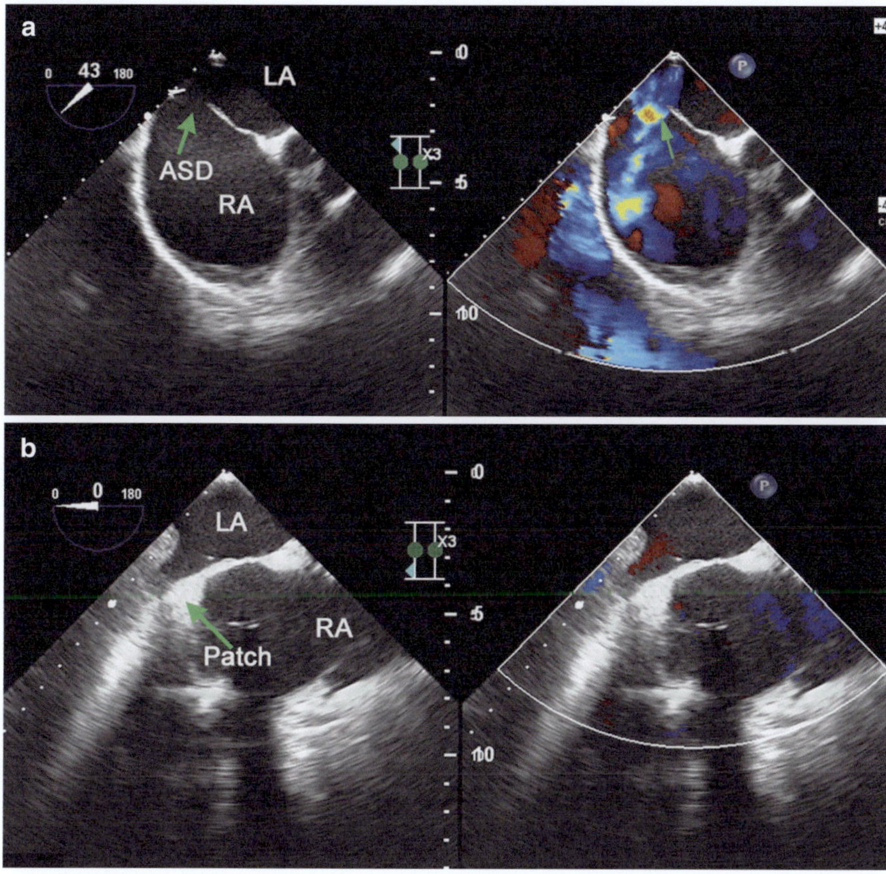

Fig. 3.3 A child with secundum atrial septal defect underwent surgical repair. (**a**) Preoperative TEE in the ME AV SAX view showing an ostium secundum defect with dilated RA (left diagram). Color Doppler flow image demonstrates a left to right shunt flow (arrow in right diagram). (**b**) Postoperative TEE in the same patient showing successful patch repair without any residual shunt (right diagram)

condition usually generally associated with an anomalous pulmonary venous connection. It accounts for about 5–10% of all ASD cases.

4. Unroofed coronary sinus ASD (as shown in Figs. 3.6, 3.7, and 3.8): This rare type of ASD (less than 1% of all ASD) occurs when there is a defect (complete or incomplete) on the wall between the coronary sinus and the left atrium, and it can occur with persistent left SVC. The complete form is also known as totally unroofed coronary sinus ASD (as shown in Fig. 3.7).

The symptoms of ASD vary depending on the size of the defect and the age of the individual. Small ASDs may not cause any symptoms and may close spontaneously during infancy. Larger ASDs can cause serious complications such as

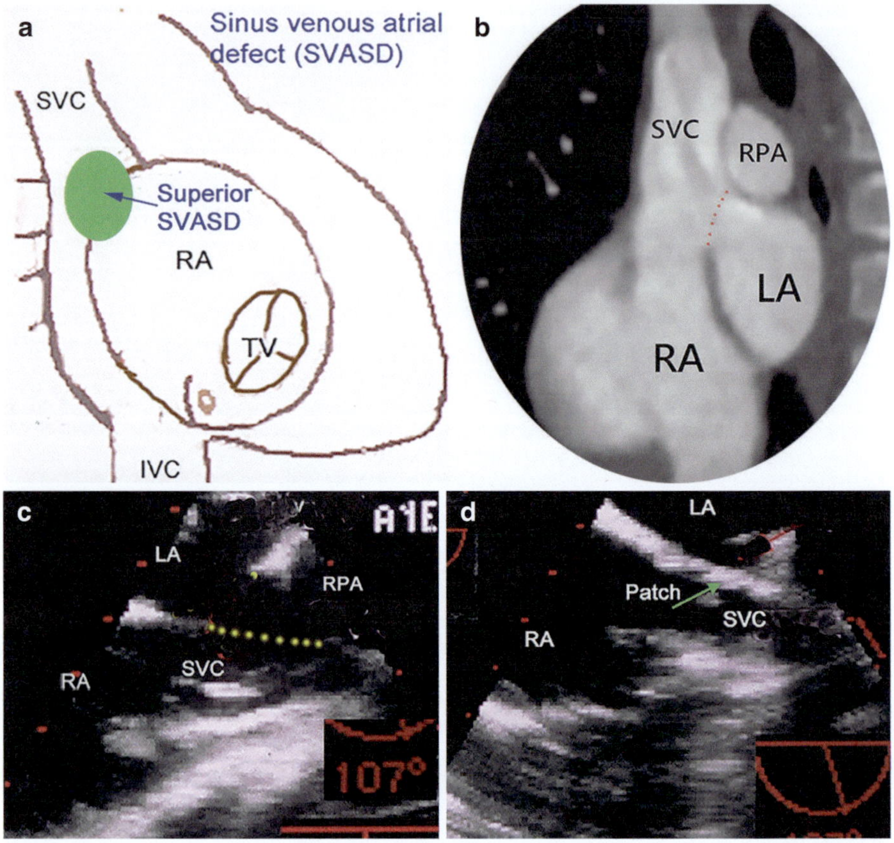

Fig. 3.4 Shows the surgical repair of a superior sinus venous atrial septal defect (SVASD) in a 6-year-old boy. A schematic drawing in (**a**) illustrates the superior SVASD (green circle) located above the superior vena cava (SVC), as viewed from the unroofed right atrium. The preoperative oblique sagittal contrast-enhanced cardiac CT (**b**) shows the SVC draining to the left atrium (LA) through the defect (red dotted line). The preoperative TEE bicaval view (**c**) demonstrates the discontinuity of the SVC-IAS (interatrial septum) junction (yellow dotted line), resulting in blood flow from the SVC into both the right and left atria and partial anomaly of pulmonary venous drainages into the right atrium. The postoperative TEE bicaval view (**d**) shows the successful repair of the defect between the SVC-IAS with a patch

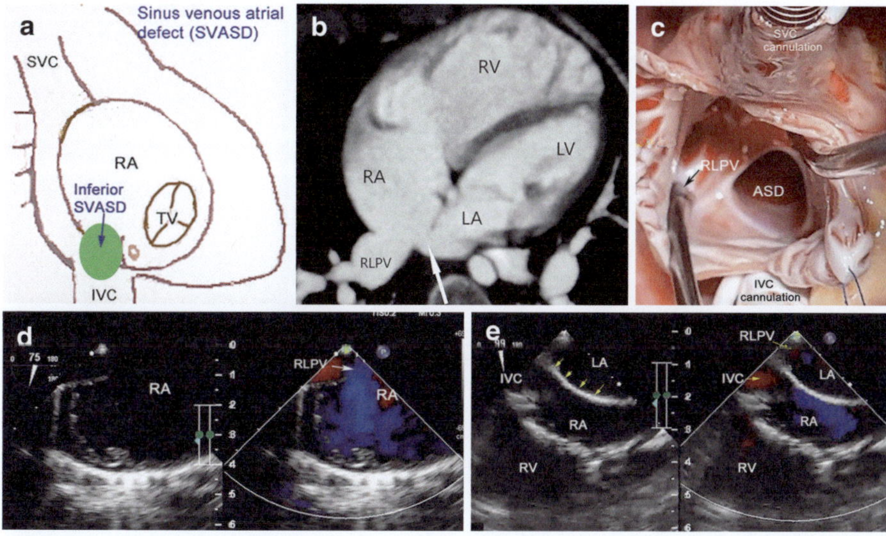

Fig. 3.5 Shows the surgical repair of an inferior sinus venous atrial septal defect (SVASD) associated with anomalous pulmonary venous drainage in a 3-year-girl. A schematic drawing in (**a**) highlights the sinus venosus defect (green circle) of the inferior vena cava (IVC) viewed from the unroofed right atrium. The preoperative cardiac CT in a four-chamber thin-slab MIP image (**b**) shows an inferior SVASD (arrow) with a right lower pulmonary vein (RLPV) draining into the right atrium (RA) and a dilated RA. Intraoperative photo taken after the right atrial incision (**c**) displays a large atrial septal defect (ASD) measuring 1.5 cm and the drainage of the RLPV into the RA, as indicated by the inserted suction tube. The preoperative TEE with color Doppler bicaval view (**d**) reveals a dilated right atrium (RA) and a discontinuity in the inferior vena cava-interatrial septum (IVC-IAS) junction. This defect could allow the flow from the RLPV returns into the RA (right diagram). The postoperative TEE bicaval view (**e**) displays the baffle rerouting of the partially anomalous venous connection to the LA and ASD repair, indicated by the small yellow arrows in the left diagram. The color Doppler image shows the blood flowing from the IVC into the RA and the RLPV into LA, without any shunt crossing the patch (right diagram)

right-sided heart failure, arrhythmias, stroke, early death or pulmonary hypertension. Larger ones may require percutaneous repair (will be discussed in Sect. 8.3) or surgical repair [3, 4] under the TEE monitoring (see Figs. 3.2, 3.3, 3.4, 3.5, 3.6, 3.7, 3.8, 3.9, and 3.10).

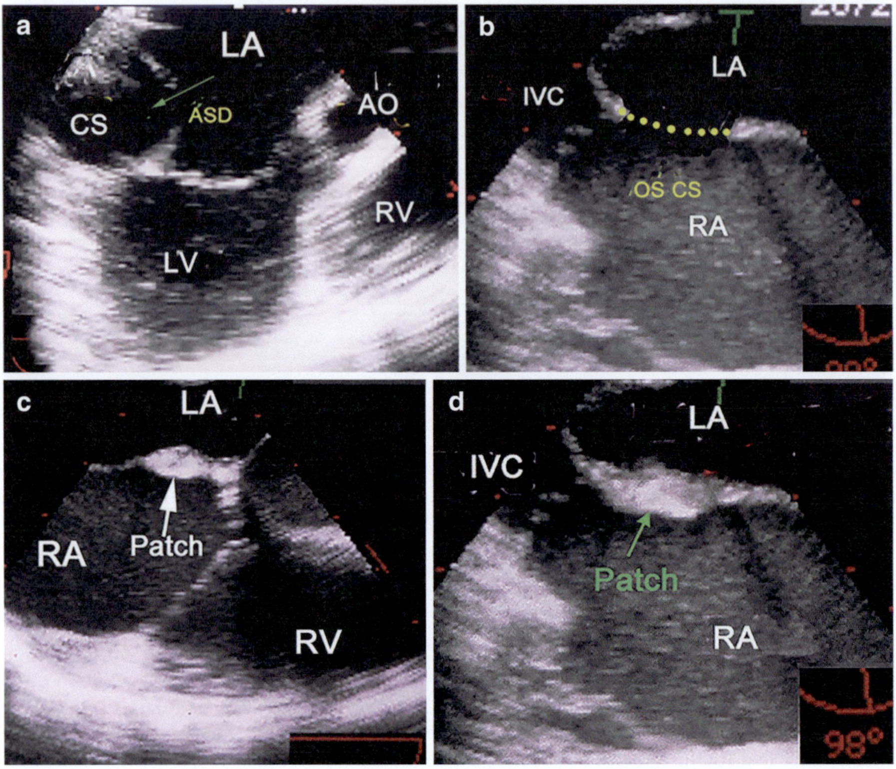

Fig. 3.6 An 8-year-old boy with a history of an atrial septal defect underwent surgical repair. The preoperative TEE ME AV LAX view (**a**) depicted a defect located in the terminal portion of the coronary sinus (CS), indicated by an arrow, as well as the lack of the left superior vena cava (LSVC), also known as an isolated coronary sinus atrial septal defect (ASD). The preoperative bicaval view (**b**) showed a dilated right atrium (RA) and wide-opened ostium of the CS (OS CS) with an unroof part (dots line) connecting directly to the LA. The postoperative TEE ME four-chamber view (**c**) showed the surgical repair with a patch closure of the ostium of the CS. The postoperative bicaval view (**d**) showed the surgical closure of the ostium of the CS with a patch

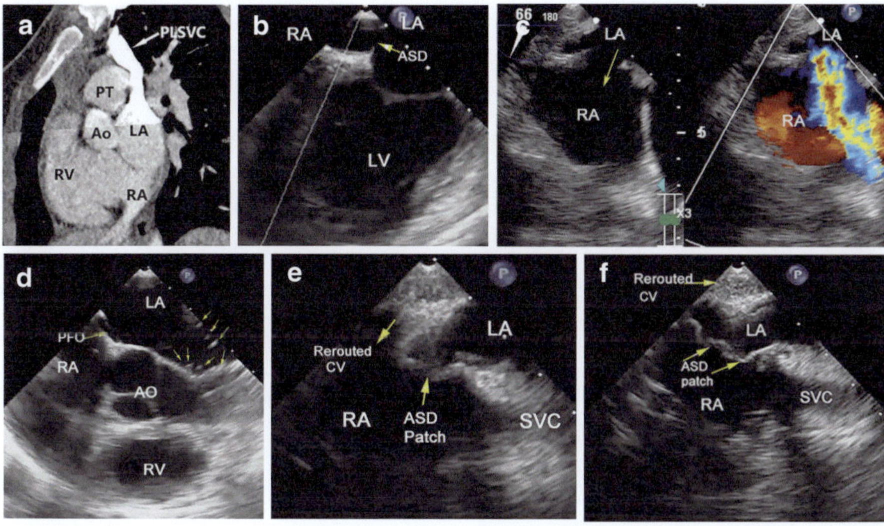

Fig. 3.7 A 5-year-old boy presenting with symptoms of exertional dyspnea underwent surgical repair for a totally unroofed coronary sinus (CS) atrial septal defect. Preoperative double-oblique-sagittal CT (**a**) showed blood in the persistent left superior vena cava (PLSVC) draining directly into the left atrium (LA) instead of the right atrium (RA). Intraoperative TEE (**b**) revealed an interatrial defect (ASD) and complete absence of the roof of CS. The intraoperative color Doppler TEE (**c**) demonstrated a small LA and large RA, with a left-to-right shunt clearly visible across the atrial septal defect (arrow). Bubble study (**d**) demonstrated bubbles (small yellow arrows) in the LA via PLSVC and a patent foramen ovale (PFO) defect between the RA and LA. Postoperative TEE (**e**, **f**) showed successful atrial septal defect repair with patch by closure of the opening of the native coronary sinus. And rerouted coronary venous return to the RA. The four-chamber view (**f**) showed the spiral repair with patch and reconnection of the LSVC to the right atrial appendage (RAA). However, the reconnection of the LSVC to the RAA is not visible in this figure (Abbreviation: CV, Coronary vein)

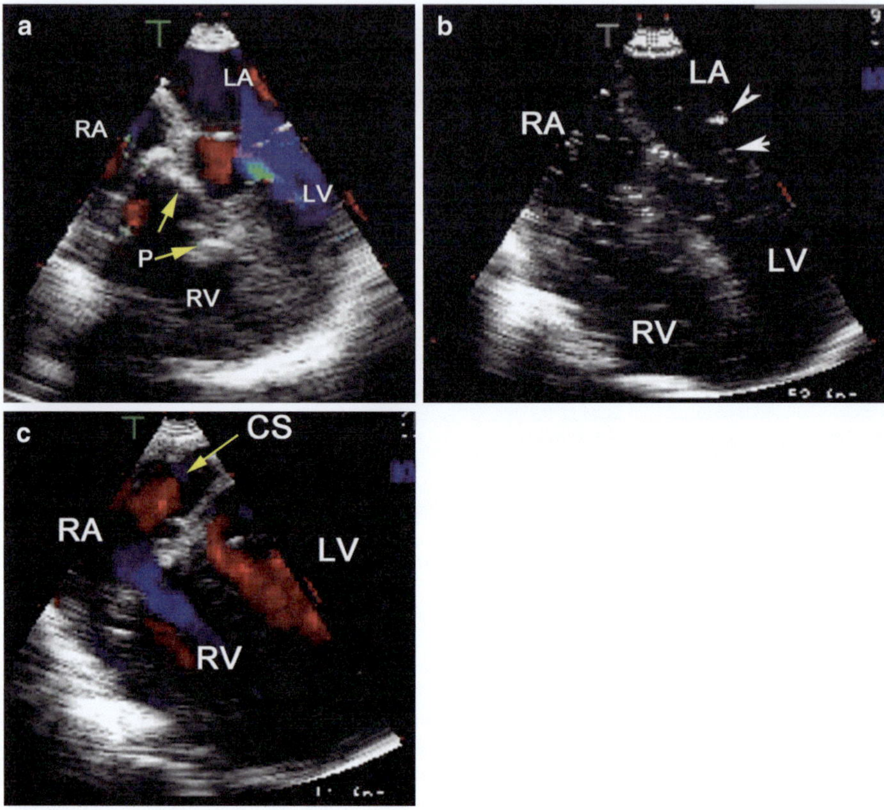

Fig. 3.8 A 4-year-old boy experienced hypoxemia after TOF repair, which was caused by an undiagnosed coronary sinus (CS) atrial septal defect (ASD). This was revealed through: (**a**) TEE with a ME four-chamber view displaying the repaired VSD patch (p, yellow arrows), (**b**) TEE with contrast injection showing a partial CS ASD, by identifing some bright echogenity bubbles (arrowheads) in LA and (**c**) ME four-chamber view demonstrating a large CS, right-to-left shunt, and elevated RA pressure. As a result, the partial CS ASD was repaired again

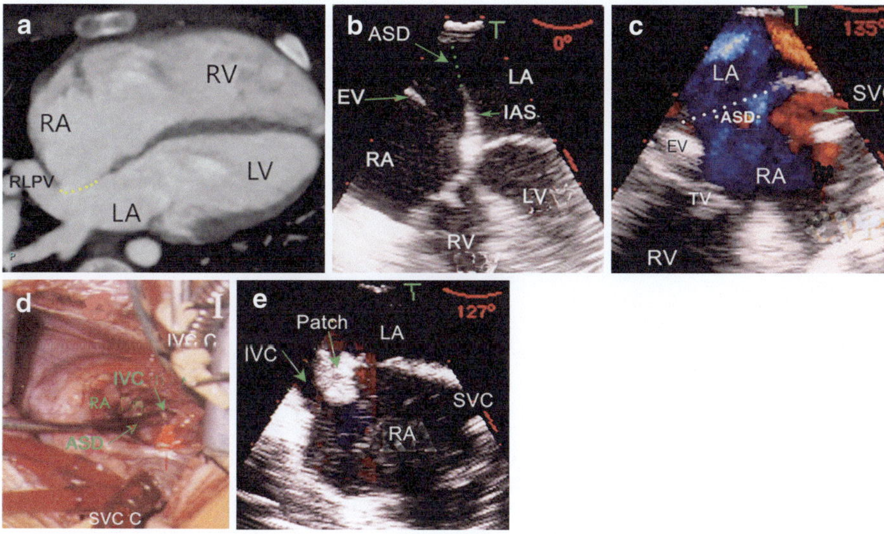

Fig. 3.9 A girl underwent surgical repair for ASD and persistent Eustachian valve. (**a**) The cardiac CT scan revealed an inferior sinus venous atrial septal defect (ASD), indicated by a red dotted line, in which all the right pulmonary veins open into the RA. (**b**) Preop TEE showed large interatrial defect (green dotted line) and a giant Eustachian valve (EV). (**c**) Color Doppler showed a 2.2 cm diameter ASD with left-to-right shunt and discontinuity of IVC-IAS. (**d**) Intraoperative photo showed an inferior sinus venous ASD, with the suction tube pointing toward it. (**e**) Postoperative TEE showed removal of Eustachian valve and surgical repair of inferior sinus venous defect by a patch

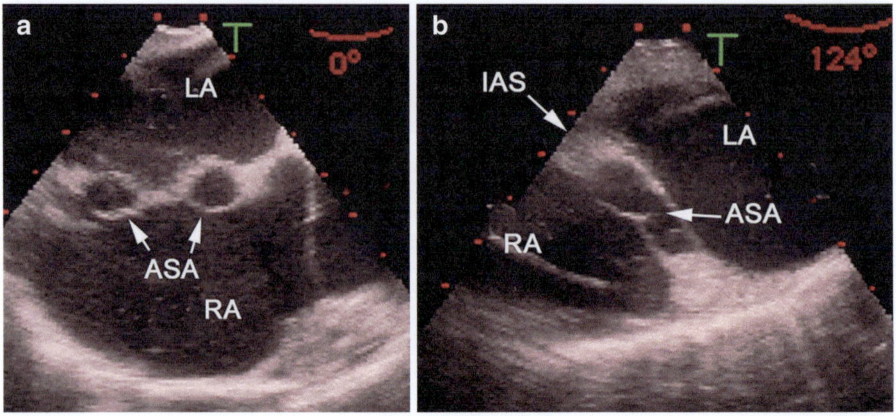

Fig. 3.10 A 12-year-old boy with an atrial septal aneurysm (ASA) during routine follow-up. (**a**) TEE with ME four-chamber view showed two localized saccular deformities in the atrial septum (eye glass appearance). (**b**) LAX view showed the ASA without shunting flow or septal defect

References

1. Naqvi N, McCarthy KP, Ho SY. Anatomy of the atrial septum and interatrial communications. J Thorac Dis. 2018;10:S2837–47.
2. McCarthy K, Ho S, Anderson R. Defining the morphologic phenotypes of atrial septal defects and interatrial communications. Images Paediatr Cardiol. 2003;5:1–24.
3. Murphy JG, Gersh BJ, McGoon, et al. Long-term outcome after surgical repair of isolated atrial septal defect. Follow-up at 27 to 32 years. N Engl Med. 1990;323:1645–50.
4. Cho YH, Jun TG, Yang JH, et al. Surgical strategy in patients with atrial septal defect and severe pulmonary hypertension. Heart Surg Forum. 2012;15:E111–5.

3.2 Ventricular Septal Defect (VSD)

Ventricular septal defect (VSD) is a common congenital heart defect that involves a hole or holes in the septum between the two ventricles.

There are four types of VSD based on the location of the defect within the septum [1, 2] (Fig. 3.11).

- Perimembranous (Pm) VSD, accounting for approximately 80% of cases, occurs in the region of the membranous septum, which is located near the aortic and tricuspid valves (Fig. 3.12).
- Muscular VSD, also known as trabecular VSD, accounts for approximately 5–20% of cases. This type of VSD primarily affects the muscular septum, which will be further explained in Figs. 8.35, 8.36, and 8.37 in the context of catheter interventions.

- Inlet VSD, also known as AV canal type VSD, accounts for approximately 5–8% of cases. It occurs in the inlet muscular septum. Inlet septum defects often involve abnormalities in the tricuspid and mitral valves, collectively known as common atrioventricular canal defect (Figs. 3.18 and 3.20).
- Outlet VSD occurs in the infundibular region of the ventricular septum and can be classified into two subtypes: muscular outlet VSD or doubly committed juxtaarterial (subarterial) VSD. It accounts for approximately 5–7% of cases. Please refer to Figs. 3.13 and 3.15 for visual representations of these subtypes of VSDs.

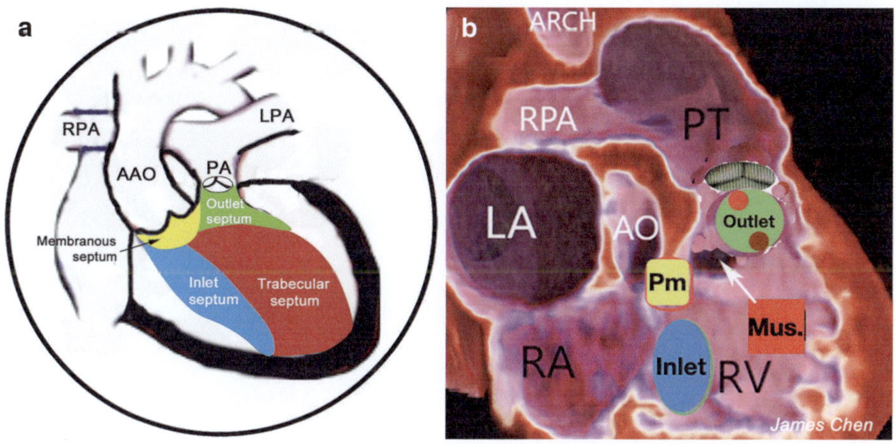

Fig. 3.11 Describes the various types of ventricular septal defect (VSD) based on their location. (**a**) This schematic illustration shows the various segments of the ventricular septum as viewed from the unroofed right ventricle. It displays the length of the interventricular septum, including the membranous septum (yellow), outlet septum (green), inlet septum (blue), and trabecular septum (brown). (**b**) This 3D virtual image model displays various types of VSDs in a baby's heart. The image shows different types of VSDs, including the muscular VSD indicated by the white arrow. Other types of VSDs depicted in the image include the outlet type (green) with a red dot indicating a doubly committed subarterial (juxtaarterial) VSD and a brown dot indicating a muscular outlet VSD. Additionally, the perimembranous (pm) type is shown in yellow, the inlet type (also known as atrioventricular septal defect or AVSD) is shown in blue, and the muscular type is depicted in red-brown. (**c–e**) Show schematics of different types of VSDs in TEE images: (**c**) displays the ME five-chamber view with a pmVSD in membranous septum (yellow) and a muscular VSD in trabecular septum (brown), (**d**) ME AV SAX view shows the presence of a pmVSD (yellow) and an outlet VSD (green), with a brown arrowhead indicating muscular outlet and a red arrowhead indicating doubly committed subarterial (juxtaarterial) VSD along ventricular septum, (**e**) AV LAX view shows the presence of a pmVSD (yellow) and an outlet VSD (green) along ventricular septum. (**f–h**) TEE images corresponding to the VSD diagrams (**c–e**). In (**f**), the ME four-chamber view shows a muscular VSD (arrow) with left-to-right shunt confirmed by color Doppler. In (**g**), ME AV SAX view displays a perimembranous (pm) VSD (arrow) with turbulent flow toward the tricuspid valve (TV) also demonstrated by color Doppler. (**h**) The same view as (**d**) displays an outlet VSD (arrow) with a turbulent flow toward the pulmonary valve (PV) confirmed by color Doppler

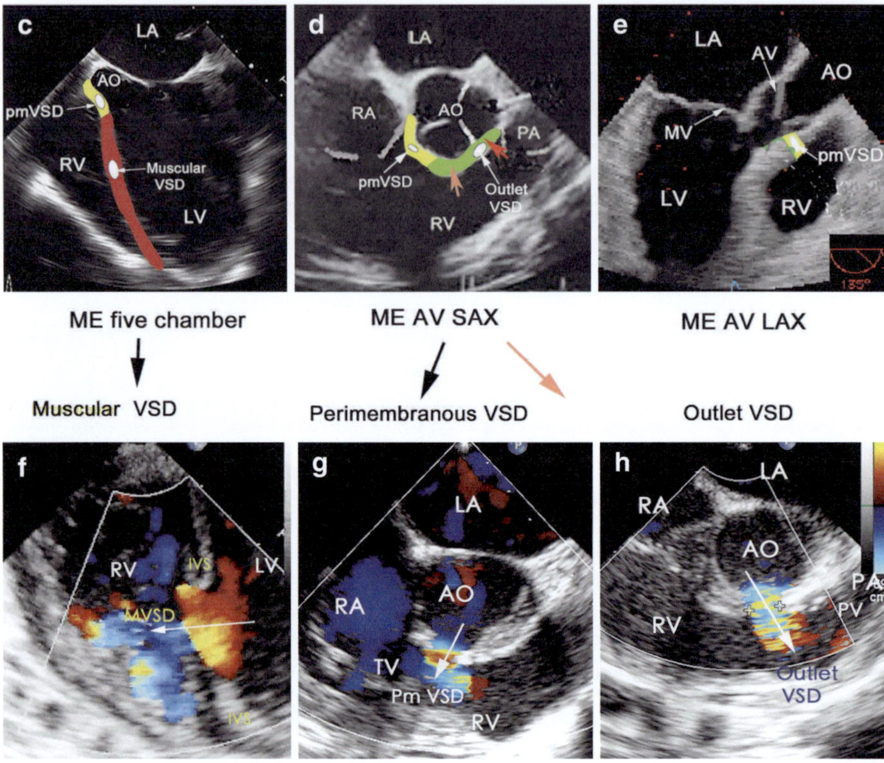

Fig. 3.11 (continued)

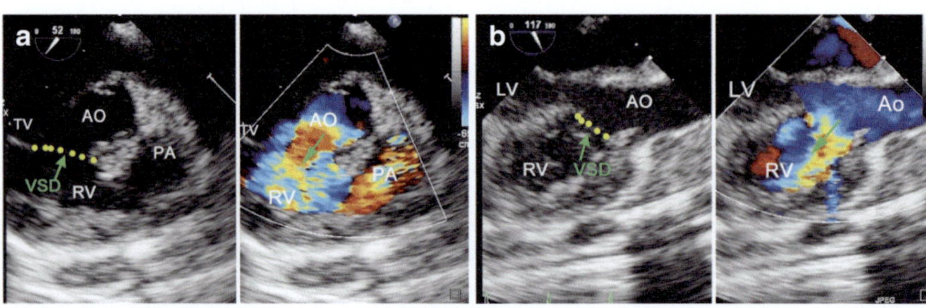

Fig. 3.12 Depicts a significant perimembranous ventricular septal defect (VSD) in children, as observed through intraoperative transesophageal echocardiography (TEE) with the mid-esophageal aortic valve short-axis (ME AV SAX) view (**a**) and the mid-esophageal aortic valve long-axis (ME AV LAX) view (**b**). The TEE images illustrate a VSD with a diameter of 1.3 cm (indicated by the yellow dotted line), and the color Doppler TEE demonstrates the flow of blood from the left to the right heart chamber and toward the tricuspid valve (TV)

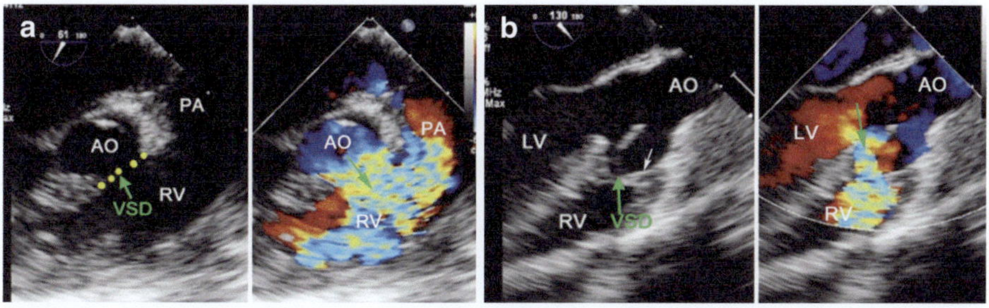

Fig. 3.13 Shows outlet VSD in children as seen on: (**a**) Intraoperative TEE with ME AV SAX view displays a 1 cm outlet ventricular defect (yellow dotted line) and VSD jet flow from left to right heart chamber toward PV as seen in color Doppler TEE (right diagram). (**b**) TEE with ME AV LAX shows a partial prolapse of the aortic valve (white arrow) with outlet ventricular defect and VSD jet flow from left to right heart chamber (RV) as seen in color Doppler TEE (right diagram)

The clinical course for pediatric patients with VSD depends on the size and location of the defect, as well as the age and overall presence of any other heart conditions.

Small VSDs may not require any treatment and may close on their own over time. However, large symptomatic VSDs (calculated pulmonary to systemic shunt larger than 1.5 or increased pulmonary vascular resistance, poor weight gain, exercise intolerance, associated aortic valve prolapse, associated double-chambered right ventricle, infective endocarditis) usually require catheter-based intervention (will be discussed in Sect. 8.4) or surgical repair under the TEE monitoring (as shown in Figs. 3.11, 3.12, 3.13, 3.14, 3.15, 3.16, 3.17, 3.18, 3.19, and 3.20).

The complication of residual VSD following surgical repair:

Following the repair procedure, it was found that the majority of children exhibited a small, asymptomatic residual ventricular septal defect (VSD) [3–5]. In cases where the diameter of the residual VSD was less than 3 mm, spontaneous healing was observed (Fig. 3.16). However, certain children presented with larger VSDs, which resulted in volume overload, heart failure, and reduced cardiac output. These cases necessitated further surgical or catheter intervention (Please refer to Chap. 10, Sect. 10.2).

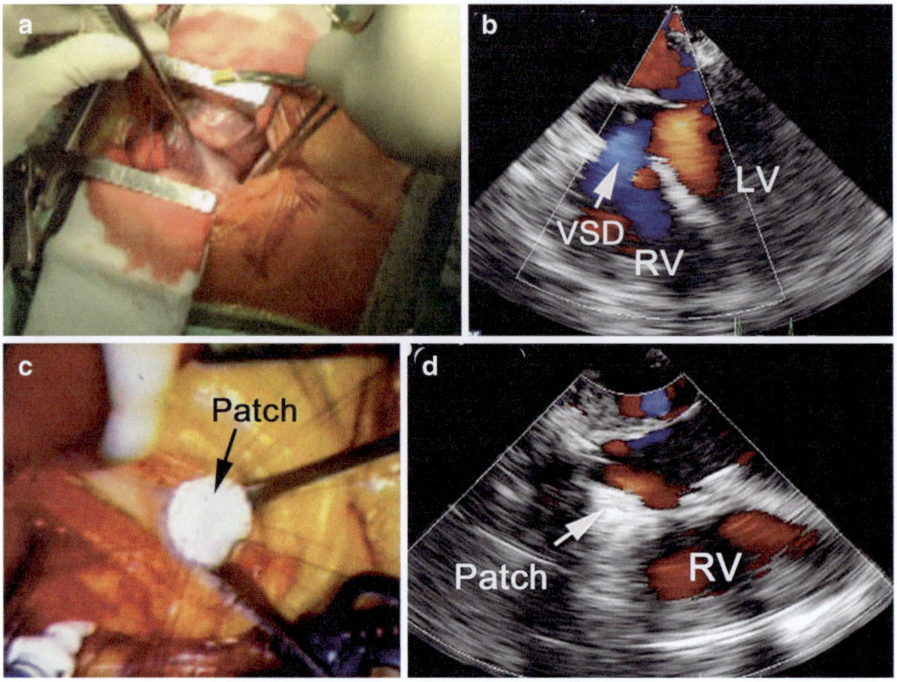

Fig. 3.14 A 3-month-old baby with heart failure due to a large VSD underwent surgery. (**a**) Intraoperative photo of open-heart surgery. (**b**) Preop color Doppler TEE shows a large perimembranous VSD with a L-R shunt. (**c**) VSD repaired with patch during surgery. (**d**) Postop TEE displays a successful patch repair without any residual shunt

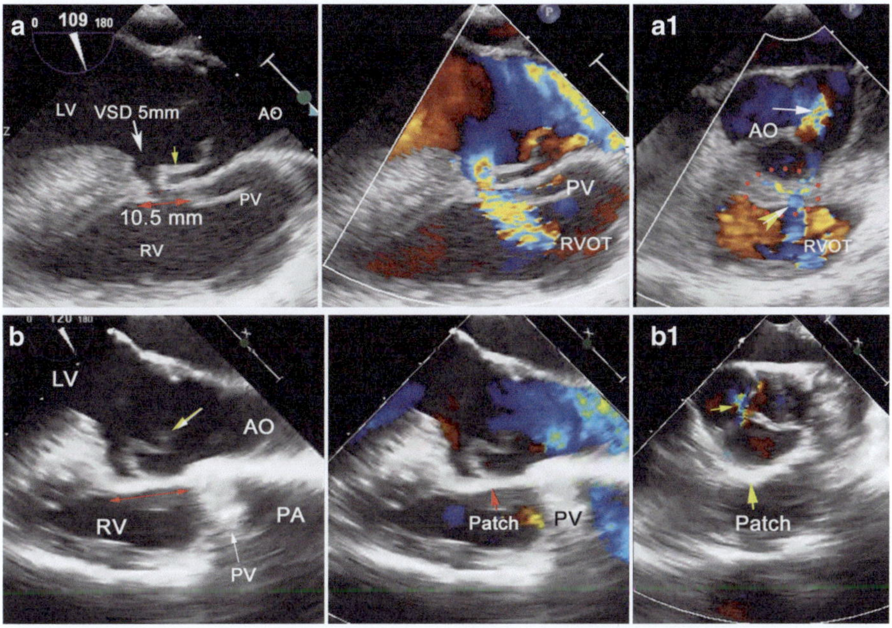

Fig. 3.15 A 7-year-old boy with an outlet-type ventricular septal defect (VSD) and aortic valve prolapse underwent surgical repair. (**a**) Preop TEE image with ME AV LAX view displays a 5 mm VSD partially obstructed by prolapsed right coronary cup (yellow arrow). The defect has a diameter of 10.5 mm from the RV side and there is a left-to-right shunt visible on color Doppler image. (**a1**) ME AV SAX color TEE image displays a VSD (red dotted circle) with a small jet flow of left-to-right shunt (yellow arrowhead) obstructed by right coronary cup prolapse, and mild aortic regurgitation (white arrow) during diastole. (**b**) Postop TEE image with ME AV LAX view displays surgical closure of VSD using a 1.5 cm patch (double-head red line) and without any residual shunt is visible on the right diagram. (**b1**) ME AV SAX color TEE image shows trivial aortic regurgitation during diastole after VSD closure with patch

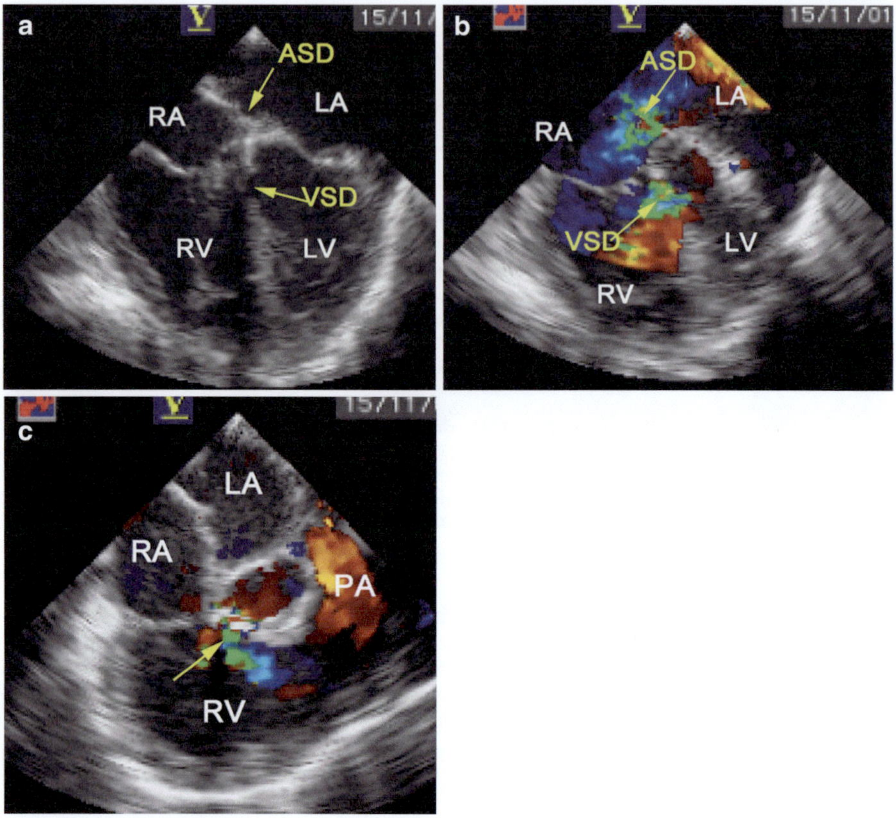

Fig. 3.16 Residual shunts after VSD repair in children. (**a**) Preoperative transesophageal echocardiography (TEE), ME five-chamber view showing a ventricular septal defect (VSD) and an atrial septal defect (ASD). (**b**) Color Doppler TEE showing left-to-right shunts in both atrial and ventricular septal defects. (**c**) Postoperative color Doppler TEE showing a residual shunt (arrow) after a patch repair. According to a report by Bibevski S, et al. (2020. World J Pediatr Congenit Heart Surg) [5], it was found that the majority of children who underwent repair had a small, asymptomatic residual ventricular septal defect (VSD). It was further noted that residual VSDs with a diameter of less than 3 mm would heal spontaneously

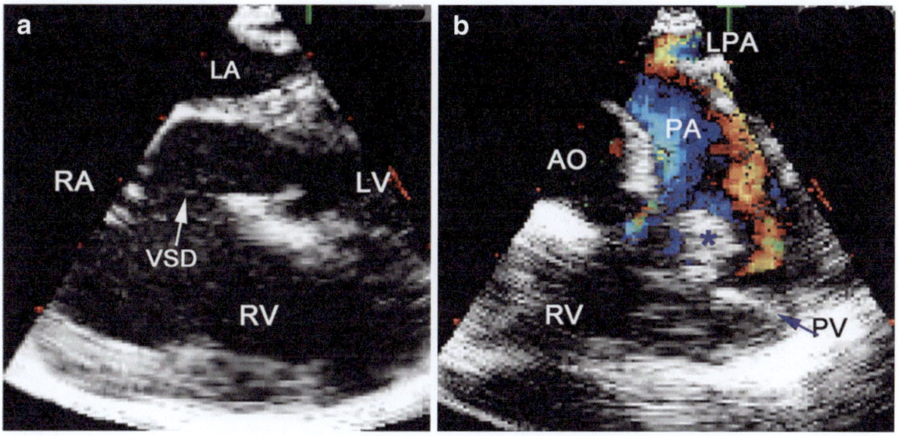

Fig. 3.17 Large VSD presenting with pulmonary insufficiency due to infective endocarditis in children. (**a**) TEE in ME 5-chamber view showing a large ventricular septal defect. (**b**) Color Doppler transesophageal echocardiography (TEE) revealed a significant vegetation (*) on the pulmonic aspect of the pulmonary valve, leading to severe pulmonary insufficiency. Additionally, a high-speed turbulent blood jet was observed, originating from the right ventricular outflow tract and flowing into the pulmonary artery. The patient underwent 6 weeks of antibiotic treatment, which was followed by surgical closure of the ventricular septal defect (VSD)

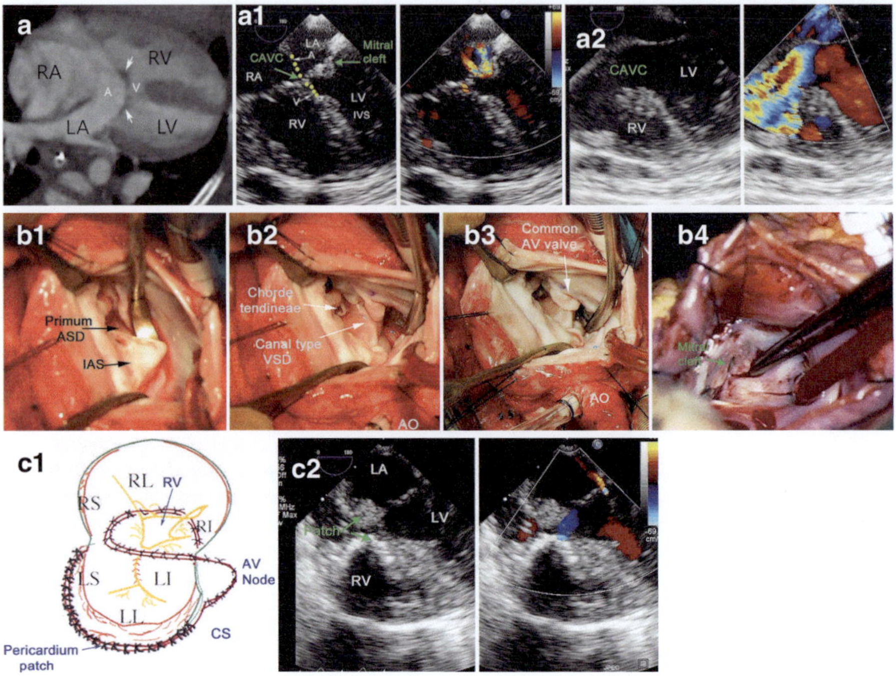

Fig. 3.18 A 5-month-old girl with a complete atrioventricular canal defect (CAVC also known as atrioventricular septal defect or endocardial cushion defect) presented with heart failure and underwent surgical correction. (**a**) A four-chamber CT image displays a CAVC consisting of a primum ASD (indicated by A) and an inlet VSD (indicated by V). The image also shows that the RA and RV are enlarged, and the atrioventricular valve can be seen (indicated by two white arrows). (**a1**) Preoperative TEE four-chamber view displays CAVC (yellow dotted line) consisting of a primum ASD (indicated by A) and an inlet VSD (indicated by V), with the atrioventricular valve leaflets inserted on the crest of the interventricular septum. A mitral cleft and regurgitation are also shown on the color Doppler TEE (right diagram). (**a2**) Transgastric view: a large inlet VSD is shown in the left diagram, consistent with a large left-to-right shunt as shown in the right diagram. (**b**) Intraoperative photography displays a large primum ASD as depicted in (**b1**); a large canal-type VSD as illustrated in (**b2**); a common atrioventricular (AV) valve with a single opening and no inlet ventricular septum, as shown in (**b3**); and a cleft in the anterior leaflet of the mitral valve (MV), as demonstrated in (**b4**). (**c1**) Diagram of the surgeon's view from the patient's right for the double-patch surgical technique to repair a CAVC. The technique involves closing the ASD and VSD with a pericardial membrane, suturing the cleft in the mitral valve leaflet, and reconstructing the tricuspid and mitral valves. Abbreviations: *L* Left, *R* Right, *S* Superior, *I* Inferior, and *L* Lateral. (**c2**) Postoperative TEE in a four-chamber view demonstrates a two-patch (also known as the sandwich technique) repair of the defect (arrows). Color Doppler imaging reveals no residual shunt crosses the patches and only mild mitral regurgitation observed in the right diagram

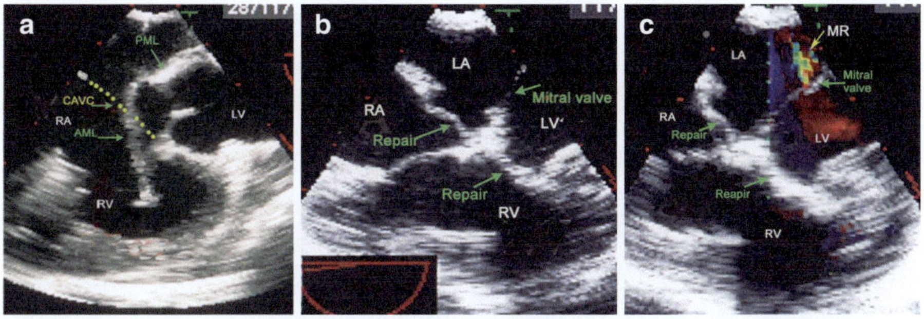

Fig. 3.19 A child with heart failure and an unusual presentation of a type B CAVC defect underwent surgical correction. (**a**) A preoperative TEE four-chamber view revealed a large primum ASD and a small inlet VSD indicated by the yellow dotted line. The anterior mitral leaflet (AML) was found to bridge the ventricular septum and attach to an anomalous papillary muscle on the right side of the ventricular septum. (**b**) A postoperative TEE four-chamber view shows repair of the defect with a double-patch technique (arrows). (**c**) A color Doppler TEE image showed no residual shunt crossed the patches and only minor mitral regurgitation (MR)

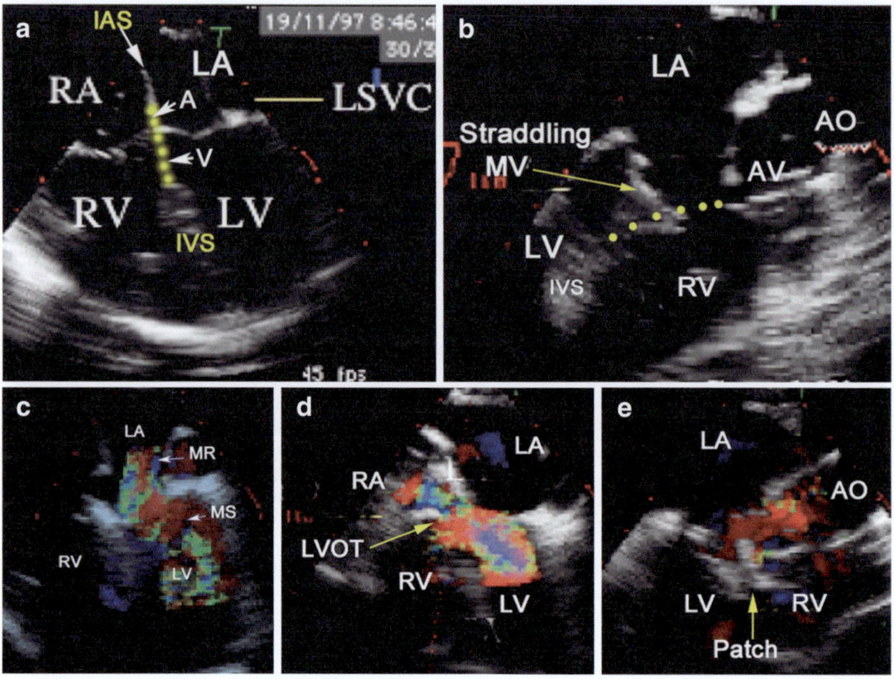

Fig. 3.20 An infant suffering from heart failure and having a complete atrioventricular canal (CAVC) defect underwent surgical correction, but needed to be reoperated twice after the initial repair. (**a**) Preoperative TEE four-chamber view revealed a large primum ASD (A) and an inlet VSD (V), indicated by the yellow dotted line. The left superior vena cava (LSVC) was also noted. (**b**) TEE in a ME AV LAX view showed a large inlet VSD, indicated by the yellow dotted line. There was absence of an atrioventricular septum, anterior displacement of the aortic valve (AV), and straddling of the mitral valve. (**c**) Postoperative color Doppler TEE four-chamber view showed severe mitral stenosis (MS) and mitral regurgitation (MR) after the surgical correction. (**d**) The patient underwent a repeat procedure to correct the MS and MR. The postoperative color Doppler in the ME five-chamber view revealed a left ventricular outflow tract (LVOT) obstruction with a pressure gradient of 50 mmHg (arrow). (**e**) Following another reoperation for correction of the LVOT obstruction, the postoperative color Doppler ME AV LAX view showed a patent LVOT without residual obstruction

References

1. Minette MS, Sahn DJ. Ventricular septal defects. Circulation. 2006;114:2190–7.
2. Devlin PJ, Russell HM, Monge MC, et al. Doubly committed and juxtaarterial ventricular septal defect: outcomes of the aortic and pulmonary valve. Ann Thorac Surg. 2014;97:2134–40.
3. Bibevski S, Ruzmetov M, Mendoza L, et al. The destiny of postoperative residual ventricular septal defects after surgical repair in infants and children. World Pediatr Congenit Heart Surg. 2020;11:438–43.
4. Ruzmetov M, Mendoza L, Decker J, et al. The destiny of postoperative residual ventricular septal defect after surgical repair in infants and children. World J Pediatr Congenit Heart Surg. 2020;11:438–43.
5. Raap GB, Weerheim J, Kappetein AP, et al. Follow-up after surgical closure of congenital ventricular septal defect. Eur J Cardiothorac Surg. 2003;24(4):511–5.

4 Valvular Abnormalities of Atrioventricular Connections

4.1 Tricuspid Atresia (TA)

1. Tricuspid atresia (TA) is a cyanotic congenital heart defect in which the tricuspid valve fails to develop properly, as a result, the right ventricle remains underdeveloped, and blood is redirected to the left side of the heart via an atrial septal defect (ASD); and a ventricular septal defect (VSD) may also exist.

   In typical cases of TA, the right ventricle (RV) becomes hypoplastic, while the position of the great arteries can be normal or transposed. Diagnosis is typically made within the first few weeks of life through echocardiograms (TTE or TEE, as shown in (Fig. 4.1d), or cardiac CT scans (depicted in Fig. 4.1b, c).

   The Bjork procedure [1, 2] is a surgical treatment option for patients with tricuspid atresia (Fig. 4.1) that involves redirecting blood flow from the right atrium to the pulmonary arteries in order to improve oxygenation and circulation. This procedure is typically performed after the initial shunt procedure (as discussed in Fig. 4.2).

S.-K. Tsai et al., *Transesophageal Echocardiography in Pediatric Congenital Cardiac Surgery and Catheter Intervention*, https://doi.org/10.1007/978-981-99-6582-3_4

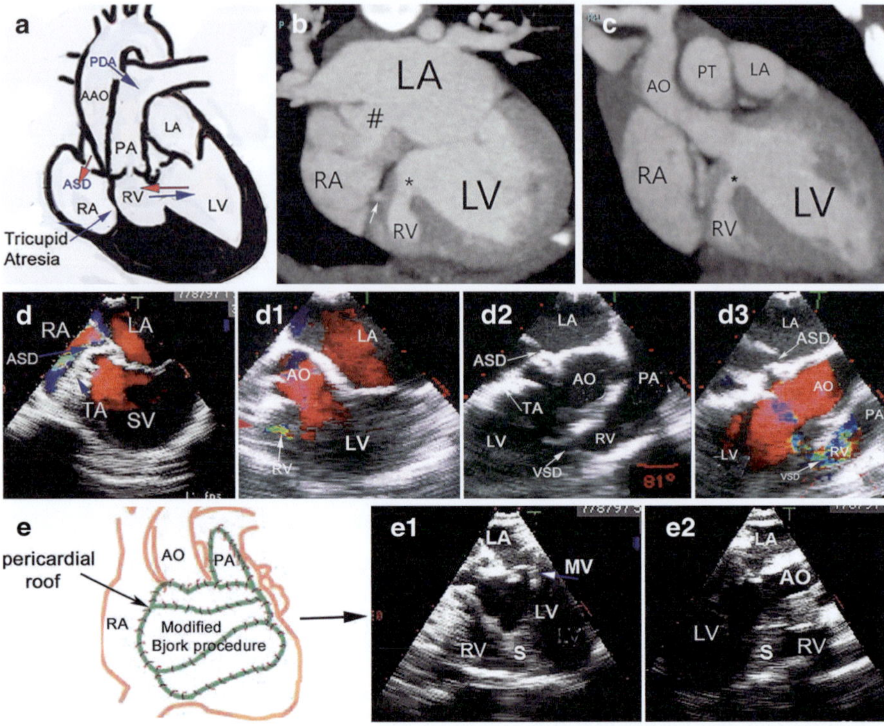

Fig. 4.1 A 2-year-old boy was diagnosed with tricuspid atresia (TA) and presented with cyanosis. He underwent surgical repair. He had a Blalock-Taussig shunt operation within the first few days of life. (**a**) A schematic drawing of TA is shown, highlighting the presence of ASD, VSD, and rudimentary RV. (**b**) A four-chamber CT image displays an interrupted connection between the RA and RV, with an invaginated right coronary artery (indicated by an arrow). The presence of an ASD (#), VSD (*), and hypoplastic RV can also be observed. (**c**) Another more cephalic section CT image depicts a normal-sized pulmonary trunk (PT) and this hypoplastic RV. The RA is dilated. (**d**) Preoperative TEE, ME four-chamber view reveals TA, a dominant LV, and an ASD. (**d1**) ME four-chamber view shows TA, ASD, a restrictive VSD, and a rudimentary RV. (**d2**) ME AV LAX view displays normally positioned major great arteries with their normal valves. The pulmonary artery (PA) is normal in size. ASD, VSD, and a small RV are well shown. (**d3**) Color Doppler TEE, ME AV LAX view displays a mosaic left-to-right jet flow through this VSD. (**e**) Surgical diagram of the modified Bjork procedure: (1) Creation of an atrioventricular connection through a direct anastomosis from the RA to the RV using a valveless conduit made from an atrial tissue flap and a large piece of pericardial roof. (2) Repair and closure of the ASD and VSD to complete a biventricular repair. (**e1**) Postoperative TEE, ME four-chamber view displays the results of this biventricular repair with patches to close the ASD and VSD. (**e2**) ME AV LAX view displays a biventricular structure with normal both ventricular outflow tracts

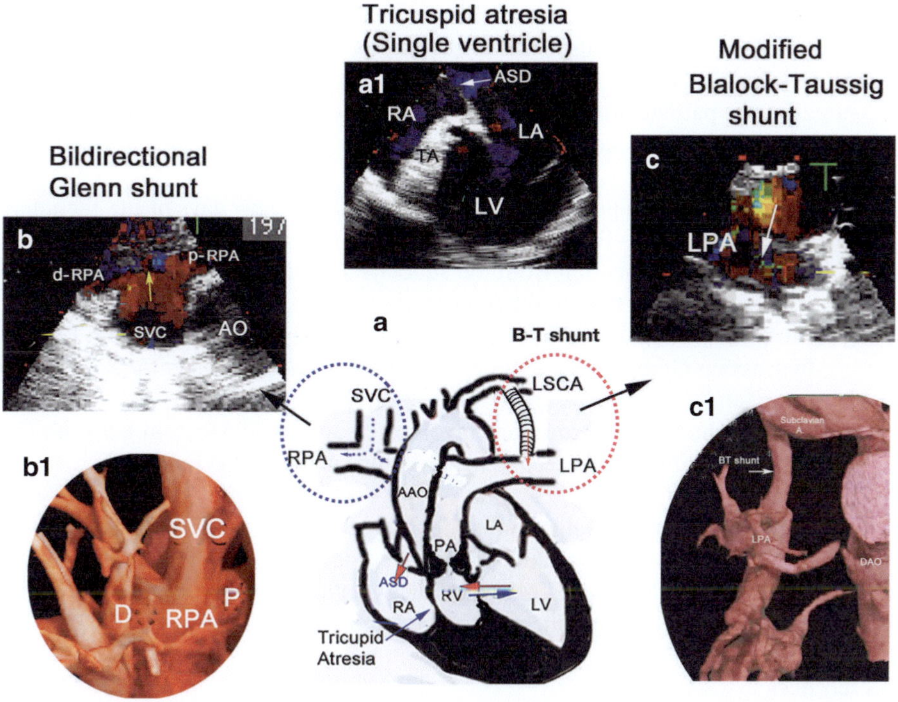

Fig. 4.2 A 4-month-old infant with cyanosis presented with tricuspid atresia (TA) and associated pulmonary stenosis (PS). The infant underwent shunt operations during the preparing stage. (**a**) A schematic representation of this case shows TA, PS, ASD, hypoplastic right ventricle (RV), and a restrictive VSD. The shunt operations performed are highlighted, including the modified left Blalock-Taussig (B-T) shunt (represented by the red dotted circle), which connects the left subclavian artery (LSCA) to the left pulmonary artery (LPA) with a graft, and the right bidirectional Glenn shunt (represented by the blue dotted circle), which connects the superior vena cava (SVC) to the right pulmonary artery (RPA). The corresponding transesophageal echocardiogram (TEE) image of TA with a dominant left ventricle (LV) is shown in (**a1**). (**b**) A color TEE image in the UE AAO view displays the bidirectional Glenn shunt, which exhibits shunt flow from the SVC into the RPA. The corresponding 3D CT image is shown in (**b1**). The abbreviations used are: P, for proximal RPA; and D, for distal RPA. (**c**) A color TEE image in the UE DAO view depicts the Blalock-Taussig shunt, which displays shunt flow into the LPA. The corresponding 3D CT image viewing from dorsally of the Blalock-Taussig shunt is shown in (**c1**)

References

1. Bjork VO, Henze A, Lillehei CW, et al. The surgical treatment of tricuspid atresia. Ann Surg. 1959;150:456–68.
2. David TE. The Ross operation for congenital aortic stenosis: update 2009. J Heart Valve Dis. 2009;18:255–261.

2. Babies born with tricuspid atresia, where the tricuspid valve is absent, underdeveloped right ventricle, also with coexisting severe pulmonary stenosis or pulmonary atresia, resulting in a functional single ventricle, require a series of surgeries to palliate this congenital heart condition. A shunt operation is a palliative surgical procedure used as a temporary measure to increase blood flow to the lungs.

   The most common palliative shunts within the first few days of life include:
   (a) Classical Blalock-Taussig (BT) shunt: This is a surgical procedure that creates a direct connection from the subclavian artery to the pulmonary artery to increase blood flow to the lungs.
   (b) Modified Blalock-Taussig (mBT) shunt: This is a variation of the BT shunt that uses a Gore-Tex tube to create the connection between the subclavian artery and pulmonary artery (refer to Fig. 4.2c, c1).
   (c) Central shunt: This procedure involves creating a connection between the aorta and pulmonary artery to increase blood flow to the lungs.

The second stage of the palliation is the bidirectional Glenn (BDG) shunt [1, 2] which is shown in Fig. 4.2b, b1, and is a surgical procedure performed at 3–6 months of age. This involves creating a connection between the superior vena cava and the pulmonary arteries, bypassing the right atrium and ventricle.

References

1. Allgood NL, Alejos J, Drinkwater DC, et al. Effectiveness of the bidirectional Glenn shunt procedure for volume unloading in the single ventricle patient. Am J Cardiol. 1994;15(74):834–6.
2. Dohain AM, Ismail MF, Elmahrouk AF, et al. The outcomes of bidirectional Glenn before and after 4 months of age: A comparative study. J Card Surg. 2020;35:3326–33.

4.2 Ebstein's Anomaly

Ebstein's anomaly is an uncommon congenital heart condition that affects the tricuspid valve, causing it to be abnormally formed and positioned lower than usual. This leads to insufficiency of tricuspid valve and blood flowing back into the right atrium, causing an enlarged right atrium, a thinned and dilated atrialized portion of the right ventricle, and usually associated with patent foramen ovale [1].

Ebstein's anomaly can be classified into four types [2]. Type A involves adequate volume of the true right ventricle. Type B has a large atrialized component of the right ventricle, but the anterior leaflet of the tricuspid valve moves freely. Type C has severely restricted movement of the anterior leaflet, leading to significant obstruction of the right ventricular outflow tract. Type D is characterized by almost complete atrialization of the ventricle, except for a small infundibular component.

The diagnosis of Ebstein's anomaly typically involves a combination of medical history, physical examination to check for abnormal heart sounds or murmurs, and

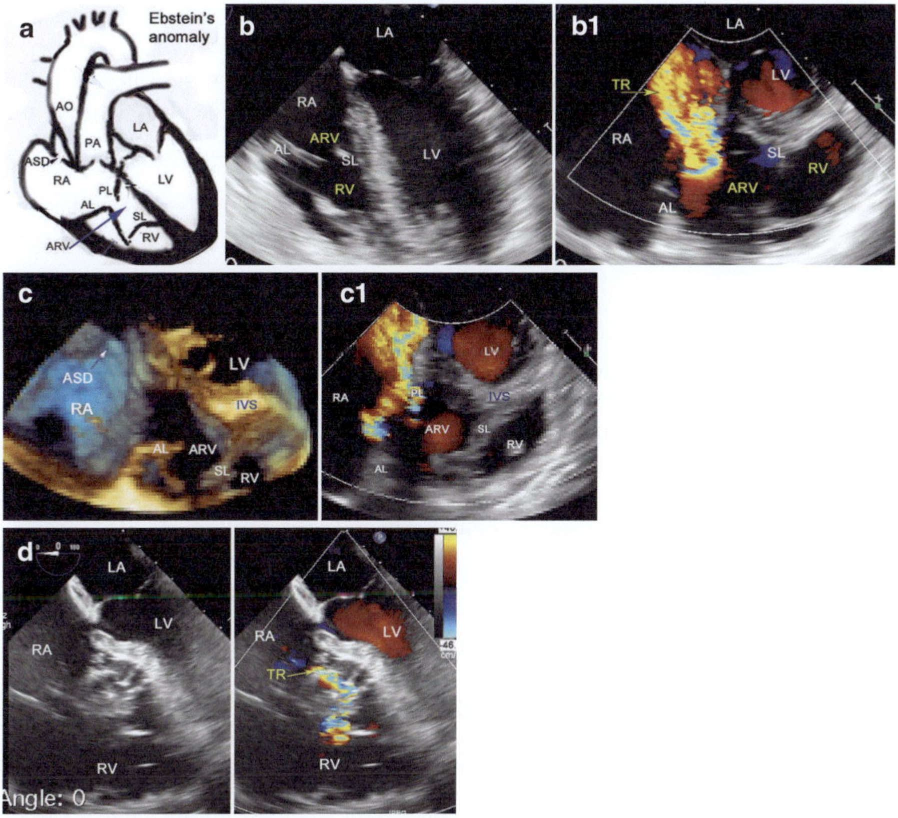

Fig. 4.3 Depicts a 16-year-old child who presented with mild cyanosis and a history of exertional dyspnea and shortness of breath. The child was diagnosed with Ebstein's anomaly and underwent surgical correction. (**a**) This diagram depicts Ebstein's anomaly, which is characterized by a malformed tricuspid valve. The septal leaflet (SL) is displaced apically, and the anterior leaflet (AL) is elongated and tethered. (**b**) The preoperative TEE image in the ME four-chamber view displays the ASD, as well as the malformed tricuspid valve with a redundant, sail-like AL and a downward attachment of the SL leading to the atrialization of the RV. The corresponding color Doppler TEE image in (**b1**) displays a moderate to severe tricuspid regurgitation and an atrialized right ventricle (ARV). (**c**) The 3D TEE image shows the ASD, a redundant sail-like AL, and a middle RV obstruction with the SL inserting directly into the interventricular septum (IVS). The corresponding color Doppler 3D TEE image in (**c1**) reveals tricuspid regurgitation, further highlighting the SL insertion into the IVS and the middle-RV obstruction. (**d**) After surgical repair, which included plication of the ARV, atrioplasty, and tricuspid valve repair with tricuspid annuloplasty, the postoperative color Doppler TEE in the ME four-chamber view shows a mild residual tricuspid regurgitation (TR) (right diagram)

diagnostic imaging tests such as an echocardiogram (TTE or TEE) may be used in confirming cases, as shown in Fig. 4.3.

The specific repair of the tricuspid valve in Ebstein's anomaly will depend on the severity and location of the valve abnormality. In some cases, the tricuspid valve may be able to be repaired using surgical techniques. The goal of surgery is to improve the function of the valve and to prevent blood from flowing backwards into the right atrium.

Surgical repair of Ebstein's anomaly may include mobilizing the anterior leaflet of the tricuspid valve, repositioning the anterior and posterior leaflets to cover the orifice area at the normal level, and remodeling and reinforcing the tricuspid annulus using a prosthetic ring, as shown in Fig. 4.3d.

Valve repair is preferred over valve replacement, if possible, because it has the potential to be more durable and avoids potential complications associated with valve replacement [3].

References

1. Van Son JA, Konstantinov IE, Zimmermann V, et al. Ebstein and Ebstein's malformation. Eur J Cardiothorac Surg. 2001;20:1082–85.
2. Carpentier A, Chauvaud S, Mace L, et al. A new reconstructive operation for Ebstein's anomaly of the tricuspid valve. J Thorac Cardiovasc Surg. 1988;96:92–101.
3. Chen JM, Mosca RS, Altmann K, et al. Early and medium-term results for repair of Ebstein anomaly. J Thorac Cardiovasc Surg. 2004;127:990–8.

4.3 Mitral Atresia (MA) with Hypoplastic Left Heart Syndrome (HLHS)

4.3.1 Mitral Atresia [1, 2]

Mitral atresia [1, 2] is a rare congenital heart defect where the mitral valve does not form correctly, causing a complete blockage of blood flow from the left atrium to the left ventricle. Mitral atresia often occurs with other congenital heart defects (atrial septal defect or ventricular septal defect).

Mitral atresia typically involves a univentricular atrioventricular connection to a dominant right ventricle via a tricuspid valve, with an imperforate or absent mitral valve and a hypoplastic underdeveloped left ventricle. In cases where there is an intact ventricular septum, the left ventricular blood inflow is obstructed, leading to a smaller, underdeveloped left ventricle (as seen in Fig. 4.4). This can affect surgical approach and outcome.

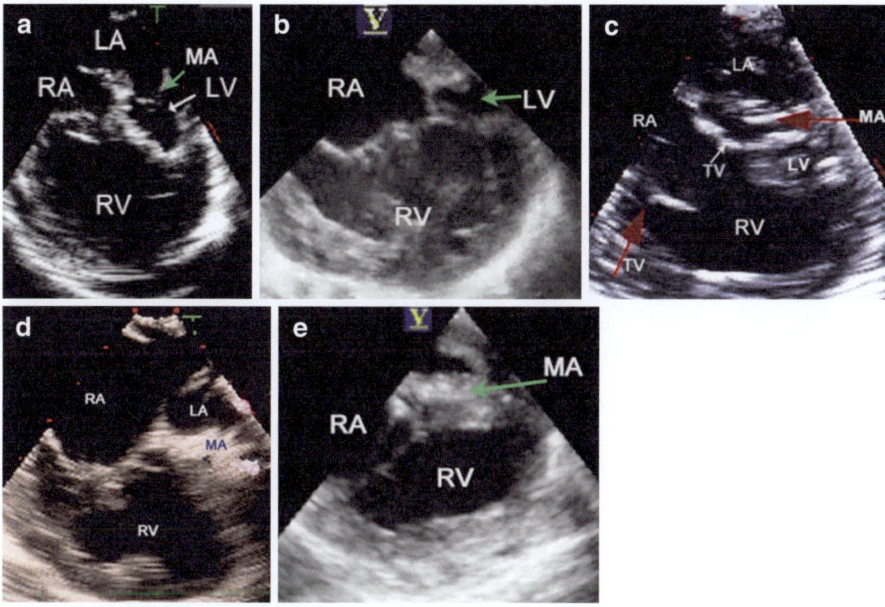

Fig. 4.4 Illustrates the different types of morphology associated with underdevelopment of the mitral valve. In neonates with congenital mitral atresia (MA) and an intact ventricular septum, blood from the left atrium (LA) is unable to flow to the left ventricle (LV), resulting in varied degree of underdevelopment of the LV. Mitral atresia is frequently accompanied by other congenital heart defects. Underdevelopment of the mitral valve is characterized by a range of features, including varying degrees of hypoplasia of the LV and the mitral valve. The TEE images above mainly depict the different morphologies of mitral valve and the accompanying LV in neonates. The TEE images of MA depict a univentricular atrioventricular connection with a dominant right ventricle through a tricuspid valve. This condition is associated with an intact ventricular septum, and the aorta arises from the rudimentary LV. MA is often part of hypoplastic left heart syndrome (HLHS), which affects the surgical approach and outcome. The LV can exhibit varying degrees of hypoplasia (**a**–**c**) or may appear as a blind pouch (**d**, **e**)

Types of mitral atresia are based on the anatomy of the heart and include:

- Isolated Mitral Atresia: The mitral valve is completely blocked, and there are no other significant structural abnormalities in the heart.
- Mitral Atresia with Hypoplastic Left Heart Syndrome (HLHS): In addition to mitral atresia, there is also underdevelopment or hypoplasia of the left ventricle, aortic valve, and ascending aorta (will be discussed in Fig. 4.5).

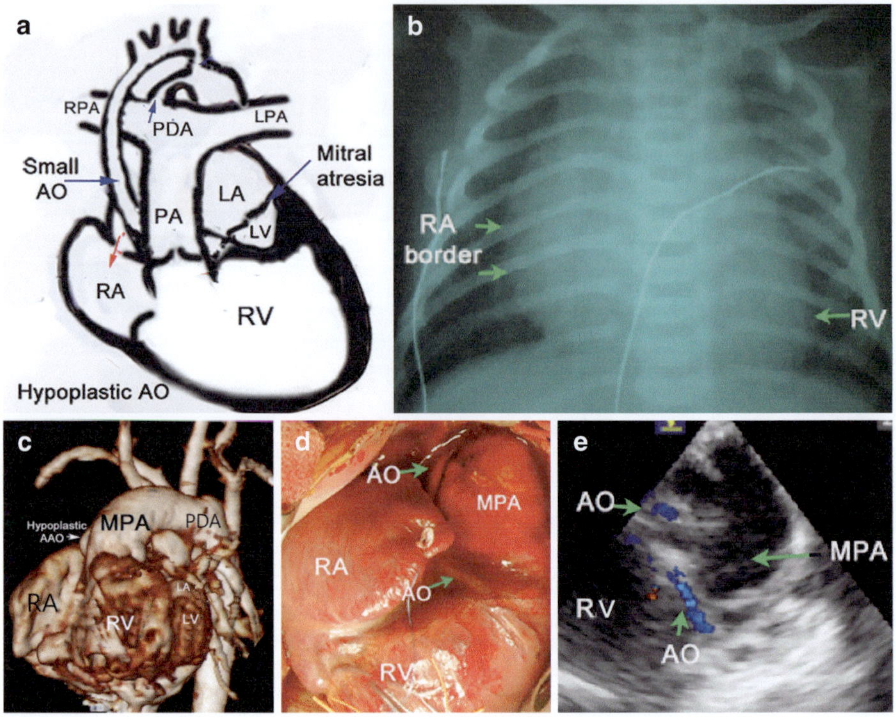

Fig. 4.5 Shows a 1-day-old male neonate who developed respiratory distress and cyanosis a few hours after birth. He was diagnosed with hypoplastic left heart syndrome (HLHS) and pulmonary venous hypertension. (**a**) This schematic drawing shows the typical features of HLHS, including a small aorta due to hypoplasia, a large main pulmonary artery (PA), mitral atresia with a rudimentary left ventricle (LV), an atrial septal defect (ASD), and a large patent ductus arteriosus (PDA). (**b**) This chest X-ray shows an oddly shaped silhouette, an enlarged cardiac silhouette, and mild pulmonary edema. (**c**) This 3D cardiac CT image shows a very hypoplastic ascending aorta (AAO), an engorged main pulmonary artery (MPA), and PDA, as well as a rudimentary LV and dilated right ventricle (RV). (**d**) This intraoperative photograph shows an enlarged RV, a large MPA, and a small AAO indicated by the green arrows. (**e**) This intraoperative TEE, ME AV SAX view demonstrates RV dilatation, a large MPA, and a small AO

References

1. Anderson RH, Strasburger JF, Jonas RA. Mitral atresia. Circulation. 2007;115(4):442–51.
2. Geva T. Management of patients with mitral atresia. Curr Opin Pediatr. 2018;30(5):609–15.

4.3.2 Mitral Atresia (MA) with Hypoplastic Left Heart Syndrome (HLHS)

Mitral atresia with hypoplastic left heart syndrome (HLHS) is a complex congenital heart defect that affects the development of the left side of the heart. In addition to mitral atresia (as discussed in Sect. 4.3), HLHS involves hypoplasia, or underdevelopment, of the left ventricle, aortic valve, and ascending aorta. As a result, the right ventricle becomes the dominant pumping chamber for the body, and the ductus arteriosus remains open to allow blood to rescue the underdeveloped left side of the heart [1, 2].

It is important to note that HLHS is a complex and serious condition, and an accurate and timely diagnosis is crucial for ensuring the best outcomes. These tests may include a chest X-ray, echocardiogram, or a computed tomography (CT) scan. These imaging studies (refer to Fig. 4.5) can provide more detailed information about the heart and surrounding structures.

The size of the aorta is crucial for the success of the Norwood procedure in treating hypoplastic left heart syndrome. Therefore, careful preoperative evaluation and planning (as discussed in Fig. 4.6) are necessary to optimize outcomes for each patient. If the aorta is too small, the surgical complexity, duration, and risk of complications increase.

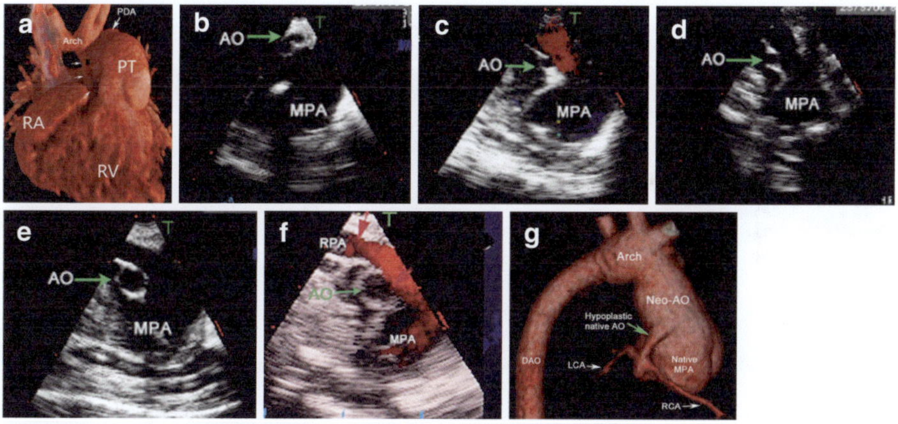

Fig. 4.6 Displays hypoplastic left heart syndrome (HLHS) with a hypoplastic aorta, as depicted in (**a**), which shows a 3D cardiac CT image with three arrows indicating the hypoplastic ascending aorta. There is a significant variation in the aortic morphology of HLHS, which is a crucial factor in determining the success of surgical intervention. Accurately identifying the morphological features and size of the aorta in the TEE image is of paramount importance in selecting the appropriate surgical option, such as the Norwood procedure. This procedure involves connecting the bottom part of the pulmonary artery to the hypoplastic ascending aorta and reconstructing it to create a larger neo-aorta, as shown in (**g**), which shows a 3D cardiac CT image of the Norwood operation with a neo-AO reconstruction. In neonates with HLHS, there are varying degrees of hypoplasia of the ascending aorta, indicated by the green arrow. Intraoperative TEE images, specifically the ME AV SAX view, in cases (**b**), (**c**), and (**d**) show a small ascending aorta with a diameter of less than 3 mm. In contrast, case (**e**) exhibits a larger aorta with a diameter of 5 mm, while case (**f**) shows an even larger diameter of 6 mm

Balloon septostomy is an initial treatment option for newborns with hypoplastic left heart syndrome (HLHS). During this procedure, as described in Fig. 4.7, a balloon catheter is used to create or enlarge an opening in the interatrial septum, allowing oxygenated blood from the lungs to mix with deoxygenated blood from the body.

The Norwood procedure is a complex staged surgery used to treat hypoplastic left heart syndrome (HLHS) in newborn. It involves three stages: (as shown in Figs. 4.8, 4.9, 4.10, and 4.11).

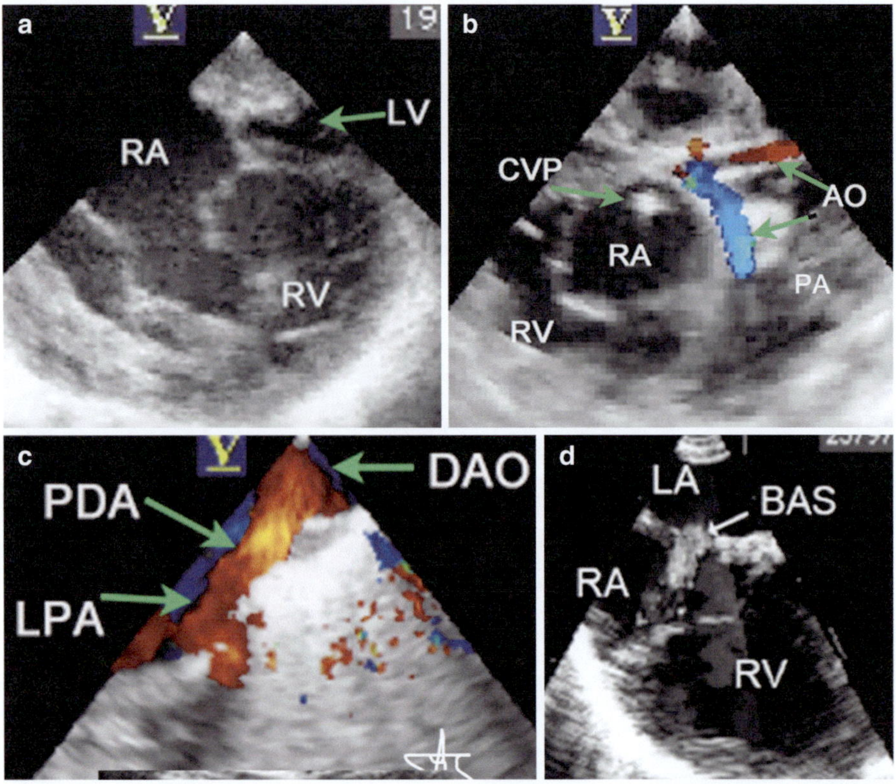

Fig. 4.7 Shows the initial stage of treatment for hypoplastic left heart syndrome (HLHS), which involves the early introduction of prostaglandin E1 to maintain ductal patency and performing balloon atrial septostomy (BAS). However, this procedure can be challenging in infants with HLHS and a small atrial septal defect (ASD). (**a**) This is an intraoperative TEE image showing a four-chamber view, which demonstrates mitral atresia with a hypoplastic left ventricle and a large right ventricle. (**b**) A color Doppler TEE image reveals a small and underdeveloped ascending aorta (AO), as well as a large pulmonary artery (PA). (**c**) The color Doppler TEE image from the UE left pulmonary artery view confirms the patency of a PDA flow with the use of prostaglandin E1 infusion. (**d**) Following the BAS procedure, the ME four-chamber view shows a blood flow across the interatrial septum from the LA to the RA, allowing for unobstructed mixing of blood between the two chambers

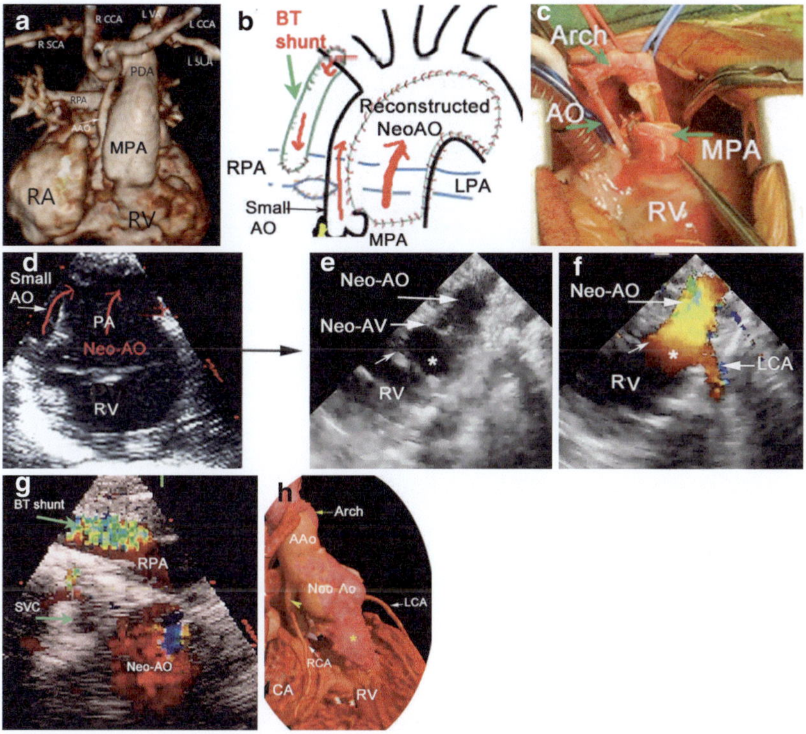

Fig. 4.8 Shows the staged Norwood procedure being performed on a neonate with hypoplastic left heart syndrome (HLHS). (**a**) This 3D cardiac CT image of a neonate with HLHS shows a large main pulmonary artery (MPA) and patent ductus arteriosus (PDA) originating from the RV and directly connecting to the descending aorta, along with severe hypoplasia of the ascending aorta and (AAO, white arrow) connecting to the aortic arch. (**b**) This illustration shows the anatomic changes made during the modified Norwood procedure for HLHS, which include joining the bottom part of the pulmonary artery with the ascending aorta to create a larger neo-aorta (neo-AO) (also known as the Damus-Kaye-Stansel procedure) divided distal MPA, creating a shunt graft between the innominate and pulmonary arteries (known as the modified Blalock-Taussig shunt), and excising the atrial septum. Red arrows indicate the direction of blood flow. (**c**) Intraoperative photograph illustrates the transection of the distal MPA, a diminutive ascending aorta (AO), the aortic arch, and the vascular allograft used to reconstruct a neo-aorta (neo-AO). (**d**) During the intraoperative TEE, a UE AAO view demonstrated a small aorta and a large pulmonary artery (PA) arising from a functional single right ventricle (RV). The large PA and small AO will fuse side by side to create a neo-aorta (red arrows). (**e**) Postoperative TEE after Norwood procedure showing neo-aorta (neo-AO) connecting to the aortic arch. (Asterisk indicates original PA; white small arrow indicates the original small AO). (**f**) Color Doppler TEE showing blood flow directly from functional RV to neo-AO without obstruction and the blood flowing very clearly to left coronary artery (LCA). Right coronary artery is not shown in this view. (Asterisk indicates original PA; white small arrow indicates the original small AO). (**g**) The color Doppler TEE of the UE AV SAX view revealed a turbulent blood flow in the modified Blalock-Taussig shunt, which connects the subclavian artery to the RPA. (**h**) This postoperative 3D volume-rendered CT image shows the neo-AO formed by the jointing of the MPA trunk to the side of the original AAo (yellow arrowhead) after the Norwood procedure (DKS procedure). This new connection allows blood from the RV to communicate directly into the AAo, with the left coronary artery (LCA) and right coronary artery (RCA) are clearly visible. The asterisk indicates the original MPA arising site. The common atrium (CA) is also visible

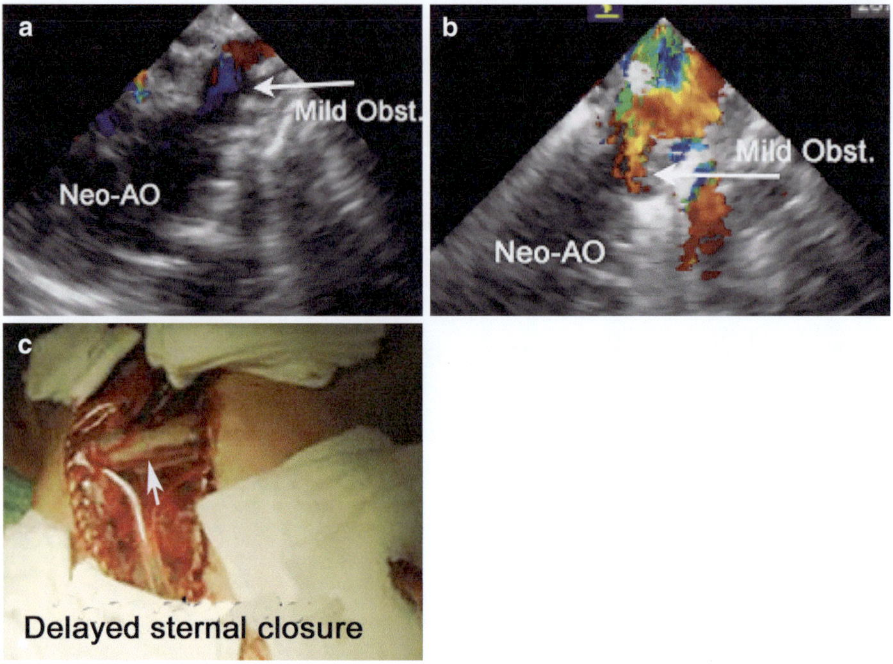

Fig. 4.9 Shows a delayed closure of sternotomy in a patient who underwent the Norwood procedure, as seen in Fig. 4.8. This complication may result from a variety of factors and can have implications for the patient's recovery and overall outcome. (**a**) This postoperative TEE image shows the neo-aorta (neo-AO) after the Norwood procedure, as viewed from the UE with a focus on the ascending aorta (AAo). Mild arch obstruction was noted during sternotomy closure, which may have implications for the patient's recovery. (**b**) This color Doppler TEE image, taken after the Norwood procedure, shows turbulence at the junction of this neo-AO to the aortic arch (indicated by the arrow). This stenosis is caused by extrinsic compression from the sternal closure resulting in a junctional kinking. (**c**) To prevent external compression or excessive tension on the neo-AO following the Norwood procedure, delayed sternal closure can be achieved by using a small piece of plastic tube (arrow) and sterile dressing to cover the wound temporally opened

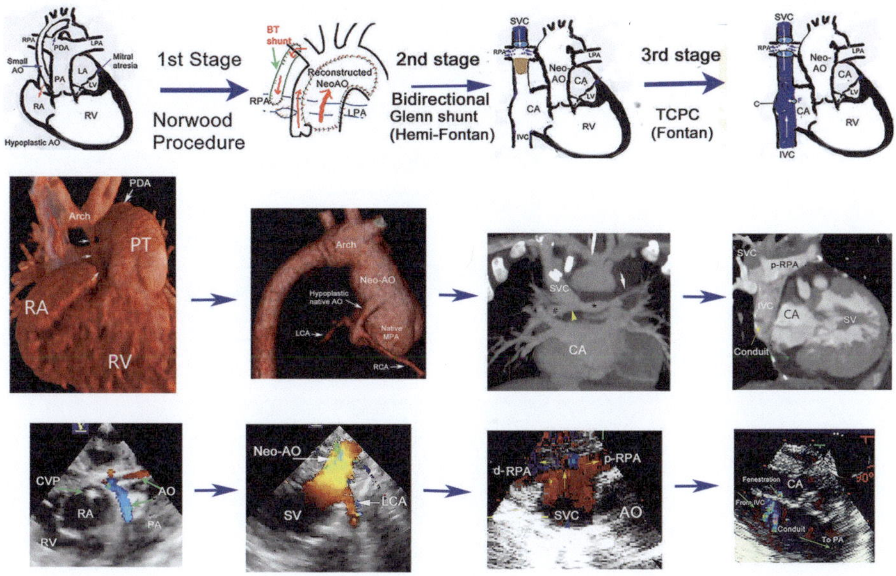

Fig. 4.10 Shows the staged surgical palliation procedure for a hypoplastic left heart syndrome (HLHS). Managing HLHS remains one of the greatest challenges in congenital heart surgery. The three-stage surgical palliation procedure remains the most common treatment for patients with HLHS. Without surgical intervention, 95% of children with HLHS die within the first month of life (ref 2, 3). (1) **The upper panel of the diagram** shows the three stages of surgical palliation for a HLHS from left to right. Stage I of the modified Norwood procedure involves aortic arch reconstruction through a side-to-side anastomosis of the main pulmonary artery (MPA) to the ascending aorta (AAO), an atrial septectomy, and a modified Blalock-Taussig shunt. The Norwood stage I procedure is best be completed during the neonatal period. Stage II is the Hemi-Fontan procedure (bidirectional Glenn shunt-superior cavopulmonary anastomosis), which is highly suggested to be completed when the child is between 4 and 6 months of age. Stage III is the Fontan procedure (TCPC-total cavopulmonary connection), which is better to be completed when the child is between 2 and 3 years of age. (2) **The middle panel** are photos demonstrating the corresponding cardiac CT images at different stages of this palliative surgery. (3) **The lower panel** are diagrams illustrating the corresponding TEE images at different stages of this surgery

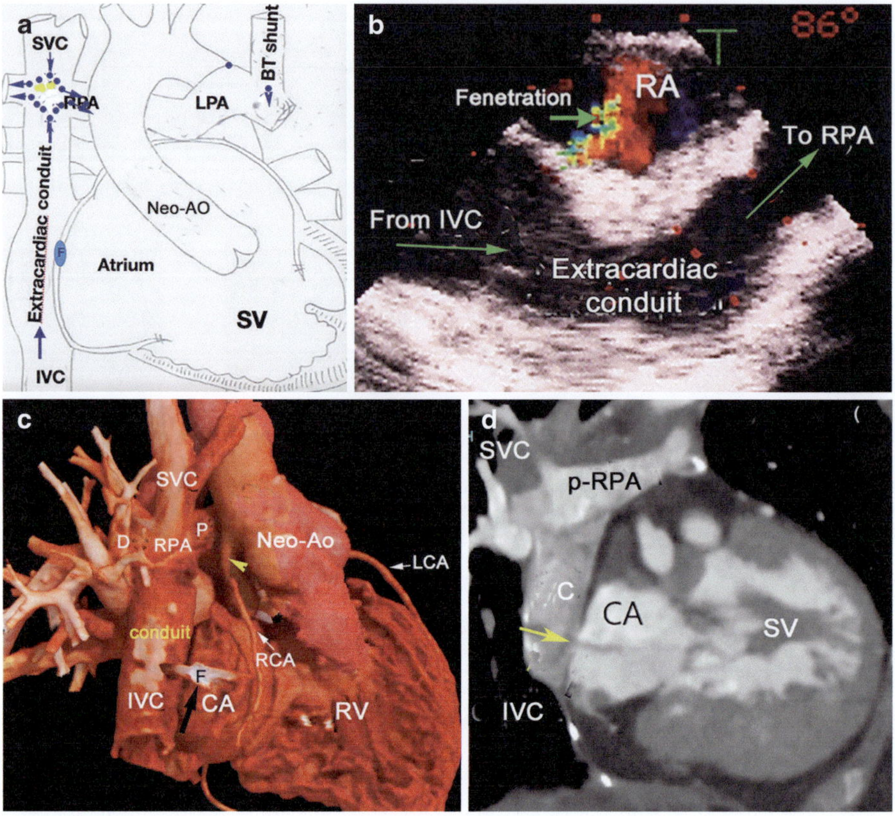

Fig. 4.11 Shows the staged operation of the Fontan procedure that was scheduled for a 5-year-old female patient diagnosed with hypoplastic left heart syndrome (HLHS) who had previously undergone the Norwood procedure and bidirectional Glenn shunt. (**a**) A Fontan procedure with an extracardiac conduit and fenestration (F) is depicted in a schematic drawing. This procedure involves the use of an extracardiac conduit with a fenestration (F) to divert blood flow from the inferior vena cava (IVC) combined with the superior vena cava (SVC) to RPA create a blood flow circuit called total cavopulmonary connection (TCPC). (**b**) The intraoperative color TEE in the bicaval view shows an extracardiac conduit connecting the IVC and RPA, with a fenestrated blood flow from the conduit to the right atrium (RA). (**c**) The postoperative 3D volume rendering CT image in frontal view shows a successful TCPC with a fenestration jet flow (F) into the common atrium (CA). The proximal and distal ends of the RPA are labeled as P and D, respectively, and the arrowhead points to the original hypoplastic ascending aorta. (**d**) The postoperative contrast-enhanced CT in oblique-coronal section also shows a patent dark jet flow (indicated by a yellow arrow) into the lumen of the CA. The major blood from IVC flows upward to RPA through this fully patent conduit, bypassing intracardiac structures, is demonstrated. The abbreviation CA refers to the common atrium; P-RPA refers to the proximal end of the RPA

1. The first stage (Norwood procedure) involves reconstructing the aorta to create a neo-aorta for blood flow to the body and creating a modified BT shunt for blood to the lung circulation, as shown in Figs. 4.8 and 4.9.
2. The second stage, called the bidirectional Glenn shunt, is usually performed when the child is a few months old (as discussed in Sect. 4.1: Fig. 4.2, Sect. 5.1.6: Fig. 5.35).
3. The third stage, known as the Fontan procedure [2, 3], is typically performed when the child is 2–3 years old, as described in Fig. 4.10. However, the complete procedure will be detailed in Fig. 4.11.

References

1. Wernovsky G, Ghanayem N, Ohye RG. Hypoplastic left heart syndrome. Lancet. 2016;387:2193–204.
2. Cohen MS. Survival and quality of life for hypoplastic left heart syndrome patients after the Fontan procedure. J Am Coll Cardiol. 2019;73:3078–87.
3. Khairy E, Poirier N, Mercier LA. Hypoplastic left heart syndrome: current considerations and expectations. J Am Coll Cardiol. 2010;56(10):793–800.

Anomalies of the Great Vessels & Ventriculoarterial Connections

5

5.1 (A). Abnormal Connections between Great Arteries and Ventricles

5.1.1 Transposition of the Great Arteries (TGA)

Transposition of the great arteries (TGA) is a congenital heart defect in which the two major arteries leaving the heart are switched, meaning that the aorta arises from the right ventricle and the pulmonary artery arises from the left ventricle, as illustrated in Fig. 5.1.

- The classification of TGA is important for determining the appropriate treatment plan for each individual patient. The most common types of TGA are (Fig. 5.2):
  - Dextro-Transposition of the Great Arteries (d-TGA): This is the most common type of TGA, accounting for about 90% of cases. In d-TGA, the aorta arises from the right ventricle and the pulmonary artery arises from the left ventricle, while the right ventricle is right to the left ventricle in situs solitus.
  - Levo-Transposition of the Great Arteries (L-TGA, also known as corrected transposition of the great arteries): In situs solitus and levocardia L-TGA, the aorta arises from the right ventricle and the pulmonary artery arises from the left ventricle, while the right ventricle is left to the left ventricle. Therefore, inflow and outflow of ventricles are both switched, and it is so called corrected TGA. This is a rare condition and is often associated with other cardiac abnormalities, such as a ventricular septal defect (VSD) or atrioventricular (AV) block.

S.-K. Tsai et al., *Transesophageal Echocardiography in Pediatric Congenital Cardiac Surgery and Catheter Intervention*, https://doi.org/10.1007/978-981-99-6582-3_5

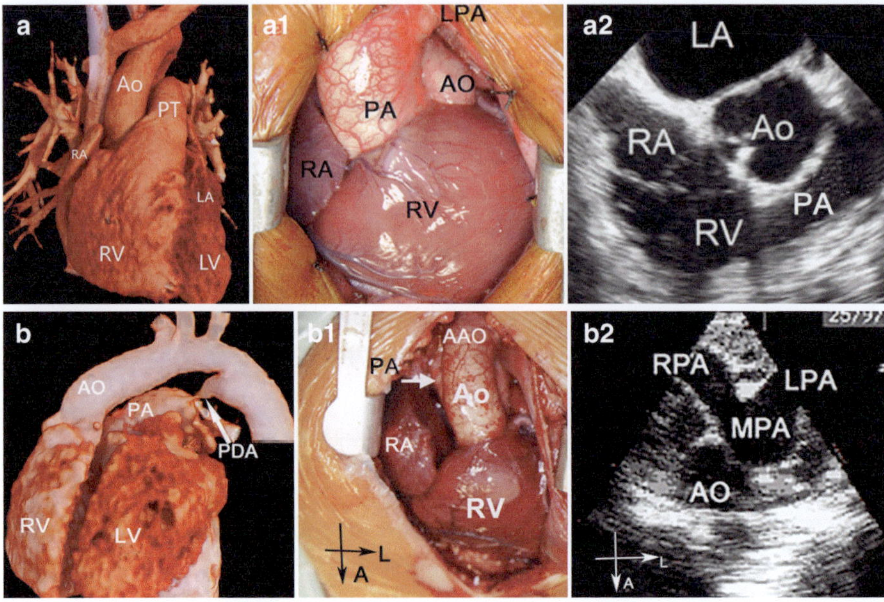

Fig. 5.1 Transposition of the great arteries (TGA) is a rare, yet serious congenital heart defect. With TGA, the two main arteries of the heart—the aorta and pulmonary artery—are switched, so that they arise from the wrong ventricles. This can lead to significant cardiac and pulmonary complications and can't survive typically, requiring surgical intervention in their life. (**a**) Normal 3D spatial relationship between the great arteries: The pulmonary artery (PA) arises from the right ventricle (RV) and is located anterior to the aorta (AO). (**a1**) Intraoperative surgical photo of a normal heart shows the PA leaving the RV and the AO leaving the LV. The AO is located posterior to the PA. (**a2**) The corresponding TEE image of a normal heart, as viewed from the ME AV SAX view, shows the normal position of the PA in front of and to the left of the AO. (**b**) Three-dimensional volume rendered CT image in left lateral view of a dextro-transposition of the great arteries (D-TGA) shows the AO arising from the RV and PA arising from LV. (**b1**) Intraoperative surgical photo of a D-TGA shows the AO leaving the RV and the PA leaving the LV (not shown). The AO is located left-anterior to the PA. (**b2**) The corresponding TEE image of a D-TGA, as viewed from the ME AV SAX view, shows the transposed position of the AO in front of the PA

– Double outlet right ventricle (DORV) with hemodynamic mimic of TGA: In this type of DORV, both the aorta and the pulmonary artery arise from the right ventricle. Pulmonary artery is adjacent to the left ventricular outflow tract and VSD (also known as Taussig-Bing anomaly). This is a rare condition and is often associated with other cardiac abnormalities, such as coarctation of aorta or pulmonary stenosis.

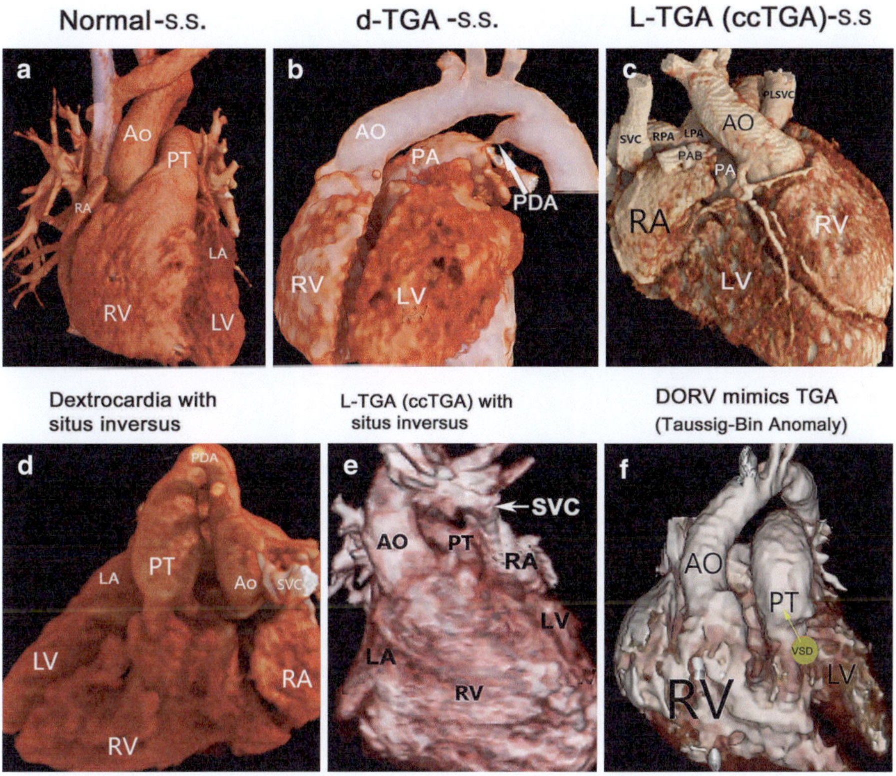

Fig. 5.2 Shows types of the transposition of the great arteries (TGA). TGA in **situs solitus** (SS) can be classified into: (**a**) normal relation of the great vessels. Atrioventricular concordance and ventriculoarterial concordance. (**b**) d-TGA: aorta arising from RV and PA arising from LV. Atrioventricular concordance but ventriculoarterial discordance. (**c**) Congenitally corrected TGA (ccTGA), also known as L-TGA (Levo-looped), in which both the atrioventricular and the ventriculoarterial connections are discordant. This “double reversal” allows the body to receive oxygen-rich blood and the lungs to receive oxygen-poor blood. The **situs inversus** shown in (**d**), inverted arrangement of the viscera and atria, with a left-sided RA and a right-sided LA, as if in a mirror-image of the normal arrangement in situs solitus. The tip of the heart points toward the right side of the chest instead of the left side, known as a dextrocardia. (**e**) In case of a L-TGA with situs inversus, the aorta originates from the morphological right ventricle. (Please refer to Figs. 5.16 and 5.17 for more details). (**f**) Hemodynamical TGA but anatomical DORV with a subpulmonary VSD (also called Taussig-Bing anomaly) consists of both great arteries that arise from the RV, and also have malpositions. Aorta (AO) is located parallelly to the right of the pulmonary artery (PA) (please refer to Figs. 6.5 and 6.7 for more detail)

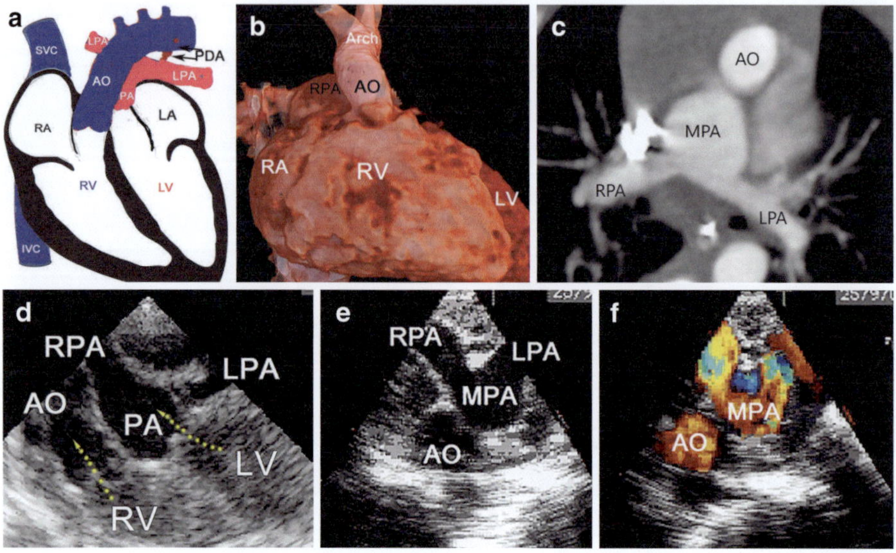

Fig. 5.3 Shows perioperative various diagnostic multimodality imaging for D-TGA. (**a**) Diagram of a TGA illustrating that the main pulmonary artery (PA) and aorta (AO) are switched in position, or transposed. The right ventricle (RV) bringing deoxygenated blood to the aorta and the left ventricle (LV) bringing oxygenated blood to the PA. (**b**) A 3D volume-rendered cardiac CT image shows that the AO arises from the RV and the PA arises from the LV. In the image, the AO is clearly positioned in front of the PA. (**c**) A cardiac CT study in axial section shows that the AO is located anterior to the main pulmonary artery (MPA). (**d**) The corresponding TEE image shows that the AO arises from the RV, and the PA arises from the LV. (**e**, **f**) Intraoperative color TEE in the UE AAO SAX view shows that the AO is located anterior and a little right of the MPA

- Diagnosis of TGA is typically made through multiple imaging studies, including transesophageal echocardiography (TEE, Fig. 5.3d–f), and CT scan (Fig. 5.3b, c).

  In Transposition of the Great Arteries (TGA), the positions of the aorta and pulmonary artery are switched, as shown in Fig. 5.3. This abnormal positioning of the great arteries in TGA can complicate the arterial switch operation (ASO), as illustrated in Fig. 5.4.
- Balloon arterial septostomy (BAS) is a medical procedure used as a temporary measure to treat d-TGA with intact ventricular septum in newborns who are not yet suitable candidates for early surgical correction (Fig. 5.5).
- The surgical treatment of d-TGA typically involves an arterial switch operation (ASO) to correct the abnormality. There are two types of ASO that may be used:

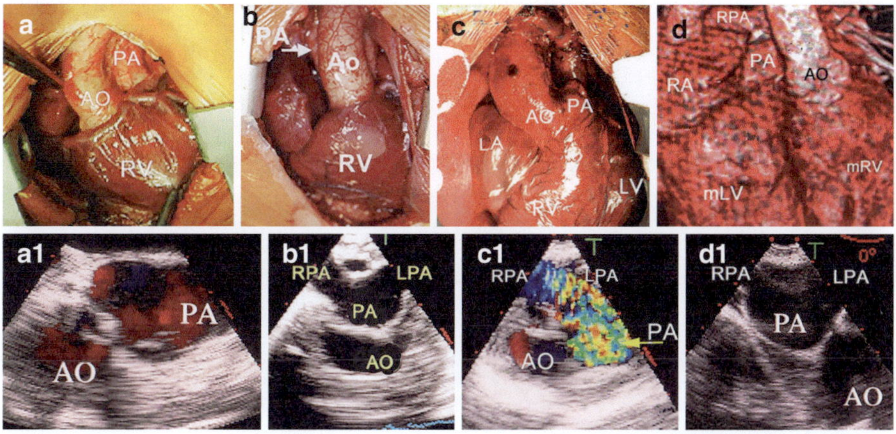

Fig. 5.4 Shows the spatial relationships of the great arteries in abnormalities of ventriculoarterial connections. Correct identification of the morphology and spatial relationship of the great arteries is essential for proper planning of an arterial switch operation (ASO). Furthermore, this can assist in assessing the potential for pulmonary artery stenosis following ASO with a LeCompte maneuver. There are four main types of spatial relationships between the great vessels in these cases. Type I is characterized by the AO (aorta) being located anterior to the right of the PA (pulmonary artery) which is a typical D-TGA (transposition of the great artery), as shown in **a** (surgical photograph) and **a1** (corresponding TEE image). Type II is characterized by the AO lying directly in front of the PA, as shown in **b** (surgical photograph) and **b1** (corresponding TEE image). Type III involves a side-by-side transposition of the AO and the PA. This is illustrated in **c**, which is a surgical photograph of a patient with the double outlet of right ventricle (DORV) mimicking TGA, and in **c1**, which shows the corresponding TEE image. Type IV is characterized by the AO positioned anteriorly and to the left of the PA which is a typical L-TGA, as illustrated in **d** (a 3D volume-rendered CT image, "m" indicating morphologically) and **d1** (the corresponding TEE image). Additionally, according to Paladini et al., it was reported that Type I comprises 56.5%, while Type II and Type III account for 26.1% and 17.4% of these cases, respectively

the Jatene procedure with LeCompte maneuver (Figs. 5.6, 5.7, and 5.8) and physiological spiral reconstruction [2, 3], which involve creating a common wall shared between the great arteries (as shown in Figs. 5.6, 5.7, and 5.8).

- Postoperative complications after ASO:

  Although most patients have successful outcomes after surgery for d-TGA, there is a possibility of postoperative complications. These include leaks or residual narrowing (stenosis) of the arteries [4], which may require immediate correction (as shown in Fig. 5.9) or later balloon dilatation (as shown in Figs. 5.10 and 5.11).

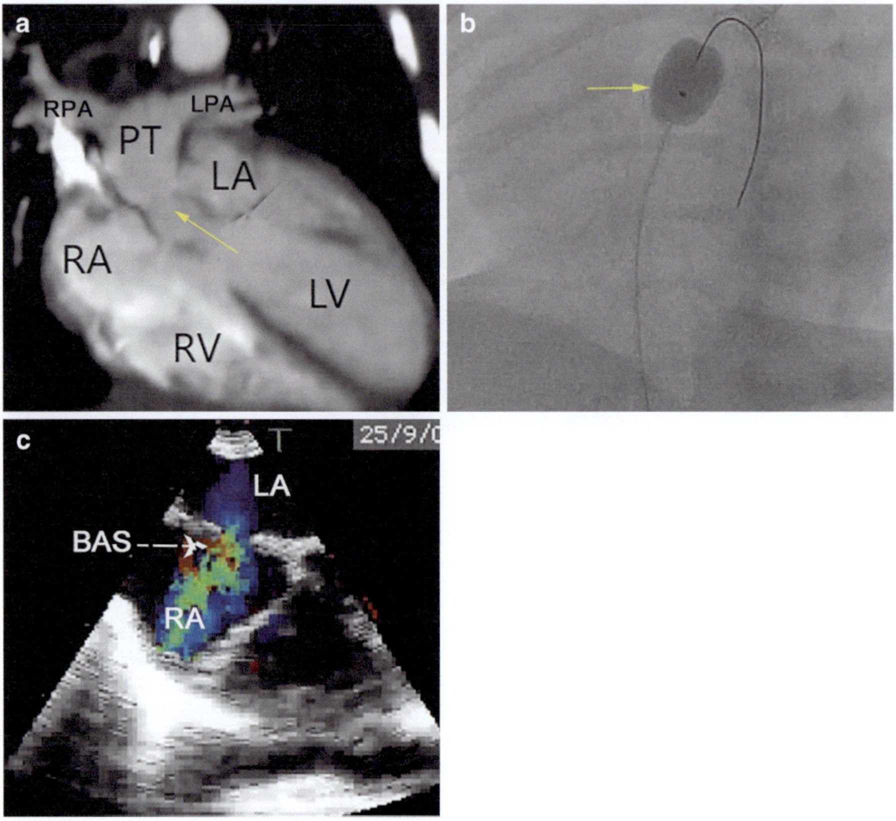

Fig. 5.5 Shows the use of balloon atrial septostomy (BAS) to improve oxygenation in a newborn with a transposition of the great arteries (TGA) who has severe cyanosis. (**a**) The oblique coronal view on the preoperative cardiac CT scan shows that the pulmonary trunk (PT) arises from the left ventricle, which is indicative of a TGA. (**b**) The fluoroscopy image shows a catheter with a fully inflated balloon (yellow arrow) in the left atrium, which via the foramen ovale. The balloon is then forcibly pulled back into the right atrium, creating an atrial septostomy. (**c**) After the BAS procedure, a color TEE in the ME four-chamber view reveals a significant left-to-right shunt resulting from the enlarged defect created by the procedure, which allows for mixing of blood flow between the atria

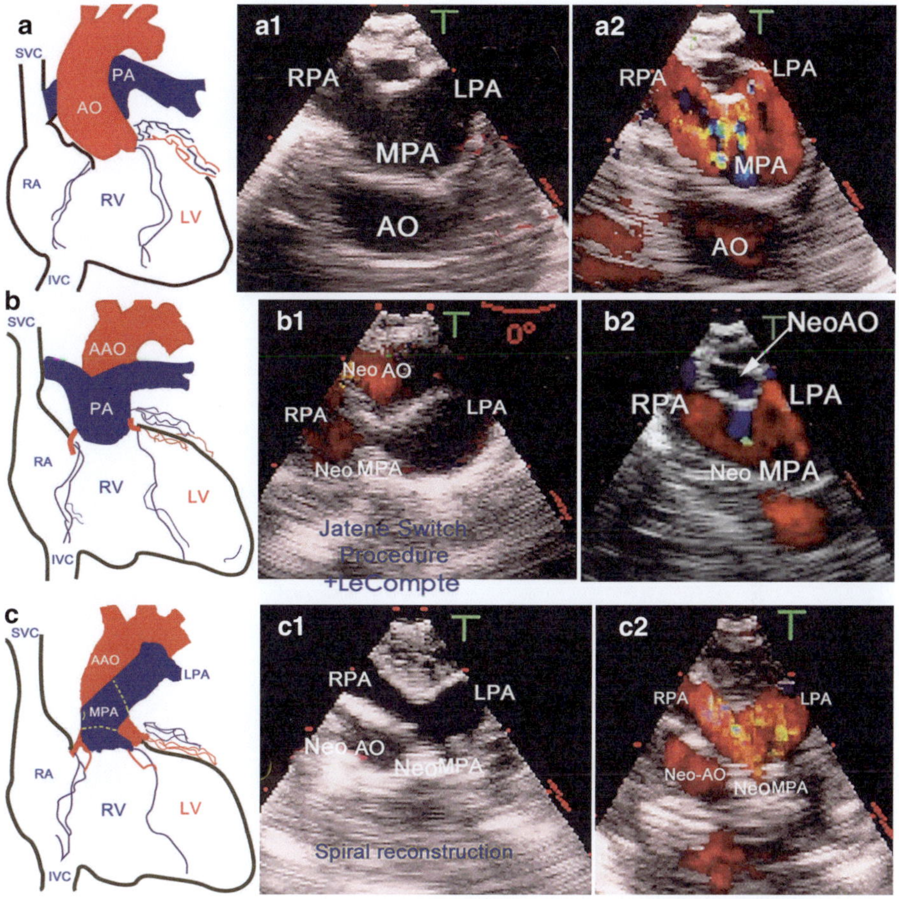

Fig. 5.6 Shows the intraoperative transesophageal echocardiography (TEE) images of standard arterial switch operation (ASO) with either the Jatene procedure with LeCompte maneuver or physiological spiral reconstruction, with a common wall shared between the great arteries. (**a**) This diagram illustrates a typical case of a dextro-looped transposition of the great arteries (TGA) in situs solitus which the aorta (AO) is transposed to the right ventricle (RV), causing deoxygenated blood to flow to the AO, while the pulmonary artery (PA) is transposed to the left ventricle (LV), resulting in oxygenated blood flowing to the PA. (**a1**) The intraoperative TEE image shows the ME AV SAX view of a TGA, with the AO located a little right anteriorly to the PA. The color Doppler image (**a2**) shows blood flow from MPA to the RPA and LPA. (**b**) This diagram shows the standard operation for ASO of Jatene with the LeCompte technique, depicting the PA being switched and connected to the native RV while the AO is switched and connected to the native LV. (**b1**) The postoperative TEE image displays the location of the neo-MPA, which is repositioned anteriorly to the neo-AO. (**b2**) The color Doppler TEE image shows normal blood flow without any focal stenosis in the neo-AO and neo-PA. (**c**) This diagram illustrates the operative technique for physiological spiral reconstruction, with a common wall shared between the great arteries, in which the neo-MPA is placed in the left anterior position, achieving a closer to normal anatomical position of the great arteries and restoring the originally transposed great arteries to their physiological position. (**c1**) The postoperative TEE image displays the neo-MPA in the left anterior position. (**c2**) The color Doppler TEE image shows the restoration of blood flow without any focal stenosis to the neo-AO and neo-MPA

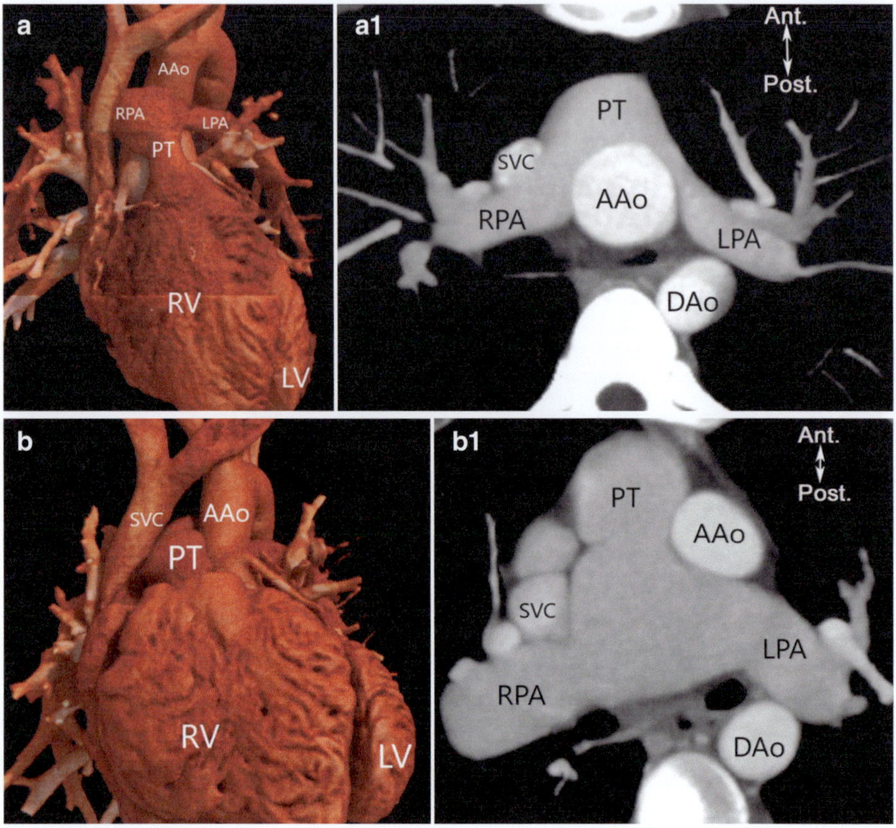

Fig. 5.7 Represents the continuation of Fig. 5.6, showing the use of 3D CT imaging to track the results of the arterial switch operation (ASO) performed using two techniques: the Jatene operation versus Chiu's method (known as a sharing common wall or party wall) technique with arterial spiral reconstruction. A CT study with a 3D (**a**) and sectional (**a1**) images confirmed that a male patient, who is 18-years-old, underwent the ASO via the Jatene procedure with LeCompte maneuver during infancy. The Jatene operation involves creating a "new anatomical configuration" for the heart and great vessels, wherein the pulmonary artery is brought anterior and draped over the neo-aorta during the procedure. A CT study with a 3D (**b**) and sectional (**b1**) images confirmed another male patient, currently 13-years-old, underwent the ASO using the Chiu's method by a spiral reconstruction with the sharing common wall technique during infancy. The sharing common wall technique is used to preserve the "original anatomical configuration" of the great vessels by fusing the pulmonary artery and aorta. With this technique, the neo-aorta is formed by utilizing the original pulmonary valve as the aortic valve

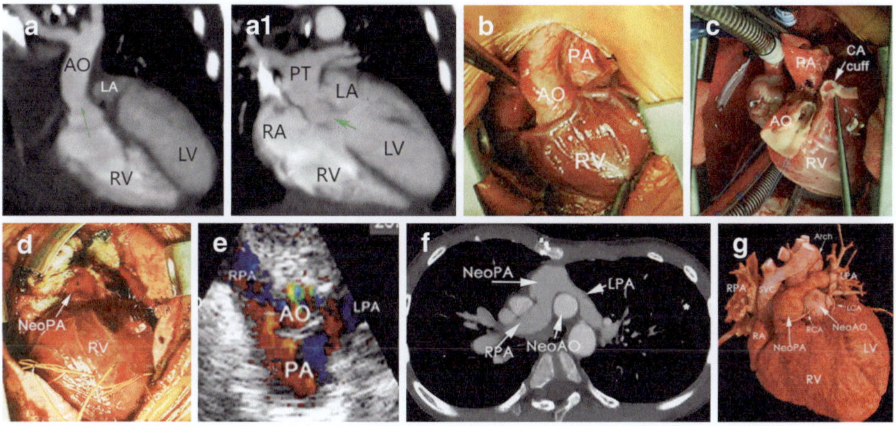

Fig. 5.8 Shows a 2-day-old newborn weighing 2.7 kg who has transposition of the great arteries (TGA) and is undergoing an arterial switch operation (ASO) using the Jatene procedure with a LeCompte maneuver. (**a**) A contrast-enhanced cardiovascular CT study reveals that the aorta (AO) originates from the right ventricle (RV), while the pulmonary artery (PA) originates from the left ventricle (LV) (see **a1**). (**b**) This intraoperative photograph, taken from the surgeon's perspective, shows that the AO originates from the RV, while the PA originates from the LV. Additionally, the aorta is located anteriorly and to the right of the PA. (**c**) This intraoperative photo shows the Jatene switch procedure being performed, with the aorta (AO) being cut from the RV and switched to the LV posteriorly, while the main PA is connected to the RV anteriorly. The coronary arteries are excised and then reimplanted onto the neo-aorta (small white arrow, CA cuff indicating coronary artery cuff), which was formerly the proximal main pulmonary artery. (**d**) The Jatene switching procedure and the LeCompte maneuver, have been completed, as shown in this image. The neo-pulmonary artery (neo-PA) is connected to the RV anteriorly, while the neo-aorta (neo-AO), which is not visible in the image, is connected to the LV posteriorly. (**e**) This TEE image was taken immediately after weaning from cardiopulmonary bypass following the Jatene switch procedure, showing the completed ASO with the neo-PA located anteriorly and connected to the RV. Color Doppler imaging reveals reduced blood flow from the neo-PA to the LPA compared to the RPA flow, with no evidence of focal stenosis in the neo-PA and neo-AO. (**f**) This postoperative cardiac CT image was taken after an ASO with LeCompte maneuver. The great arteries are positioned in direct anteroposterior relation, with the neo-PA located anteriorly and the neo-AO located posteriorly. (**g**) This image depicts a 3D reconstruction of the heart after an ASO, demonstrating that the great arteries are positioned in a direct anteroposterior relation. The neo-PA has been brought to the anterior and is draped to the neo-AO

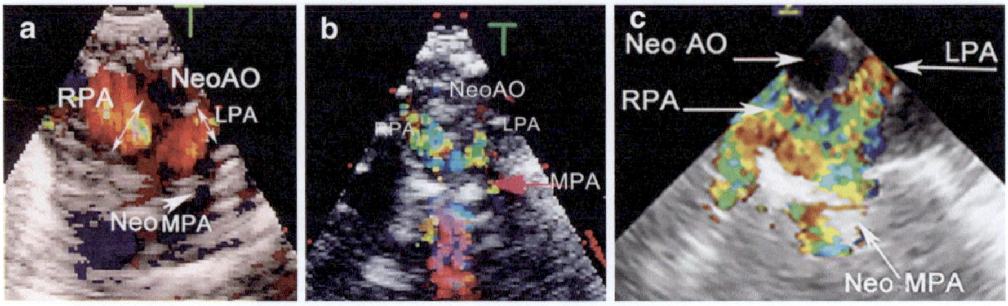

Fig. 5.9 Residual pulmonary stenosis immediately after arterial switch operation (ASO) for a TGA (transposition of the great arteries) with an intact ventricular septum. Anatomical repair is the standard surgical technique for neonates with TGA. However, pulmonary stenosis remains a frequent complication. Therefore, intraoperative TEE (transesophageal echocardiography) and color Doppler assessment play crucial roles in evaluating early acute residual pulmonary stenosis following ASO. If severe residual pulmonary stenosis or a pressure gradient >50 mmHg (EM Delmo Water et al., 2011) is detected, immediate surgical intervention can be performed without delay. Images (**b**–**h**) obtained through intraoperative TEE with color Doppler, illustrate residual focal pulmonary stenosis detected immediately after weaning from cardiopulmonary bypass (CPB) following ASO. In the case of late complications from pulmonary stenosis, catheter intervention with balloon angioplasty can serve as an initial treatment, which will be discussed in Figs. 5.10 and 5.11. (**a**) The color TEE image shows normal blood flow in the neo-AO (neo-aorta), neo-PA (neo-pulmonary artery), and both pulmonary arteries, indicating successful ASO in neonates with TGA without any artery stenosis. Additionally, the left pulmonary artery (LPA) appears smaller than the right pulmonary artery (RPA), and the neo-AO has shifted toward the left side. More information will be provided in subsequent subchapter sections. (**b**) The color TEE image demonstrates turbulent flow over both pulmonary arteries, suggesting the presence of focal stenosis located at the bifurcation of the pulmonary artery (PA). (**c**) The color TEE image demonstrates turbulent flow within the left pulmonary artery, indicating the presence of focal stenosis in close proximity to the bifurcation of the main pulmonary artery (MPA). (**d**) The color TEE image reveals mild turbulent flow in the LPA in close proximity to the bifurcation of the MPA, suggesting the presence of extrinsic compression. (**e**) The color TEE image reveals significant turbulence within the LPA, suggesting the potential presence of focal stenosis near the bifurcation of the MPA. Moreover, there is an observable difference in size between the LPA and the RPA, with the LPA appearing smaller. (**f**) The color TEE image demonstrates a slight turbulent flow in the posterior region of the neo-AO (indicated by the arrow), indicating the possible presence of focal narrowing or kinking at the ascending aorta. (**g**) The color TEE image displays turbulent flow within the main pulmonary artery (PA), suggesting the presence of pulmonary stenosis (PS). Additionally, there is an aortopulmonary (AP) window formation (arrow) observed between the aorta and the LPA after ASO. (**h**) The color TEE image reveals turbulent flow within the neo-MPA and LPA, suggesting the presence of focal stenosis at the pulmonary bifurcation near the LPA. Additionally, there is an aortopulmonary (AP) window formation (arrow) observed from the aorta (AO) to the LPA after ASO. Furthermore, based on reports by EM Delmo W et al., the most frequently observed complication is residual stenosis of the pulmonary artery at the level of the pulmonary trunk or pulmonary bifurcation. However, the primary stenosis affecting the LPA is commonly found near the pulmonary bifurcation. This stenosis occurs due to external compression caused by the neo-AO (neo-aorta) exerting pressure on the LPA during the Jantene switching procedure. Please see Figs. 5.10 and 5.11 for more detailed analysis

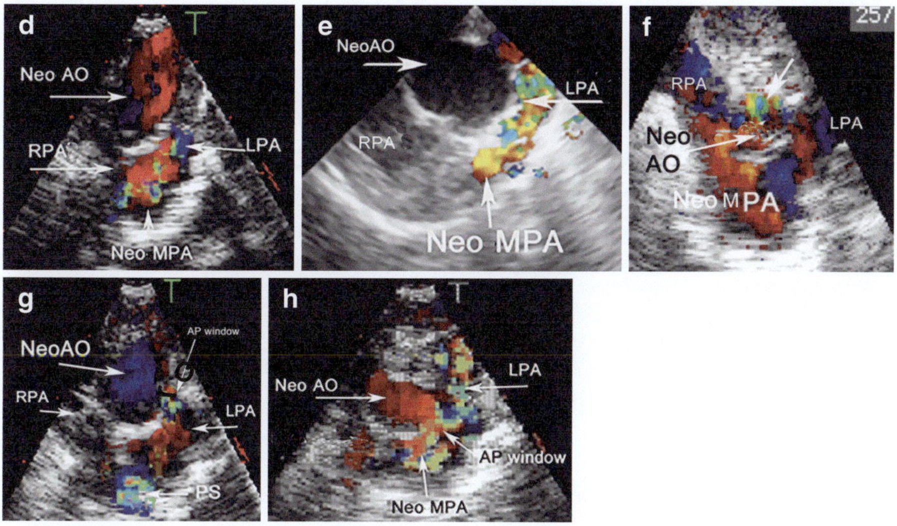

Fig. 5.9 (continued)

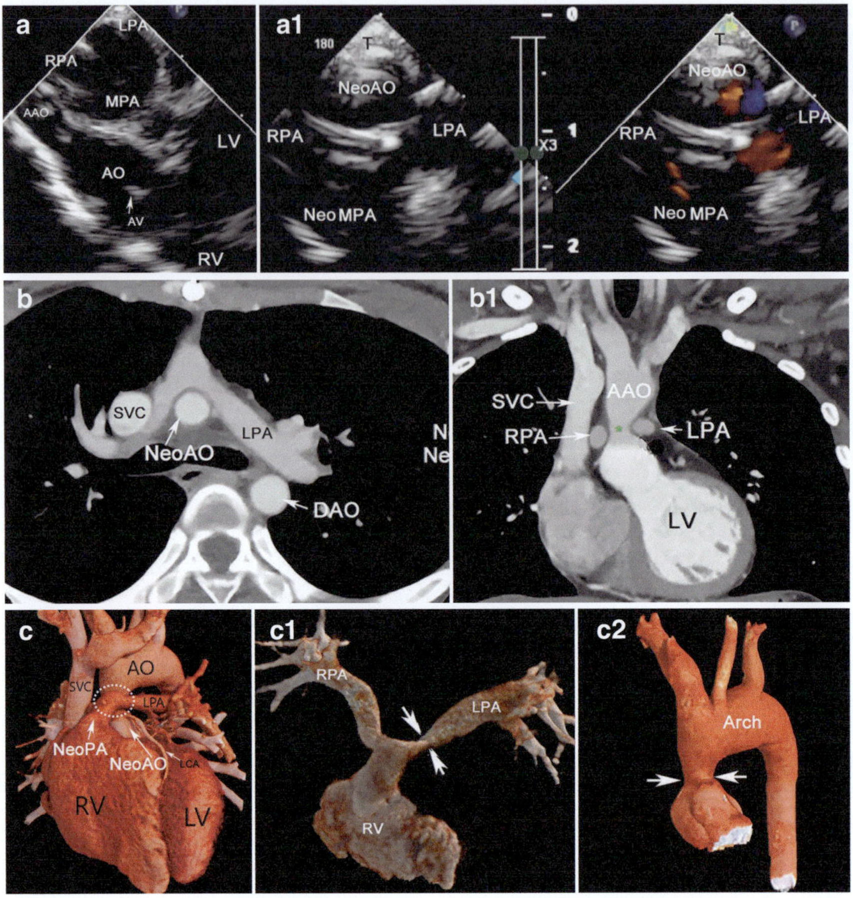

Fig. 5.10 Shows a case of late complications of supravalvular aortic stenosis and left pulmonary artery (LPA) stenosis, occurring after arterial switch operation (ASO) for transposition of the great arteries (TGA) during infancy. This case involves a 13-year-old girl who underwent a routine check-up that included a cardiac CT study. (**a**, **a1**) During infancy, intraoperative TEE was performed for TGA, revealing the aorta (AO) arising from the RV and positioned on the right anterior of the PA. The PA, in turn, arose from the LV and was located on the posterior of the aorta, as depicted in **a**. After the ASO using the Jatene procedure with the Lecompte maneuver, postoperative TEE image showed the PA switched in front of the neo-aorta (neo-AO). Furthermore, the color Doppler image revealed no turbulent flow in the neo-aorta and the pulmonary artery, as illustrated in **a1**. These findings suggest a successful outcome of the ASO procedure, which effectively corrected the TGA anomaly. (**b**, **b1**) Thirteen years after the ASO, a cardiac CT scan revealed that the diameter of the neo-aorta (neo-AO) was smaller (1.33 cm) than that of the descending aorta (DAO) (1.45 cm), as shown in **b**. Coronal plane of the cardiac CT scan demonstrated stenosis (marked with a green asterisk) at the supravalvular region near the bifurcation of the neo-PA, with the neo-AO originating from the LV, as depicted in **b1**. (**c**, **c1**, **c2**) A 3D cardiac CT image taken 13 years after ASO shows the neo-PA arising from the RV and neo-AO arising from the LV. The PA is located anterior to the AO (as shown by the white circle). The LCA was reimplanted without any focal stenosis, as depicted in **c**. Another 3D image (**c1**) depicts the PS (double arrows) at the junction of the pulmonary artery (PA) and left pulmonary artery (LPA), where it is being compressed by the adjacent ascending aorta (AAO). Furthermore, another 3D image (**c2**) of the aorta demonstrates supravalvular stenosis (double arrows). The stenosis at the junction of the LPA was treated with catheter balloon dilatation

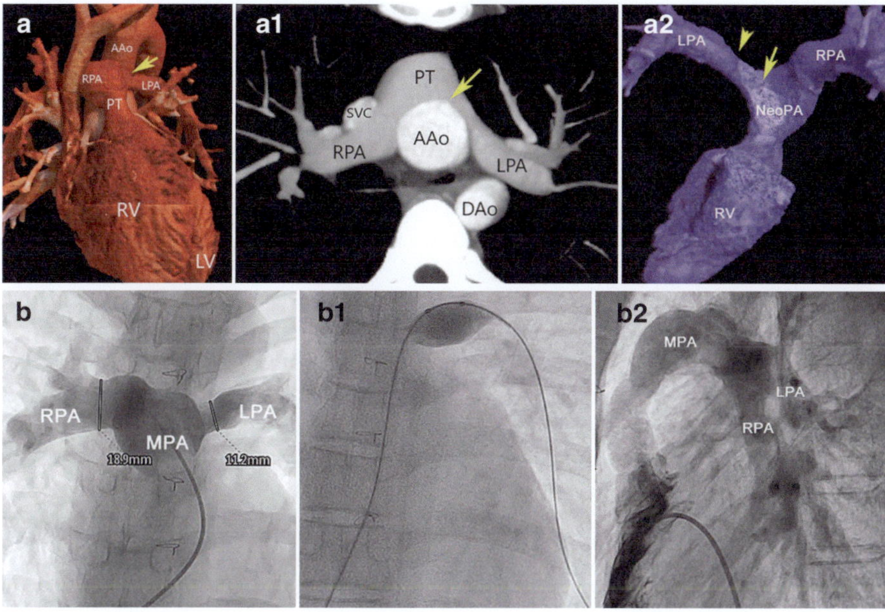

Fig. 5.11 Shows an 18-year-old male patient who received an atrial switch operation (ASO) using the Jatene procedure with LeCompte maneuver in infancy. During a routine postoperative check-up, stenosis was discovered at the junction of the left pulmonary artery (LPA) to the bifurcation of the pulmonary trunk (PT). To address this issue, the patient underwent catheter intervention with balloon dilation and experienced relief. (**a**) The 3D cardiac CT image reveals compression of the junctional LPA and PT bifurcation by the posterior ascending aorta (AAO), as indicated by the yellow arrow. Additionally, a smaller diameter of the LPA compared to the right pulmonary artery (RPA) was also observed. (**a1**) A cardiac CT scan shows that the PT was positioned anteriorly and straddling over the AAO, causing focal stenosis (arrow). (**a2**) The dorsal view of the 3D CT demonstrates the imprint of compression on the neopulmonary artery (neo-PA) (indicated by the yellow arrow) and the junction to LPA (indicated by the arrowhead). (**b**) A pulmonary angiogram shows stenosis at the junction of the LPA, with a diameter of 11.2 mm, which is smaller than the 18.9 mm diameter observed in the right pulmonary artery (RPA). (**b1**) The balloon dilation was performed at the site of this stenosis. (**b2**) Following the balloon dilation, the diameters of the RPA and LPA were nearly equal

References

1. Paladini D, Volpe P, Sglavo G, et al. Transposition of the great arteries in the fetus: assessment of the spatial relationship of the arterial trunks by four-dimensional echocardiography. Ultrasound Obstet Gynecol. 2008;31:271–6.
2. Tang T, Chiu IS, Chen HC, et al. Comparison of pulmonary arterial flow phenomena in spiral and Lecompte models by computational fluid dynamics. J Thorac Cardiovasc Surg. 2001;122(3):529–34.
3. Chiu IS, Huang SC, Chen YS, et al. Restoring the nature spiral flow in transposed great arteries. Eur J Cardiothorac Surg. 2010;37(6):1239–45.

4. Delmo WE, Miera O, Nasseri B, et al. Onset of pulmonary stenosis after arterial switch operation of transposition of great arteries with intact ventricular septum. HSR Proc Intensive Care Cardiovasc Anesth. 2011;3:177–87.
5. Tang T, Chiu IS, Chen HC, Cheng KY, Chen SJ. Comparison of pulmonary arterial flow phenomena in spiral and Lecompte models by computational fluid dynamics. J Thorac Cardiovasc Surg. 2001;122(3):529–34.
6. Chiu IS, Huang SC, Chen YS, Chang CI, Lee ML, Chen SJ, Chen MR, Wu MH. Restoring the nature spiral flow in transposed great arteries. Eur J Cardiothorac Surg. 2010;37(6):1239–45. https://doi.org/10.1016/j.ejcts.2009.12.032.

5.1.2 Transposition of the Great Arteries (TGA) with Ventricular Septal Defect (VSD)

This condition is rare, occurring in approximately 33.5% of all cases of TGA [1]. TGA with VSD can either be a "simple" or "complex" heart condition. In the case of a simple TGA with VSD, the VSD must be closed as part of the arterial switch operation (ASO), unless there are complicating factors. However, in the case of a complex heart condition with TGA and VSD including DORV (double outlet of right ventricle) or DOLV (double outlet of left ventricle), the ASO procedure carries a higher risk of mortality [2–4]. The location and size of the VSD, as well as other associated heart defects, can influence treatment and prognosis. The anatomy of complex TGA with VSD was described by TEE in Fig. 5.12

The most common type of VSD seen in TGA is perimembranous type. A DORV with a TGA-liked hemodynamics is associated with a subpulmonary VSD [4] which also recognized as a Taussig-Bing anomaly (DORV, see Fig. 6.7). Taussig-Bing anomaly is characterized by the malpositioning of the pulmonary artery and aorta, with both great arteries arising from the right ventricle, and the pulmonary artery originating from the left lateral aspect of the aorta. The surgical management under TEE monitoring will be discussed in Fig. 5.13.

Congenitally corrected transposition of the great arteries (CCTGA), as depicted in Fig. 5.2c, typically requires surgical intervention for treatment of the associated VSD and to switch the malposition of the great arteries (and atria), which performed under TEE monitoring, will be discussed in further detail in Figs. 5.14 and 5.15.

CCTGA with situs inversus is a complex congenital heart defect as depicted in Fig. 5.2e. In this condition, the pulmonary artery and aorta are transposed, as in CCTGA, and the internal organs are also malpositioned, with the heart and other organs in a mirror-image orientation from normal. The surgical intervention to repair the VSD and double switch procedure (atrial switch-arterial switch), which performed under TEE monitoring, will be discussed in Figs. 5.16 and 5.17.

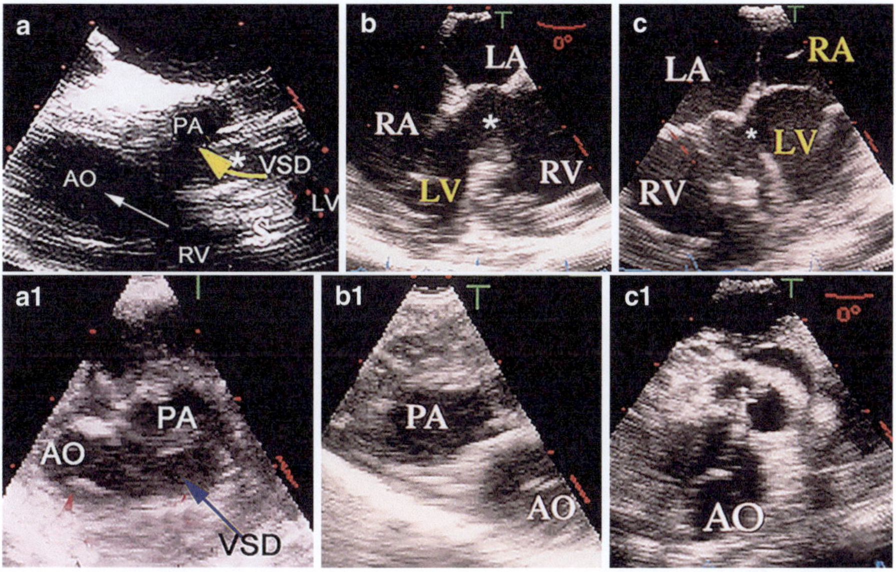

Fig. 5.12 Illustrates the various types of transposition of the great arteries (TGA) associated with ventricular septal defect (VSD) in a child using TEE imaging. The following intraoperative TEE images depict VSDs in different types of TGA-liked hemodynamics: (**a**, **a1**) Taussig-Bing anomaly. A cyanotic CHD with DORV and a subpulmonary VSD (*) may mimic TGA with a VSD between the subaortic and the subpulmonary portion. In this condition, blood from the LV preferentially flows to the PA via the VSD (asterisk), while blood from the RV flows mainly to the aorta (AO) by default. The AO is located to the right of the PA as shown in **a1**. The management of this condition will be discussed in Fig. 5.13. (**b**, **b1**) L-TGA (CCTGA) with VSD (*) in situs solitus. In this condition, both atrioventricular and the ventriculoarterial connections are discordant. The systemic venous blood flows from the RA to the LV and then to the PA circulation with the deoxygenated blood. This is also illustrated in Fig. 5.2c. Babies born with this condition are usually not cyanotic because blood is normally routed, but the right ventricle (RV) pumping at higher pressure may cause the RV function to decline over time. (**c**, **c1**) L-TGA with VSD (*) in situs inversus. In this condition, the atrioventricular and ventriculoarterial connections are discordant at the same time, as shown in **c1**. The pulmonary venous blood flows from the LA to the RV and then to the aorta (AO), resulting in oxygenated blood flowing to the AO circulation. The management of this condition will be discussed in Figs. 5.16 and 5.17

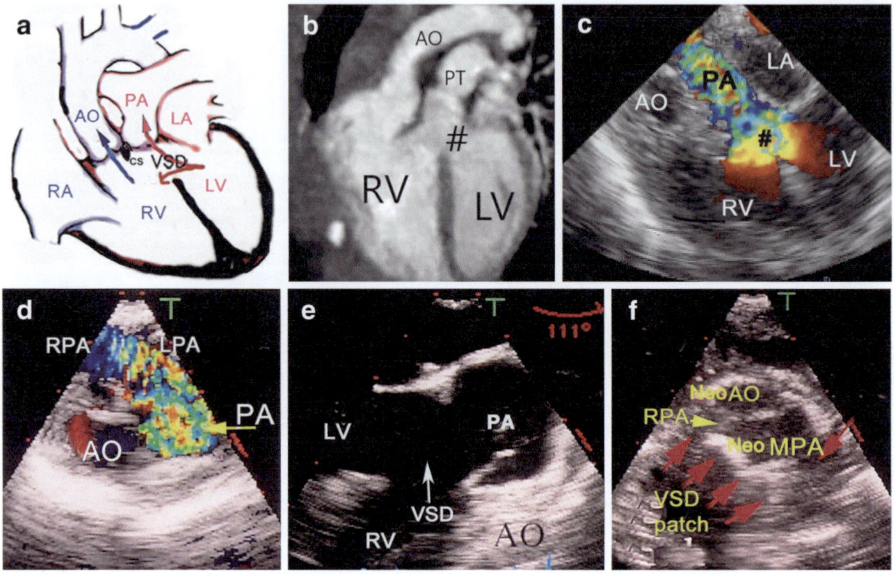

Fig. 5.13 Shows a case of Taussig-Bing anomaly in a 1-month-old infant weighing 3 kg, who underwent surgical correction with arterial switch operation (ASO) and closure of ventricular septal defect (VSD). (**a**) This diagram illustrates a Taussig-Bing anomaly, which is characterized by the arising of both aorta and puslmonary artery from the right ventricle, malposition of the pulmonary artery to the left-lateral portion of the aorta and a subpulmonary ventricular septal defect are noted. (**b**) A cardiac CT scan of a Taussig-Bing anomaly reveals the malpositioned aorta to the right-lateral aspect of the pulmonary trunk (PT) and both great arteries come from the right ventricle, a subpulmonic ventricular septal defect (#), and mild subaortic narrowing caused by hypertrophied conal septum. (**c**) This preoperative color TEE image shows turbulent color flow across the both ventricular outflow tract in the ME five-chamber view. The aorta is fully arising from the RV and away from the ventricular septal defect (#). (**d**) TEE in the ME AV SAX view shows a side-by-side arrangement of the great arteries. (**e**) This TEE image, taken in the ME AV LAX view, shows that the pulmonary artery (PA) is committed more than 50% to the RV, and there is a subpulmonic VSD with more than 50% override. Additionally, there is an absence of pulmonary-mitral fibrous continuity. (**f**) The postoperative TEE image shows the ASO with Jatene switching procedure and LeCompte maneuver. Additionally, it demonstrates the construction of an intracardiac baffle to close the VSD, redirecting the left ventricle (LV) to the neo-aorta through the original VSD (indicated by the red arrows)

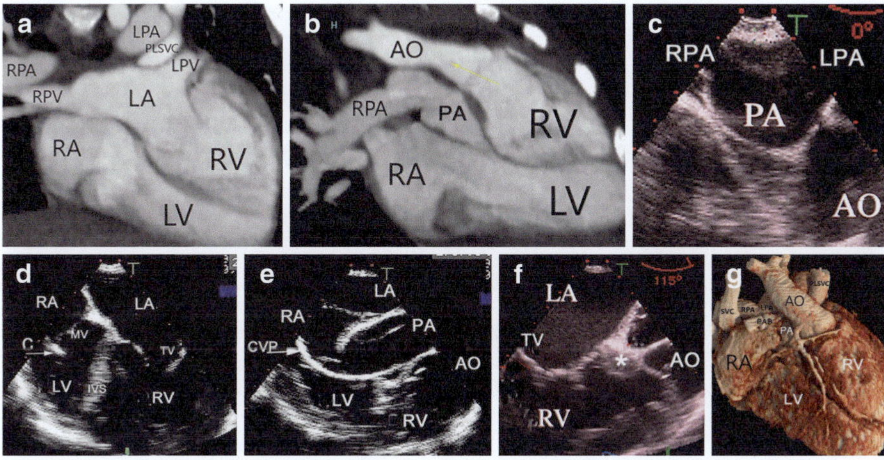

Fig. 5.14 A 6-year-old child weighing 13 kg with L-TGA (congenitally corrected TGA, ccTGA) underwent pulmonary artery banding (PAB) procedure. (**a**, **b**) Show preoperative computed tomography images of a patient with a ccTGA. The oblique coronal sections demonstrate that the RA is connected to a morphological left ventricle (LV) on the right side of the heart, while the left atrium (LA) is connected to a morphological right ventricle (RV) on the left side of the heart (**a**), The aorta arises from the left superior RV and PA comes from the right inferior LV (**b**) with the blood flow to the aorta. This double discordance results in physiologically corrected circulation. (**c**) The TEE image obtained from the UE AAO SAX view shows that the aorta (Ao) is positioned left anterior to the pulmonary artery (PA). (**d**) During intraoperative TEE in the four-chamber view of a patient with a ccTGA, both ventricles have changed their positions. The RV appeared dilated, hypertrophied, and more trabeculated. Additionally, the right atrioventricular valve (TV) was located closer to the apex than the left, and there was an abnormally lower offset of the morphological TV compared to the morphological mitral valve (MV). There was also malalignment between the interatrial septum (IAS) and interventricular septum (IVS). (C indicates central venous catheter, CVP.) (**e**) The TEE image obtained from the ME five-chamber view shows that the RA is receiving flow from the systemic veins (CVP, in situ). The RA is connected to the morphological left ventricle (MLV) by a mitral valve, but there is a discordant connection to the transposed pulmonary artery. (**f**) The LA receives blood flow from the pulmonary circulation and is connected to the morphological right ventricle (RV). During systole, the RV outflow tract (marked with an asterisk) is narrowed by a muscular bridge, which is most pronounced. (**g**) The postoperative 3D cardiac CT image displays the location of pulmonary artery banding (PAB) positioned above the pulmonary valve

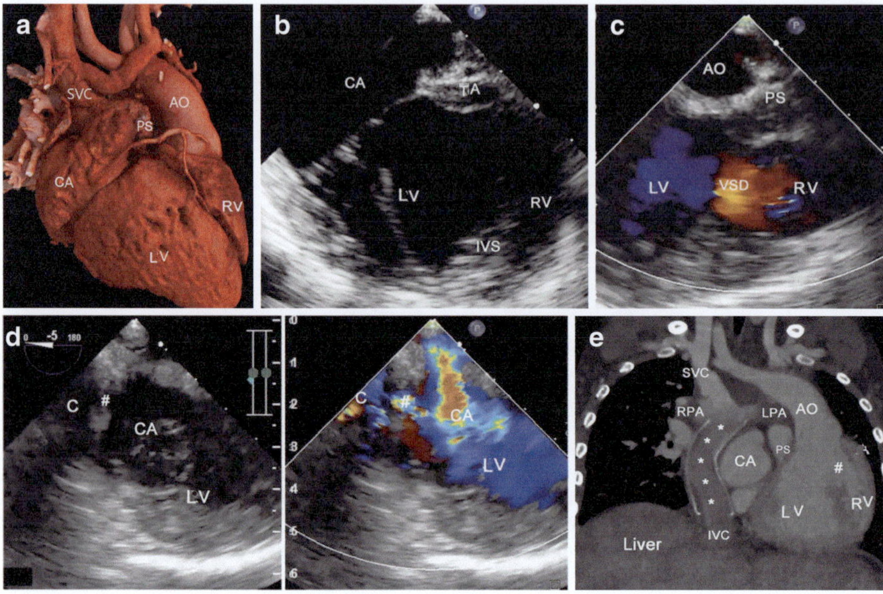

Fig. 5.15 Shows a 4-year-old girl who was diagnosed with congenitally corrected transposition of the great arteries (ccTGA), tricuspid atresia (TA), large VSD, and PS who underwent TCPC surgery. She received an enlargement of the ASD and BT shunt at her first year of age. (**a**) A 3D cardiac image shows ccTGA, TA with a hypoplastic RV ventricle (RV), pulmonary stenosis (PS), but a normal aorta. (**b**) The preoperative 2D TEE image shows a common atrium (CA), TA, a large VSD, hypoplastic RV, and an enlarged LV as seen in the ME four-chamber view. (**c**) The preoperative 2D TEE image shows a large VSD, and PS as seen in the ME five-chamber view. (**d**) The postoperative 2D color TEE image shows the extracardiac conduit (C) of the TCPC with a fenestration (#) as seen in the ME four-chamber view. The color Doppler image (right diagram) shows shunting through the 5 mm fenestration hole (#) to the common atrium (CA). (**e**) The postoperative cardiac CT, performed after TCPC with an extracardiac conduit, demonstrates full patency of the TCPC (asterisks)

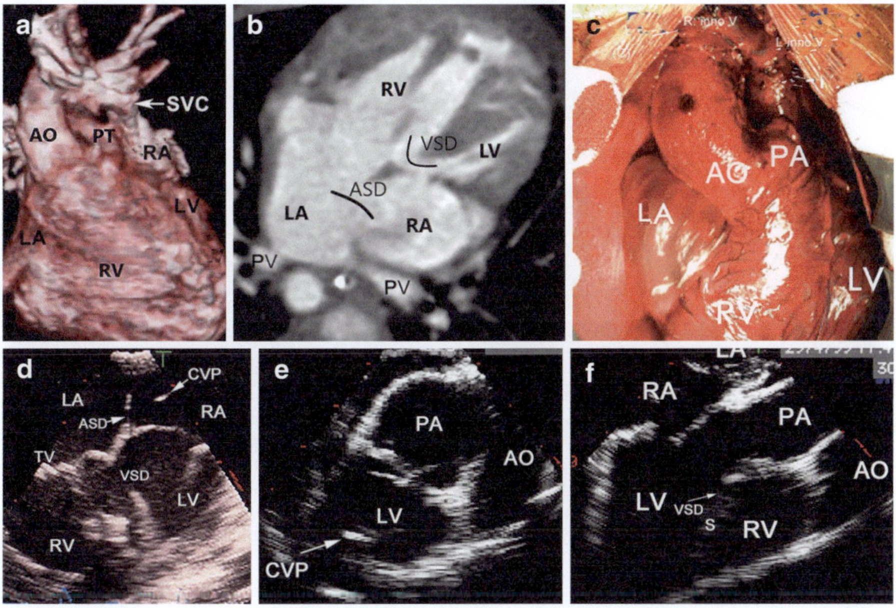

Fig. 5.16 Shows a 1.3-year-old child weighing 9.2 kg with congenitally corrected transposition of the great arteries (ccTGA), situs inversus, and VSD who underwent a double switch operation (as shown in Fig. 5.17). (**a**) The 3D volume image of the inverted ccTGA from cardiac CT shows that the right-sided left atrium (LA) connects to the right ventricle (RV) and drains into the aorta (AO), while the left-sided right atrium (RA) connects to the left ventricle (LV) and drains into the pulmonary trunk (PT). (**b**) The four-chamber view of the contrast-enhanced cardiac CT reveals atrial situs inversus, where the right-sided left atrium (LA) receives pulmonary venous return (PV) and drains into the right ventricle (RV). Additionally, a small left ventricle (LV), ASD, and VSD are also present. (**c**) The intraoperative photograph shows the aorta (AO) located in the anterior position, originating from the RV. The PA is located in the posterior position on the left side of the AO, and originates from the LV. The LA is located on the right side and drains into the RV. (**d**) The preoperative TEE shows a four-chamber view in which there is a discordant atrioventricular connection, and the LA is located on the right side and is connected to the RV. The RA is located on the left side and contains the central venous pressure (CVP) catheter, and is connected to the LV. ASD and VSD are also noted. (**e**) During the preoperative TEE, ME AV SAX view reveals that the aorta is located on the anterior and right side of the PA. The PA originates from the LV and is noted to contain central venous pressure (CVP) catheter, indicating LV originating from RA. (**f**) During the preoperative TEE, a ME AV LAX view revealed that the RA is located on the left side and is connected to LV, which in turn drains to the PA. A VSD is also noted between the LV and the RV

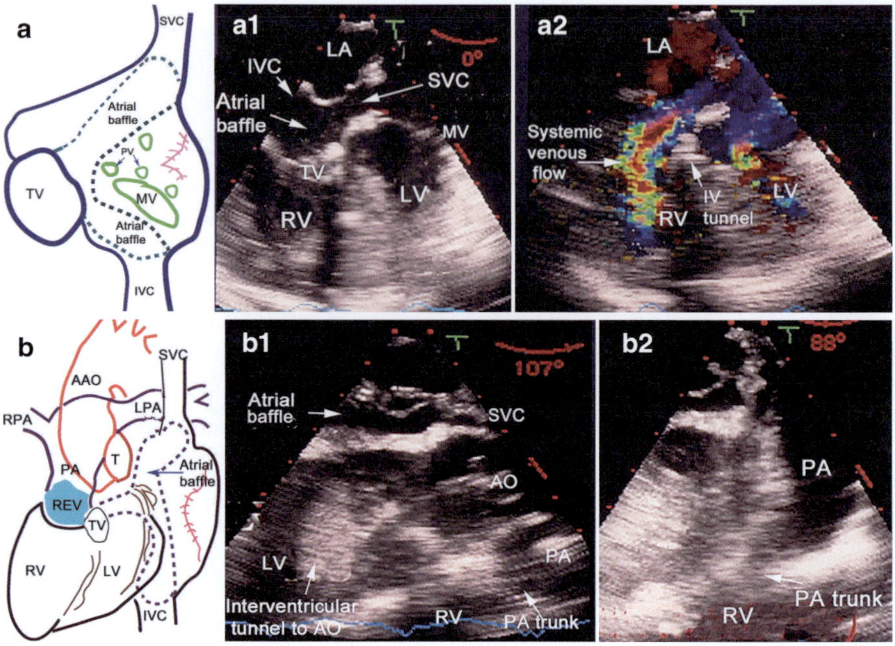

Fig. 5.17 Shows CCTGA/VSD with situs inversus in a 1.3-year-old child from the case presented in Fig. 5.16. The child underwent surgical repair with a double-switch procedure. The double-switch procedure (atrial switch-arterial switch) is performed for ccTGA with situs inversus in order to allow the right ventricle to pump deoxygenated blood to the lungs, while the left ventricle with the mitral valve pumps oxygenated blood to the body, thus supporting systemic pressure. (**a**) This is a schematic representation of the atrial switch procedure used in the Mustard procedure. The atrial septum is excised, and a pericardial baffle is used to redirect caval venous blood flow to the right ventricle via the tricuspid valve (TV). From there, the deoxygenated blood is pumped to the lungs. (**a1**) This is a postoperative TEE image from the Mustard procedure for atrial switch. The ME four-chamber view displays an atrial baffle carrying blood from the SVC and IVC and draining it to the RV via the tricuspid valve. (**a2**) Color Doppler TEE reveals systemic venous blood flow draining into the RV. (**b**) This is a schematic representation of the arterial switch procedure also known as the "LeCompte maneuver." The main PA is cut and moved anteriorly to the aorta. The PA trunk is reconstructed using the "REV procedure" (patch augmentation of the reconstructed outflow tract) to the RV. The AO is reimplanted to the LV, and the VSD is repaired using an intraventricular tunnel (T) patch to reroute the LV to the AO. (**b1**) This is a postoperative TEE image showing the ME AV LAX view. The atrial baffle can be seen in the atrial cavity. The arterial switch has been performed, with the PA reimplanted directly into the RV and anterior to the AO. The VSD has been closed using an interventricular rerouting technique with an LV-to-AO tunnel. (**b2**) This postoperative TEE image demonstrates the REV procedure. In comparison to the "Rastelli procedure," the REV procedure lets the muscular outlet septum be resected and the PA trunk is anteriorly augmented with a pericardial patch, without using a conduit

References

1. Digilio MC, Casey B, Toscano A, et al. Complete transposition of the great arteries. patterns of congenital heart disease in familial precurrence. Circulation. 2001;104:2809–14.
2. Brawn WJ, Mee RB. Early results for anatomic correction of transposition of the great arteries and double-outlet right ventricle with subpulmonary ventricular septal defect. J Thorac Cardiovasc Surg. 1998;95:230–8.
3. Wernovsky G, Mayer JE, Jonas RA, et al. Factors influencing early and late outcome of the arterial switch operation for transposition of the great arteries. J Thorac Cardiovasc Surg. 1995;109:289–302.
4. Wetter J, Belli E, Sinzobahamvya N, et al. Transposition of the great arteries associated with ventricular septal defect: surgical results and long-term outcome. Eur J Cardiothorac Surg. 2001;20:816–23.

5.1.3 Truncus Arteriosus (TrA) and Hemitruncus Arteriosus

The truncus arteriosus (TrA) is a congenital heart defect that occurs when the aorta and the pulmonary artery do not divide properly during fetal development, resulting in remaining as a single vessel known as the truncus arteriosus, where a single large vessel arises from the heart and gives rise to both the pulmonary and systemic arteries [1]. Ventricular septal defect (VSD) and truncal valvular insufficiency are commonly associated with truncus arteriosus.

Truncus arteriosus can be classified into four types (I, II, III, and IV) based on the location and number of pulmonary arteries. Type I is the most common, where a single pulmonary trunk is originating from the truncus arteriosus, and the branching pulmonary arteries arise from the pulmonary trunk. In Type II, the bilateral pulmonary arteries arise separately from the lateral aspects of truncus. In Type III, the pulmonary arteries arise from the posterior aspect of the truncus. Type IV involves the bilateral pulmonary arteries arising from the descending aorta also known as aortopulmonary collateral arteries.

With truncal valve insufficiency, a physical examination may reveal a heart murmur that is audible over the mid-left sternal border, characterized by a high-pitched diastolic decrescendo sound. Echocardiography or CT is a common imaging tool used to visualize the anatomy of the heart and great vessels, as depicted in Fig. 5.18.

The surgical repair of truncus arteriosus involves separating the single large blood vessel into two separate vessels: the main pulmonary artery and the aorta. This procedure will be discussed in detail in Fig. 5.19. Furthermore, late complications after surgical repair will be addressed in Fig. 5.20.

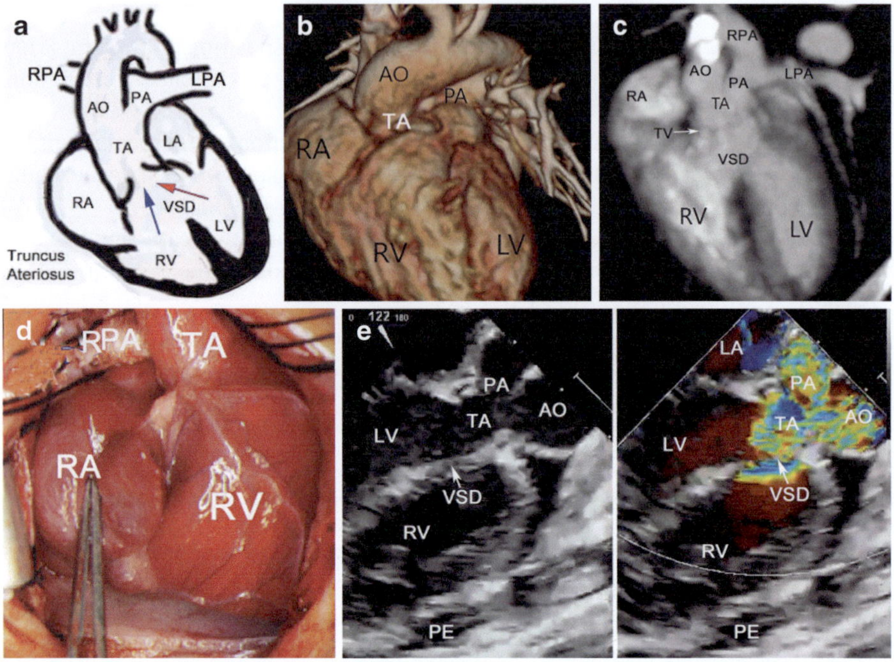

Fig. 5.18 Shows a case of truncus arteriosus (Type 1) in a 3-day-old newborn weighing 2.9 kg who presented with respiratory distress and underwent surgical correction. (**a**) Schematic diagram of truncus arteriosus illustrates a single, large, common blood vessel arising from the heart, with the pulmonary artery directly branching off from the truncus, and the common ventricular outflow tract. The systemic venous blood and pulmonary venous blood are mixed at the VSD. (**b**, **c**) Preoperative 3D volume rendering cardiac CT and oblique transverse images showing a common trunk (TA) and truncal valve (TV) arise from the both ventricular outlet with a subvalvular large VSD. Bilateral pulmonary arteries come from a very short main pulmonary artery (PA). (**d**) This is an intraoperative surgical photograph of a truncus arteriosus, which shows a common trunk (TA) arising from both ventricular outlets. There is a short pulmonary artery originating from the posterolateral aspect of the truncal root (TA), which bifurcates into the right and left pulmonary arteries. However, in this image, only the right pulmonary artery is visible. (**e**) This is a preoperative TEE with the ME AV LAX view that shows a common trunk (TA) and a common ventricular outflow tract spanning a high ventricular septal defect (VSD). There is also evidence of pericardial effusion (PE). The color Doppler (right diagram) reveals blood flow from the RV and LV entering the truncus arteriosus (TA) via the VSD with turbulent flow due to high pulmonary vascular resistance. The blood then travels to the aorta and PA

Hemitruncus is a rare subtype of truncus arteriosus where one pulmonary artery branch, typically the right, arises from the ascending aorta just above the aortic sinuses, while the main pulmonary artery and the other pulmonary branch arise normally [2]. The treatment of hemitruncus depends on the severity of the condition and any associated cardiac abnormalities. Surgical options may include reconstructing the affected pulmonary artery, as discussed in further detail in Fig. 5.21.

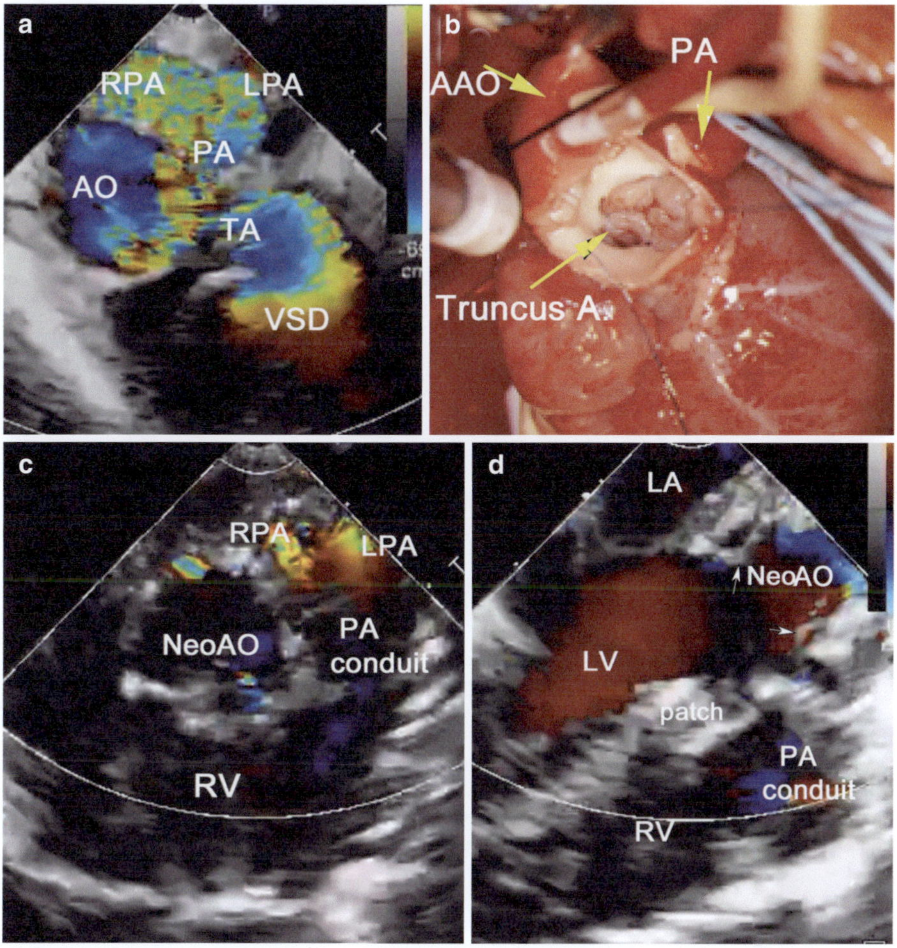

Fig. 5.19 Shows the same patient presented in Fig. 5.18. The patient underwent surgical correction of truncus arteriosus with a single-stage repair that involved reimplanting the pulmonary artery to the right ventricle (RV) and closing the large conoventricular ventricular septal defect (VSD). (**a**) This is a preoperative color Doppler TEE with the ME AV SAX view that shows a common trunk (TA) and a common ventricular outflow tract spanning a high ventricular septal defect (VSD). The flow to the aorta (AO) and bilateral pulmonary arteries is turbulent. (**b**) This is an intraoperative surgical photograph that shows a quadricuspid common semilunar valve. The image also depicts the cutting and mobilization of a short segment of the main pulmonary arteries from the truncus arteriosus (TA), which are then connected to the right ventricle (RV) using the Rastelli procedure (RV-PA conduit). (**c**) The postoperative color TEE in ME AV SAX view shows restoration of RV-to-PA continuity using the Rastelli procedure with a valved PA conduit. The neo-aorta and PA are in a normal sagittal relationship. (**d**) This is a postoperative TEE in the ME AV LAX view. The image shows the reimplantation of the PA from the truncus arteriosus to the RV using conduit-based RVOT reconstruction (Rastelli procedure). The VSD has been closed with a patch, and the LV now directly connects to the neo-aorta. The white arrows point to the aortic valve

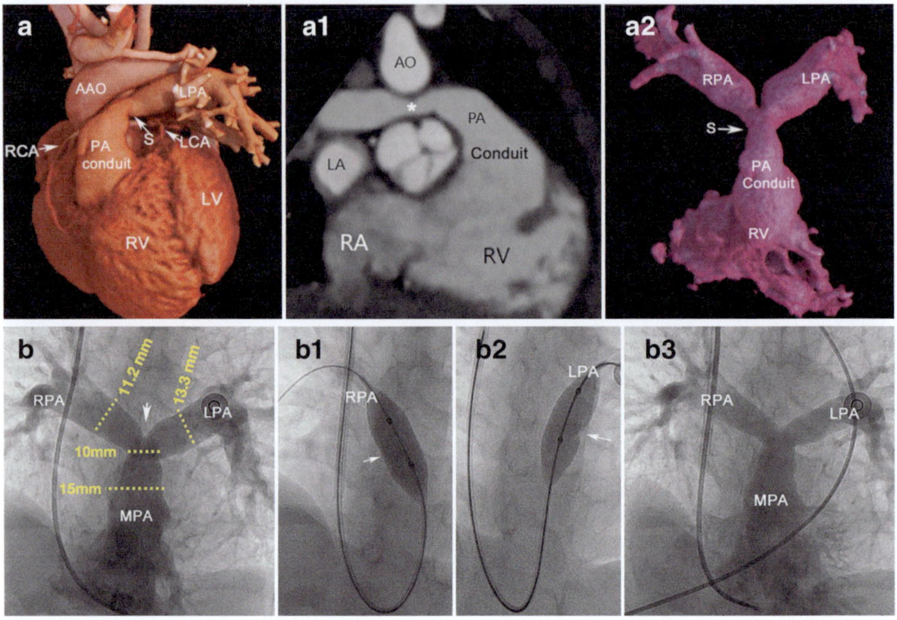

Fig. 5.20 Shows the same patient as presented in Fig. 5.19, 2 years after the total correction of the truncus arteriosus. The patient now has severe focal stenosis at the pulmonary bifurcations and underwent catheter intervention with balloon dilatation. (**a**, **a1**, **a2**) After 2 years of correcting truncus arteriosus, 3D cardiac CT images show focal stenosis at the pulmonary bifurcations (S, asterisk indicating stenosis). On thin-slab MPR cardiac CT images (**a1**), the four leaflets of the truncal valves remain visible. (**b**) Pulmonary angiogram shows preballoon dilation, and (**b1**) shows the RPA balloon dilation, (**b2**) shows the LPA balloon dilation, and (**b3**) shows the result after bilateral balloon dilatations

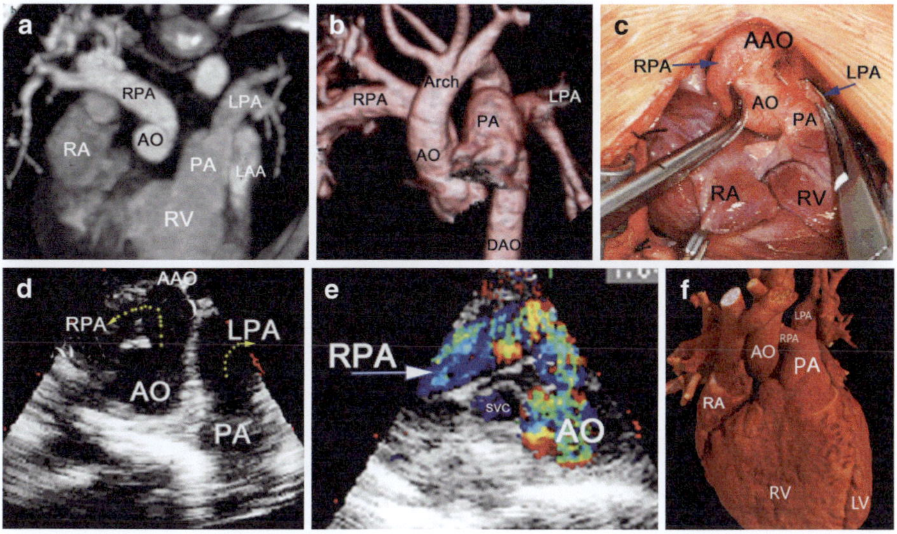

Fig. 5.21 Shows a hemitruncus arteriosus in a 1.5-month-old neonate weighing 5 kg who presented with pulmonary hypertension and respiratory distress and underwent surgical correction. (**a**, **b**) Preoperative cardiac CT and 3D images of the great arteries. (**b**) Show an isolated abnormal origin of the right pulmonary artery (RPA) from the dorsal wall of the ascending aorta (AO), and left pulmonary artery (LPA) arising directly from the main pulmonary artery (PA). (**c**) Intraoperative surgical photograph shows the LPA arising from the main pulmonary artery (PA) while the RPA has an abnormal origin from the ascending aorta (AAo). (**d**) Intraoperative TEE, UE AAO SAX view depicts the direction of LPA arising from the PA (dotted curved arrow line) and RPA originating from the ascending aorta (AO) (dotted curved arrow line), which is consistent with the surgical photograph. (**e**) Color Doppler TEE shows that the blood flow in the RPA is coming from the aorta with a turbulent flow due to high systemic pressure to the lungs. (**f**) A 3D image of the same child taken 2 years after total correction, which involved reimplanting the RPA to the main PA during infancy, shows a completely normal 3D spatial relationship between the great arteries

References

1. Marcelletti C, McGoon DC, Mair DD. The natural history of truncus arteriosus. Circulation. 1976;54:108–11.
2. Prifti E, Bonacchi M, Murzi B, et al. Anomalous origin of the right pulmonary from the ascending aorta. J Card Surg. 2004;19:103–12.

5.1.4 Congenital Aortic Stenosis (AS)

Congenital aortic stenosis (AS) is a heart condition that occurs when the aortic outflow is narrow at birth. A range of symptoms, from mild to severe, occur depending on the degree of the stenosis.

Congenital aortic stenosis can be classified based on the location of the stenosis and the severity of the narrowing. The classification and treatment options for this condition are discussed in more detail below:

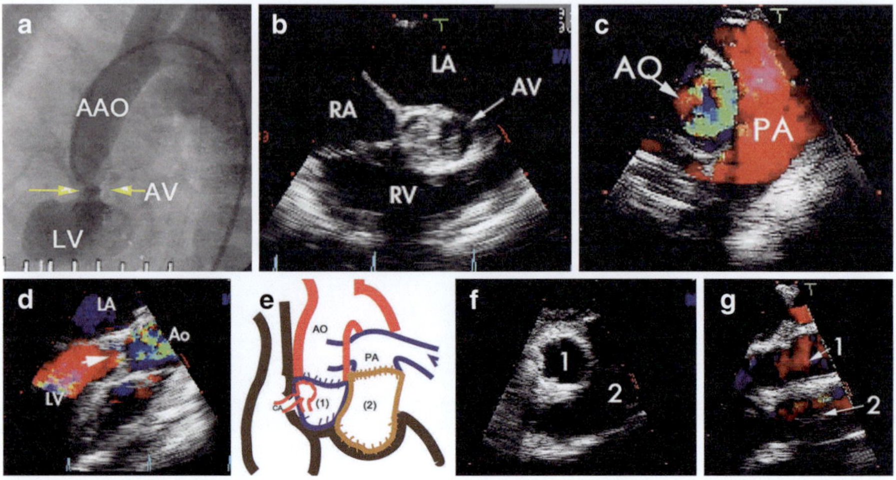

Fig. 5.22 Shows the case of a 4-year-old child who presented with exertional dyspnea, heart failure, and congenital aortic valvular stenosis. The child underwent a procedure known as the Ross procedure to address these issues. (**a**) Shows a lateral projection of an aortic root angiogram that demonstrates a significant aortic valve (AV) stenosis, indicated by arrows. (**b**) Displays an intraoperative TEE image, specifically the ME AV SAX view, which reveals a thickened and fish-mouth appearance of the calcified bicuspid aortic valve. (**c**) This color Doppler image displays a fish-mouth appearance of the valve opening during systole, as well as a mosaic turbulent blood flow through the aorta. (**d**) Presents a color Doppler TEE image, captured from the ME AV LAX view, which demonstrates critical aortic stenosis and a prominent turbulence flow across the AV. (**e**) The diagram illustrates the "Ross procedure," which involves two main steps: (1) transplanting the patient's own pulmonary valve to the aortic valve position, and (2) reconstructing a new pulmonary valve with a homograft from the right ventricle to the pulmonary artery. (**f**) Postoperative TEE, ME AV SAX view showing the neo-aorta with a pulmonary valve autograft (1) and the neo-pulmonary artery by a pulmonary homograft (2). (**g**) Postoperative TEE, ME AV LAX view showing a successful "Ross operation" with the neo-aorta, patent LVOT, and the neo-pulmonary homograft and patent RVOT

1. Valvular aortic stenosis is caused by a narrowing of the aortic valve, which can be due to thickening or fusion of the valve leaflets. Treatment options may include the Ross operation [1, 2] (pulmonary autograft), where the diseased aortic valve is removed and replaced with the patient's own pulmonary valve, as discussed in more detail in Fig. 5.22.
2. Subvalvular aortic stenosis occurs below the aortic valve, causing a narrowing in the left ventricular outflow tract. Treatment options may include surgical myectomy, which involves removing the obstructing tissue, as discussed in Figs. 5.23, 5.24, and 5.25.

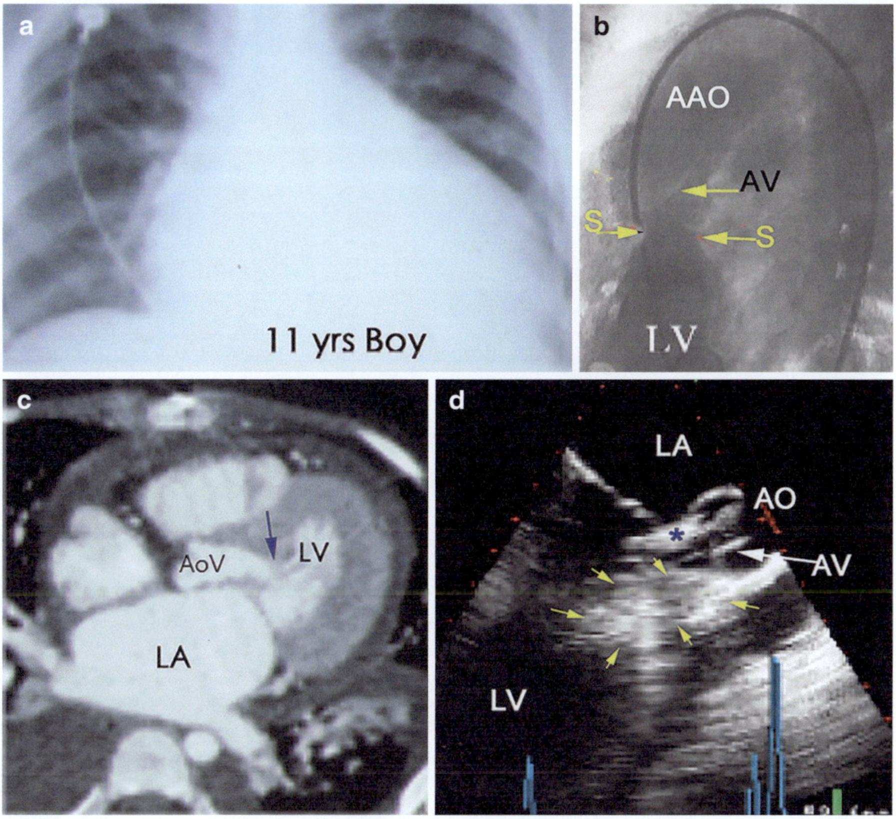

Fig. 5.23 Shows a case of a 11-year-old child who presented with exertional dyspnea, heart failure, and congenital subaortic valve stenosis, and underwent surgical correction. (**a**) Preoperative CXR shows enlarged cardiac silhouette and cardiomegaly. (**b**) Shown in the lateral projection of the aortic root angiogram is a significant subaortic valve stenosis (indicated by the arrows). (**c**) Cardiac CT image reveals an enlarged left atrium, left ventricular hypertrophy, and stenosis of the left ventricular outflow tract (arrow). (**d**) During the intraoperative TEE, the ME AV LAX view shows left ventricular hypertrophy and a fibromuscular ridge (indicated by the arrows) located below the aortic valve (AV) along the left ventricular outflow tract (LVOT), causing obstruction. The LVOT gradient is measured at 55 mmHg

3. Supravalvular aortic stenosis occurs above the valve, causing a narrowing in the ascending aorta itself, either in sinus or tubular portion. Diagnosis may include cardiac catheterization, 3D CT, and TEE imaging, as shown in Fig. 5.26.

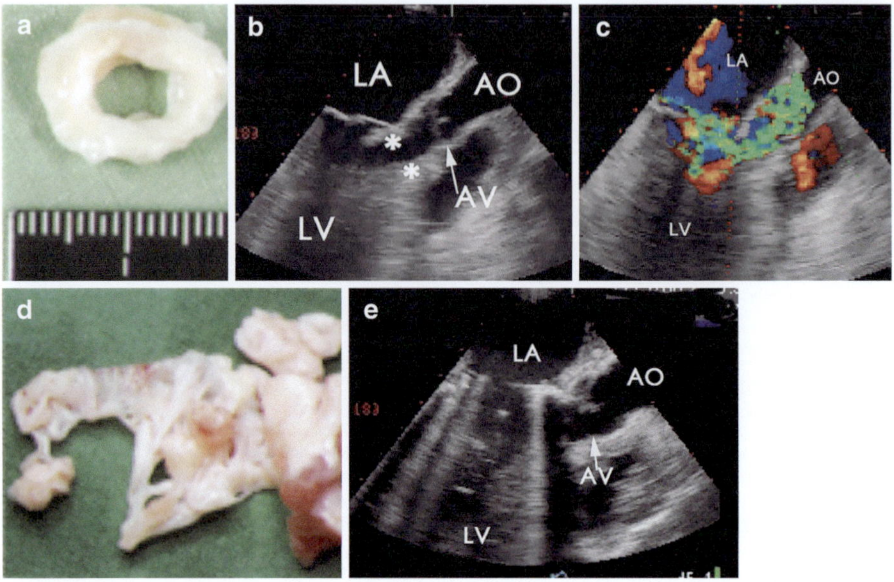

Fig. 5.24 The same patient with subaortic stenosis shown in Fig. 5.23 underwent surgical correction. (**a**) After the surgical resection of the subaortic mass, the specimen revealed a circumferential fibromuscular ridge which resulted in left ventricular outflow tract obstruction (LVOTO). (**b**) Immediately postoperative TEE, ME AV LAX view shows the presence of a residual subaortic stenosis with a visible fibromuscular tissue (*) located in the mitral valve and the subaortic region. (**c**) Color Doppler TEE shows a prominent turbulent flow across the subaortic area, as well as mitral and aortic regurgitation. These findings indicate the presence of residual stenosis. (**d**) A prompt reoperation was performed to address residual subaortic stenosis. The second and extended surgical specimen revealed the presence of the residual more fibrous tissue attached to the chordae tendineae and papillary muscle of the mitral valve. Therefore, the possibility of mitral valve replacement must be considered. (**e**) After the redo operation, TEE, ME AV LAX view shows the use of a 21 mm aortic prosthetic valve for mitral valve replacement in this 11-year-old child. No more LVOTO is detected

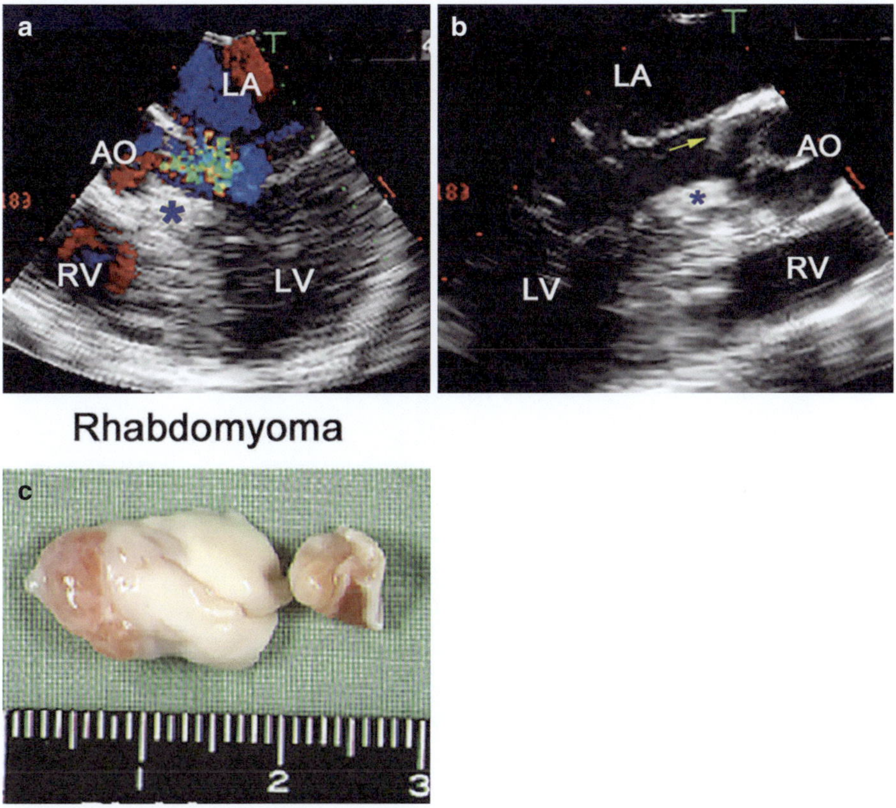

Fig. 5.25 Shows a 9-year-old child with mild exertional dyspnea and a murmur, who was found to have subaortic valvular stenosis and underwent surgical intervention. (**a**) The preoperative TEE, ME five-chamber view reveals the presence of LV hypertrophy and a subaortic mass-like lesion (*), as well as color Doppler evidence of a prominent turbulence at the left ventricular outflow tract (LVOT). (**b**) An ME AV LAX view shows a membrane (indicated by an arrow) can be traced to this mass-like lesion (*) below the aortic valve, which is causing stenosis. The LVOT gradient is 50 mmHg. (**c**) After removal of the subaortic mass, the surgical specimen reveals a 3 cm-long rhabdomyoma (as confirmed by pathology study)

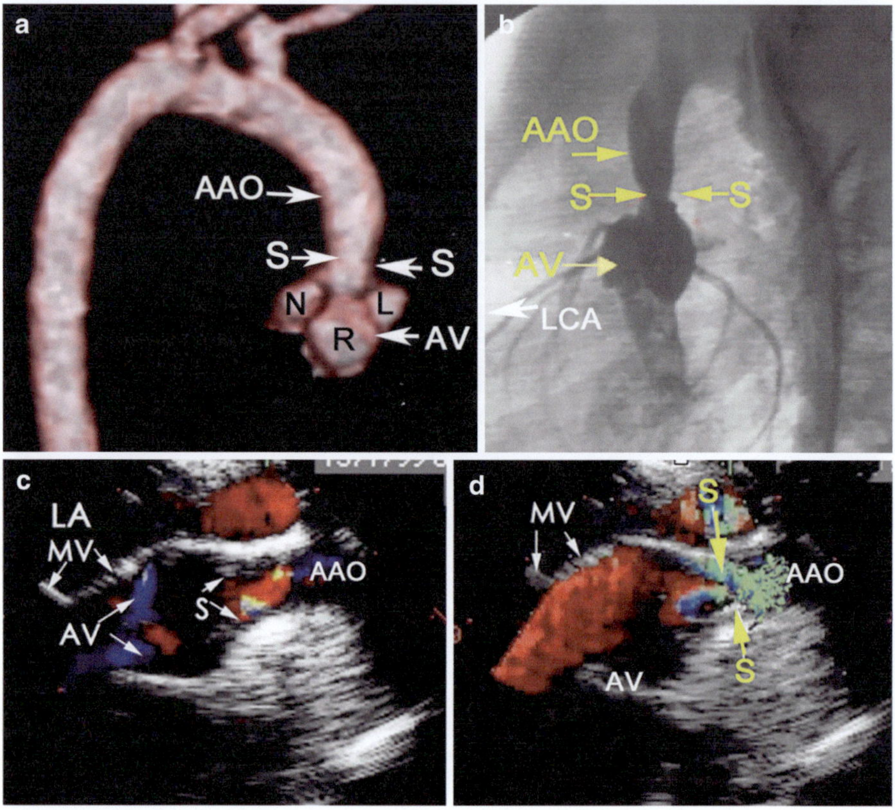

Fig. 5.26 Shows a 5-year-old child who was referred from a local hospital for evaluation due to heart murmur. (**a**) A 3D CT image shows a narrowing above the aortic valve, indicating a diagnosis of supravalvular AS (arrows). (S, stenosis; L, LCC; R, RCC; N, NCC). (**b**) This image is a lateral projection of an aortic root angiogram, which also demonstrates a diagnosis of supravalvular aortic stenosis (arrows). (**c**) This TEE, ME AV LAX view demonstrates a narrowing (S) located above the aortic valve (AV), which is compatible with a diagnosis of supravalvular stenosis. (**d**) This color Doppler TEE image demonstrates a turbulent flow across the supravalvular area, indicating the presence of supravalvular aortic stenosis (S). This case was treated with catheter balloon dilatation

References

1. David TE. The Ross operation for congenital aortic stenosis: update 2009. J Heart Valve Dis. 2009;18:255–61.
2. Etnel JRG, Elmont LC, Ertekin E, et al. Long-term outcomes after the Ross procedure in adults with congenital aortic stenosis: a systematic review and meta-analysis. Eur J Cardio Thorac Surg. 2016;50:580–7.

5.1.5 Tetralogy of Fallot (TOF)

Tetralogy of Fallot (TOF) is a critical congenital heart defect comprising four cardiac structural anomalies: ventricular septal defect, overriding aorta, pulmonary stenosis, and right ventricular hypertrophy (refer to Fig. 5.27). It can cause cyanosis while crying or feeding, commonly known as a tet spell or blue spell.

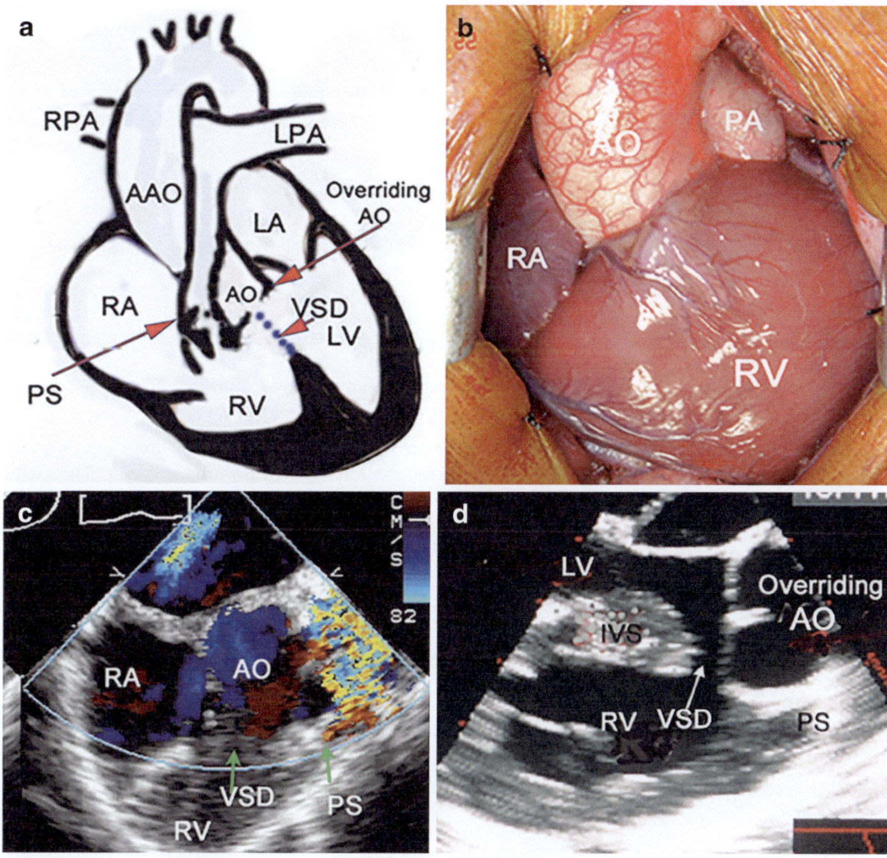

Fig. 5.27 Shows a cyanotic infant who experienced episodes of turning blue during feeding or crying, and was diagnosed with tetralogy of Fallot (TOF). The baby underwent surgical management to treat the condition. (**a**) This schematic drawing of TOF illustrates the four characteristic features of the condition: ventricular septal defect (VSD), overriding of the aorta, pulmonary stenosis, and right ventricular hypertrophy. (**b**) This intraoperative photo depicts a typical case of TOF, with hypertrophy of the right ventricle (RV), overriding of the aorta (AO), and a hypoplastic pulmonary artery (PA). (**c**) Preoperative color Doppler TEE in the ME AV SAX view shows a large VSD with bidirectional shunt, as well as severe pulmonary stenosis (PS) and right ventricular outflow tract obstruction. (**d**) Another ME AV LAX view on TEE demonstrates a VSD with an overriding AO and associated PS

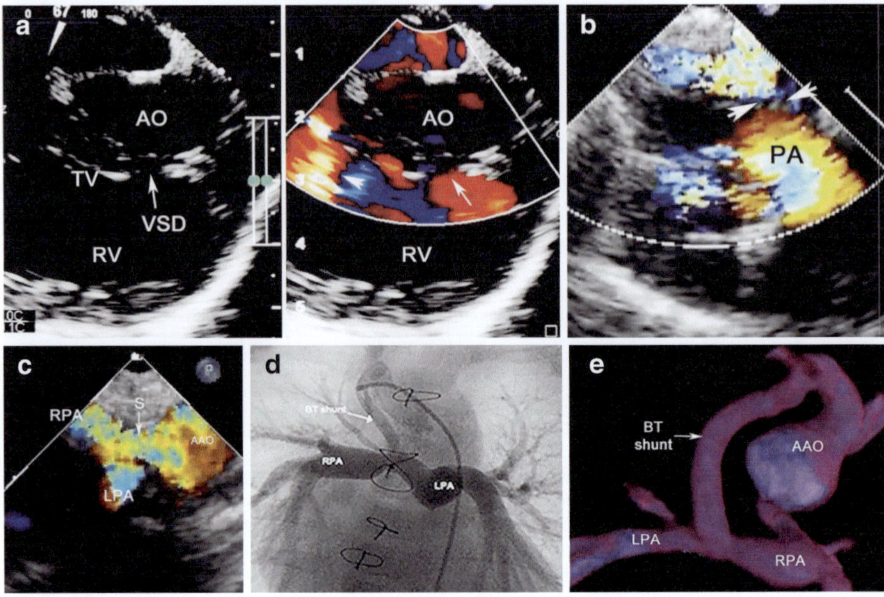

Fig. 5.28 Shows a newborn with extreme tetralogy of fallot (TOF) who underwent a primary shunt management. (**a**, **b**) Intraoperative TEE in (**a**) revealed a case of severe TOF with a dilated and thick-walled right ventricle (RV) and a ventricular septal defect (VSD). The color image (right diagram) showed TR (white arrowhead) and a right-to-left shunt flow of the VSD. The color Doppler TEE by UE PA view in (**b**) demonstrated a severe pulmonary stenosis at the bifurcation (double arrowheads). (**c**) TEE in the UE AAO view of the postoperative modified Blalock-Taussig (BT) shunt showed turbulent, patent shunt flow (S) to both the right and left pulmonary arteries (RPA and LPA). (**d**) A postoperative PA angiogram revealed a modified Blalock-Taussig (BT) shunt connecting the right subclavian artery to the RPA with a junctional stenosis and further opacifying LPA. (**e**) Shows a 3D volume image of the aortic arch and pulmonary artery, depicting a modified BT shunt connecting the left subclavian artery to the LPA

The treatment of TOF varies depending on the severity of the condition and the individual clinical presentation. Medical therapy such as beta-blockers and oxygen may be used to alleviate symptoms such as cyanosis (blue skin) and shortness of breath.

In severe cases of TOF, where the pulmonary artery is significantly narrowed, the patient may experience severe cyanosis and breathlessness. This condition is referred to as extreme or severe TOF. In such cases, a shunt operation such as a "Blalock-Taussig" shunt may be performed as a first step to create an alternative pathway for blood flow to the lungs (refer to Fig. 5.28). This helps to ensure sufficient blood flow to the lungs.

Surgical intervention is usually necessary to correct the structural abnormalities in TOF. The Rastelli operation is one of surgical procedures utilized to treat certain types of TOF that involves a large ventricular septal defect (VSD) and malposition of the aorta (refer to Fig. 5.29). After surgical repair, potential complications [1, 2] include residual VSD and pulmonary artery stenosis (refer to Fig. 5.30).

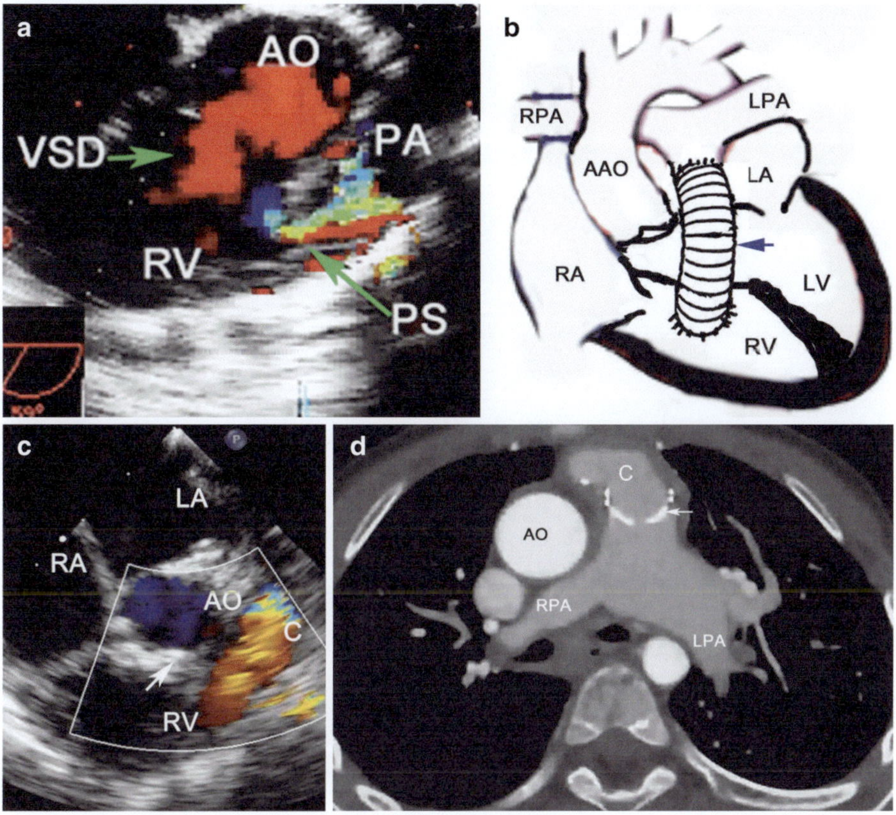

Fig. 5.29 A 1-year-old child, who presented with tetralogy of fallot (TOF) underwent total correction. (**a**) Preoperative TEE in the ME AV SAX view of a typical TOF case demonstrates a large VSD with a right-to-left shunt flow (short arrow), right ventricular hypertrophy, and severe pulmonary stenosis (PS) (long arrow). (**b**) Diagram of the Rastelli procedure for TOF repair illustrating the construction of the RV and pulmonary bifurcation using a homograft-valved conduit (arrow). (**c**) Postoperative color Doppler TEE in the ME AV SAX view shows a patch repair (arrow) for the VSD and a Rastelli procedure with a conduit (C) made of a monocuspid autologous pericardial patch for correction of the RVOTO and PS. The pulmonary flow indicates a patent conduit without focal stenosis. (**d**) Postoperative cardiac CT shows successful implantation of a conduit (C) with a monocuspid valve (arrow) between the right ventricle and the pulmonary artery

Tetralogy of Fallot with absent pulmonary valve (TOF-APV) is a rare and intricate form of TOF where the pulmonary valve is completely or nearly absent, leading to severe pulmonary regurgitation and right ventricular dilation (refer to Fig. 5.31). Surgical intervention is required, involving pulmonary artery and right ventricular outflow tract reconstruction.

In some cases of TOF with pulmonary atresia, collateral blood vessels from descending aorta called Major Aortopulmonary Collateral Arteries (MAPCAs) [3–5] may develop. The surgical repair of TOF with MAPCAs involves a staged approach to reconstruct the pulmonary artery and redirect and control blood flow to

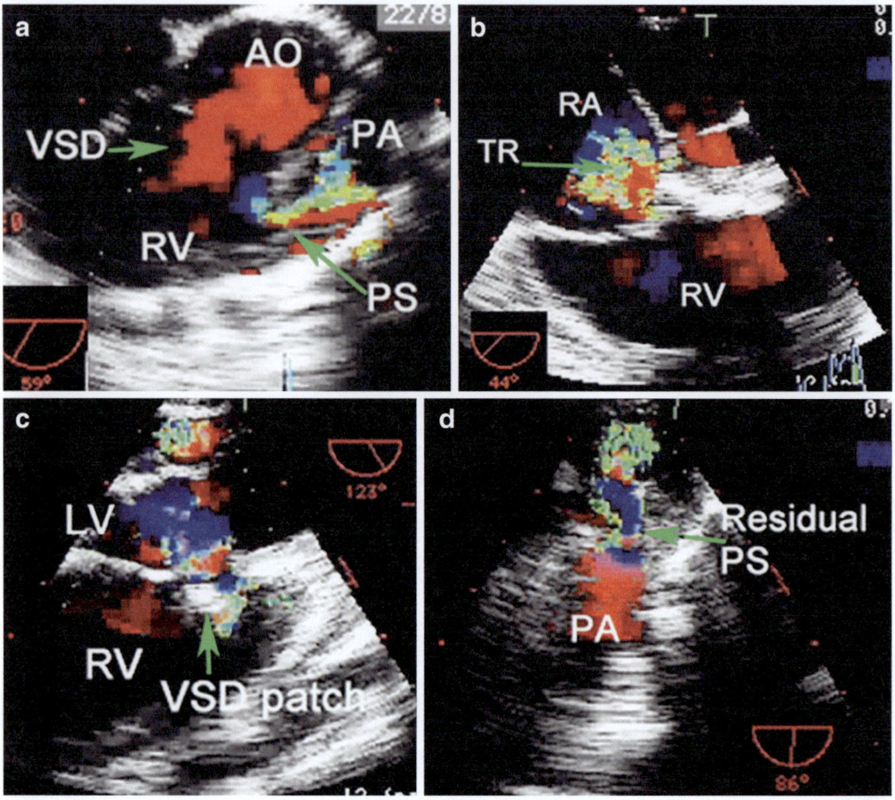

Fig. 5.30 Accurate recognition of the morphological TEE features after surgery is crucial to ensure successful surgical outcomes. Any complications that may arise after TOF repair can be promptly detected before discontinuation of cardiopulmonary bypass (CPB) and resulting redo surgery without delay. (**a**) Preoperative TEE, ME AV SUX, shows the presence of a large VSD with a right-to-left shunt and pulmonary stenosis in a child with TOF. (**b**) Four-chamber view postoperatively, showing a new mild tricuspid regurgitation (TR) after closure of the VSD using a patch. (**c**) Immediately postoperative ME AV SAX view showing the residual VSD. (**d**) Immediately postoperative ME AV SAX view showing residual pulmonary stenosis (PS). The condition in **c**, **d** is corrected by a redo surgery before discontinuation of CPB

the lungs. The first step is typically to identify and ligate (tie off) or perform transcatheter embolization of any large MAPCAs, which are dural suppling and causing excessive blood flow to the lungs. The goal of the MAPCAs operation is to create a direct connection between the heart and the lungs by bypassing the MAPCAs and reconstructing the iatrogenic native pulmonary artery. Furthermore, to ensure adequate blood flow to the lungs, a modified Blalock-Taussig shunt or a central shunt may be used to establish pulmonary flow (refer to Fig. 5.32).

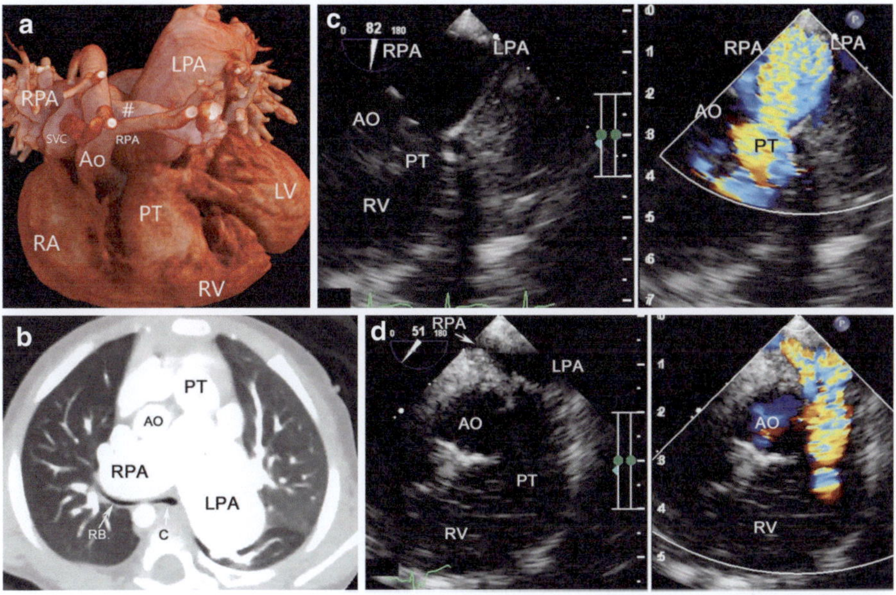

Fig. 5.31 Shows that a 10-month-old male infant, who presented with respiratory and heart failure and was diagnosed with tetralogy of Fallot (TOF) with an absent pulmonary valve, underwent surgical correction. (**a**) The 3D cardiovascular image, viewed from a frontocephalic perspective, shows a dilated pulmonary trunk (PT), exaggerated aneurysms in the bilateral pulmonary arteries, and dilation of all four chambers of the heart. (**b**) The cardiac CT scan shows bilateral pulmonary aneurysms, as well as marked compression of the carina (C) and right bronchus (RB). (**c**) The preoperative TEE in the UE AAo SAX view shows aneurysmal dilatation of the PT, right pulmonary artery (RPA), and left pulmonary artery (LPA), without a normal pulmonary valve. A multicolored mosaic flow signal is visible in the PT, RPA, and LPA (as seen on color Doppler in the right diagram). (**d**) This postoperative TEE image, taken after the pulmonary arterial plasty by plication of the RPA and LPA, shows a trend toward normal size of the pulmonary artery, but residual pulmonary regurgitation is still present (as seen on the right diagram with color Doppler)

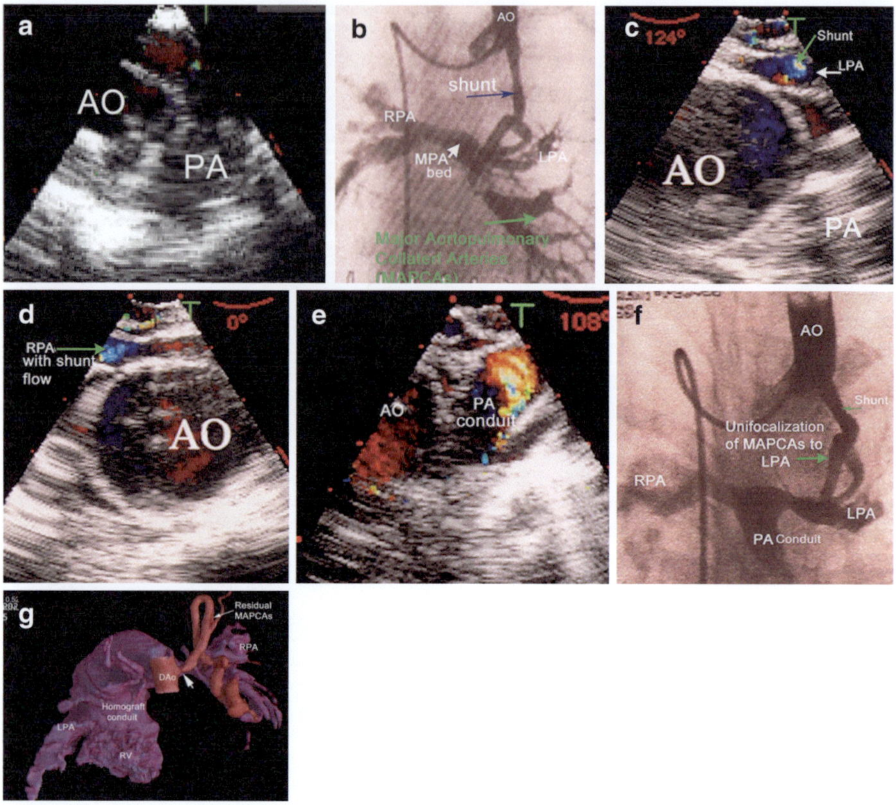

Fig. 5.32 Shows a 6-month-old child with TOF/PA/VSD and major aortopulmonary collateral arteries (MAPCAs) who was experiencing cyanosis. The child underwent shunt and unifocalization of MAPCAs surgery. (**a**) A preoperative TEE showed a case of tetralogy of Fallot (TOF) with pulmonary atresia, as seen in the ME AV SAX view. (**b**) This angiogram shows the formation of MAPCAs (indicated by a green arrow). It also shows a hypoplastic main pulmonary artery (MPA, a short white arrow) and a central shunt (thins blue arrow) between the aorta and left pulmonary artery (LPA). (**c**) After the unifocalization of MAPCAs, the modified ME AV SAX view, TEE showed shunt flow to the pulmonary artery (PA) and left pulmonary artery (LPA). (**d**) After the unifocalization of MAPCAs, the modified ME AV SAX view, TEE showed shunt flow to the right pulmonary artery (RPA). (**e**) After undergoing the Rastelli procedure to reconstruct the right ventricular outflow tract, a TEE with color Doppler in the ME AV SAX view displays the blood flow from the RV to the unifocalized pulmonary artery (PA) bed through a homograft conduit. (**f**) After the surgery, an angiogram was performed to show the placement of a central shunt (small green shunt) and homograft PA conduit from the right ventricle to the unifocalized pulmonary artery bed. (**g**) The postoperative 3D image reformatted from cardiac CT viewing dorsally revealed the presence of a residual MAPCA (as indicated by the arrow) extending from the descending aorta (DAo) to the RPA, which was later successfully treated with a coil

References

1. Sharma A, Shivaprakasha K, Kumar L, Sivasubramonian S. Early and late complications following complete surgical repair of tetralogy of fallot in infants and children. Ann Pediatr Cardiol. 2020;13(2):93–9.
2. Atallah J, Dinu IA, Ramadan R, et al. Risk factors for early and late mortality after surgical repair of tetralogy of Fallot. World J Pediatr Congenit Heart Surg. 2019;10(2):165–73.
3. Kalfa D, Belli E, Belloumi M, et al. Tetralogy of Fallot with major aortopulmonary collateral arteries: surgical strategies and outcomes. Eur J Cardiothorac Surg. 2015;47(3):e121–7.
4. Loomba RS, Geddes GC, Feinberg E, et al. A novel technique for repair of tetralogy of Fallot with absent pulmonary valve and major aortopulmonary collaterals. Ann Thorac Surg. 2018;105(3):e143–5.
5. Wielandner A, Scherr D, Beitzke D, et al. Major aortopulmonary collateral arteries in tetralogy of Fallot with pulmonary atresia: imaging features and transcatheter embolization. Radiology. 2016;279(3):962–71.

5.1.6 Pulmonary Atresia with Intact Ventricular Septum (PA-IVS)

Pulmonary atresia with intact ventricular septum (PA-IVS) is a rare congenital heart defect characterized by the complete occlusion of the pulmonary valve, which obstructs the flow of blood from the right ventricle to the pulmonary artery. The ventricular septum is intact and pulmonary blood flow is dependent on a patent ductus arteriosus after birth.

PA-IVS has various anatomical changes, such as the development of pulmonary artery, distance between pulmonary atresia and right ventricle, hypoplasia or underdevelopment of the right ventricle and tricuspid valve. Furthermore, the coronary circulation is often abnormal, with a connection between the right ventricle (RV) and subepicardial coronary arteries, known as RV-dependent coronaries or ventriculocoronary arterial communication (RCAC). This will be discussed in Fig. 5.33.

PA-IVS is usually diagnosed during fetal development or shortly after birth. Diagnostic tests such as echocardiography [1], cardiac catheterization, and CT may be used to confirm the diagnosis (Figs. 5.33b and 5.34b).

The surgical procedures for PA/IVS depend on the morphology of the RV and tricuspid valve, and are challenging to manage, with high mortality and morbidity rates [2]. The surgical management will be discussed in Fig. 5.34. In patients with an adequately sized right ventricle, transcatheter valvotomy and valvuloplasty can be performed. However, treatment for pulmonary atresia with a severely hypoplastic right ventricle usually involves a temporary procedure known as a Blalock-Taussig shunt, which creates a connection between the subclavian artery and the pulmonary artery to improve blood flow to the lungs. This is then followed by bidirectional Glenn (BDG) procedure and final Fontan procedure, if the RV is not competent to support pulmonary circulation, which aim to reroute blood flow to the lungs without passing through the right ventricle. These procedures will be discussed in Fig. 5.35.

Fig. 5.33 A 4-year-old child with cyanosis presented with type III pulmonary atresia/intact ventricular septum (PA/IVS) and a ventriculocoronary arterial communication (RCAC). The patient underwent surgical ligation of the connection between the right ventricle to the right coronary artery and right ventricular decompression. (**a**) This schematic drawing of pulmonary atresia/intact ventricular septum (PA/IVS) illustrates the relationship between the ventriculocoronary arterial communication (RCAC) and the dependent coronary circulation. (**b**) This thin-slab (2 mm) MIP reconstructed image shows an abnormally dilated right coronary artery (RCA) (indicated by white arrowheads) and a fistula (indicated by a yellow curve arrow) connecting the RCA to a hypoplastic right ventricle (RV). (**c**) In the TEE ME four-chamber view, severe tricuspid valve (TV) hypoplasia is evident, along with a diminutive and hypertrophic RV with thick myocardium. Steal blood from RCA filling into the RV may regurgitate to RA and further passes through a nonrestrictive atrial septal defect (ASD) to the left atrium (LA) (indicated by the yellow curve line). The RV is connected to an ectatic RCA by a fistula in the RV wall and is clearly demonstrated. (**d**) Color Doppler TEE reveals random color signals in the right ventricular myocardium, which confirms the diagnosis of coronary sinusoids in a condition known as a RCAC. (**e**) During the TEE examination, the ME AV LAX view reveals the hypertensive RV and dilatation of RCA

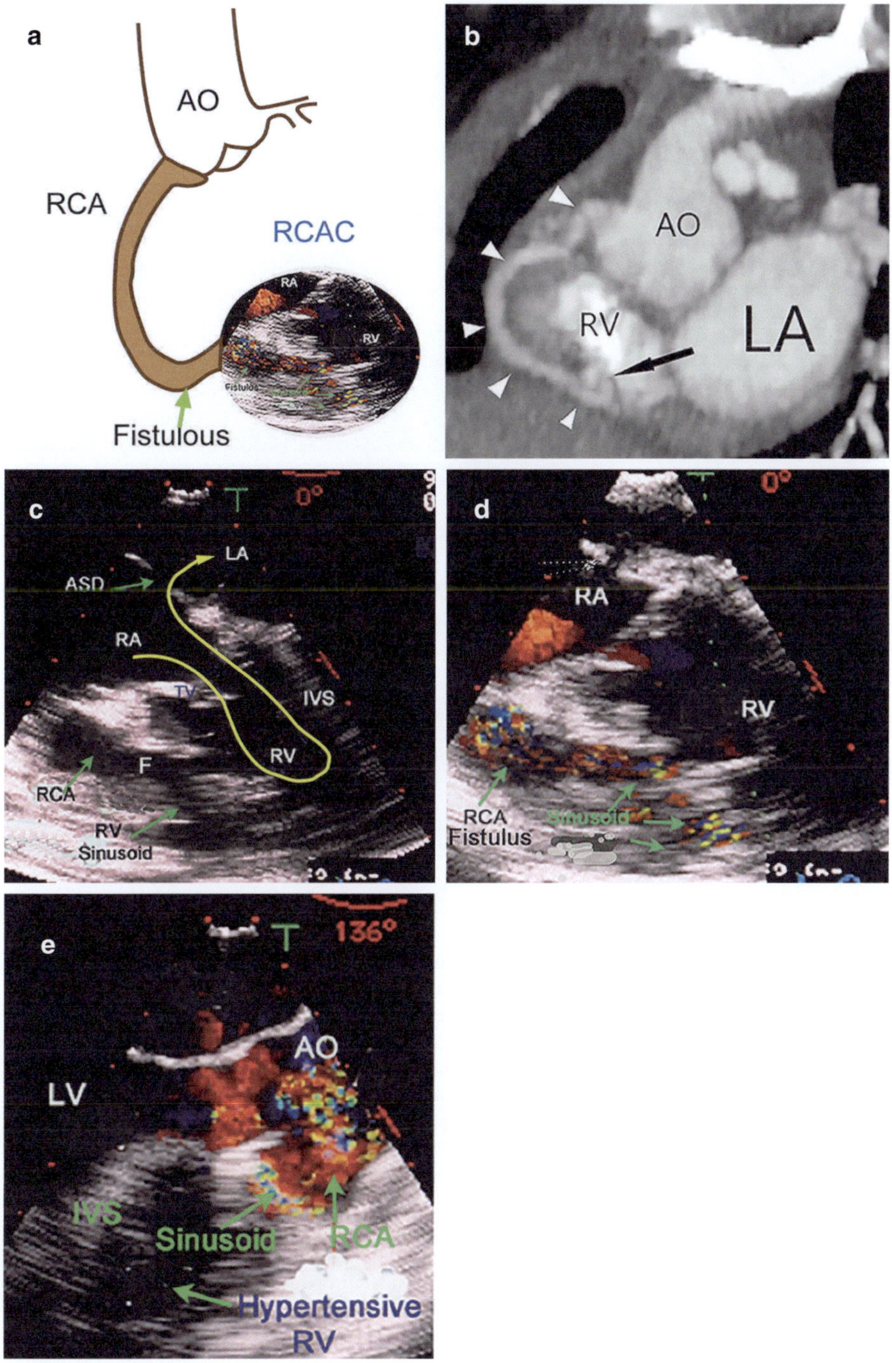
a
AO
RCA
RCAC
Fistulous
b
AO
RV
LA
c
T
0°
LA
ASD
RA
TV
IVS
RV
F
RCA
RV
Sinusoid
d
0°
RA
RV
RCA
Fistulus
Sinusoid
e
T
136°
AO
LV
IVS
Sinusoid
RCA
Hypertensive
RV

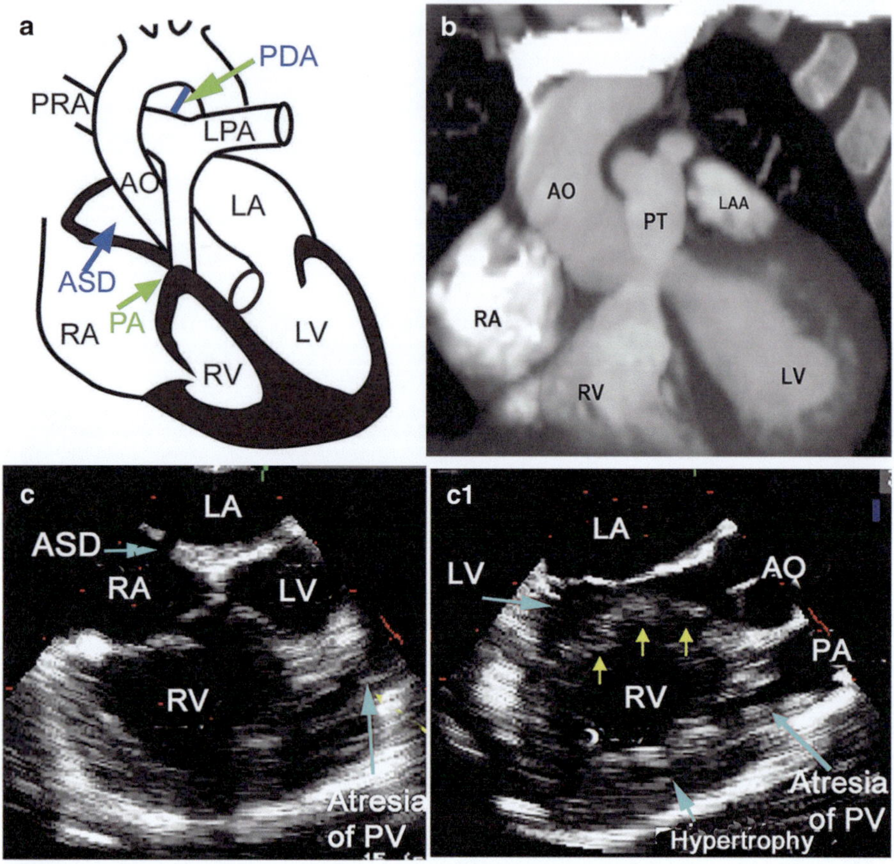

Fig. 5.34 Shows a 1-month-old girl with cyanosis, weighing 2.7 kg, who presented with a pulmonary atresia with an intact ventricular septum. She underwent surgical correction. (**a**) A schematic drawing of a pulmonary atresia with an intact ventricular septum (PA-IVS) illustrates the coexistence of an atretic pulmonary valve, right ventricular hypoplasia, as well as an atrial septal defect, patent ductus arteriosus. (**b**) Contrast-enhanced cardiac CT shows the presence of a pulmonary atresia at its valve and a dilated right atrium. There is a hypoplasia of the right ventricle. (**c**) The preoperative TEE ME four-chamber (45°) view shows a dilated right atrium with a normal-sized tricuspid valve, but the pulmonary valve is atretic. In addition, there is hypertrophy of the right ventricle and an atrial septal defect (ASD) is also present. (**c1**) The TEE, ME AV LAX view reveals severe hypertrophy of the right ventricle with elevated pressure. Membranous pulmonary valve atresia is visible. (**d**) The Rastelli procedure is depicted in a schematic drawing, which illustrates a patch repair of the right ventricular outflow tract (RVOT) and the insertion of a valved conduit (green arrow) that connects the pulmonary artery to the right ventricle. (**d1**) The postoperative TEE, ME AV SAX view demonstrates a normal appearance of the RVOT and RV-PA conduit. (**d2**) A postoperative 3D volume rendering image of the Rastelli operation shows a homograft with a valved conduit (C) positioned between the right ventricle and pulmonary artery

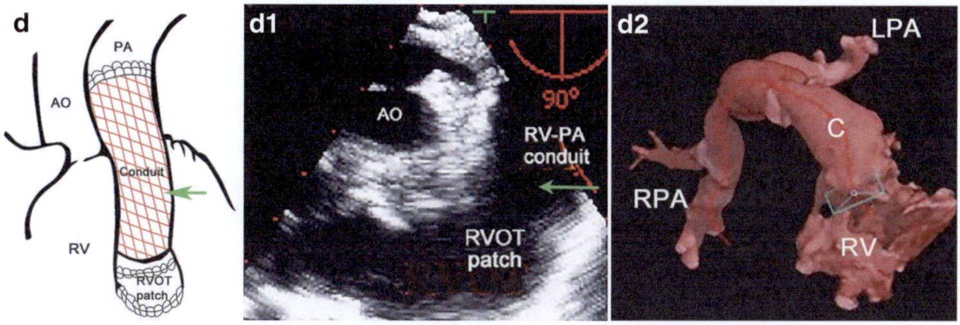

Fig. 5.34 (continued)

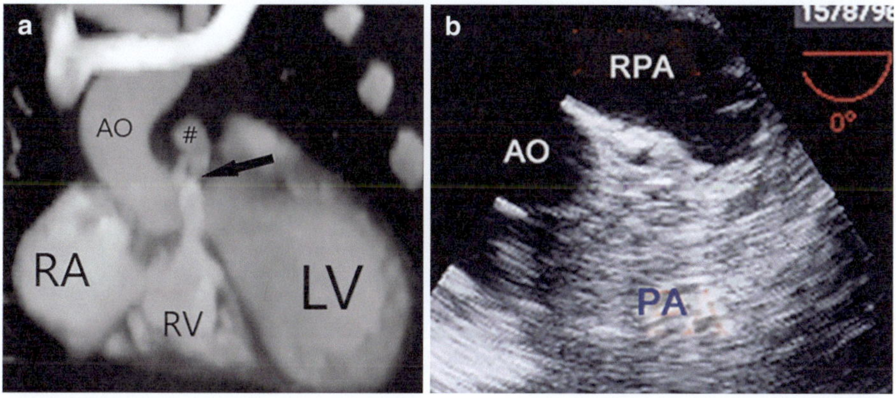

Fig. 5.35 Shows a 5-month-old child who has been diagnosed with pulmonary atresia, a large atrial septal defect (ASD), hypoplastic right ventricle (RV), and left pulmonary artery stenosis. During the neonatal period, the child received a Blalock-Taussig shunt. The child is scheduled to undergo a staged operation, starting with a bidirectional Glenn (BDG) shunt. (**a**) The preoperative cardiac CT scan shows pulmonary atresia, which indicated by a black arrow, along with a hypoplastic pulmonary trunk (indicated by #) and right ventricle. The scan also shows an intact ventricular septum and a large left ventricle (LV). (**b**) The UE AAo short-axis view shows pulmonary atresia (PA) and a dilated right pulmonary artery (RPA). (**c**) The schematic drawing of the bidirectional Glenn shunt shows the superior vena cava (SVC) connecting directly to the RPA. (**d**) The postoperative color TEE in the UE AAo view shows an anastomosis created between the SVC and RPA, with the blood flow of the SVC directly draining into the RPA (indicated by the yellow dotted arrow). P for proximal and D for distal. (**e**) The postoperative 3D volume rendering image viewing dorsally shows the SVC connecting to the RPA (indicated by the yellow arrow), the proximal site of the RPA (#), and the distal site of the RPA (*). (**f**) The postoperative contrast-enhanced CT image shows the bidirectional Glenn (BDG) shunt (indicated by yellow arrowhead) without any focal junctional stenosis. The white arrow is pointing to an area indicating stenosis (narrowing) in the LPA

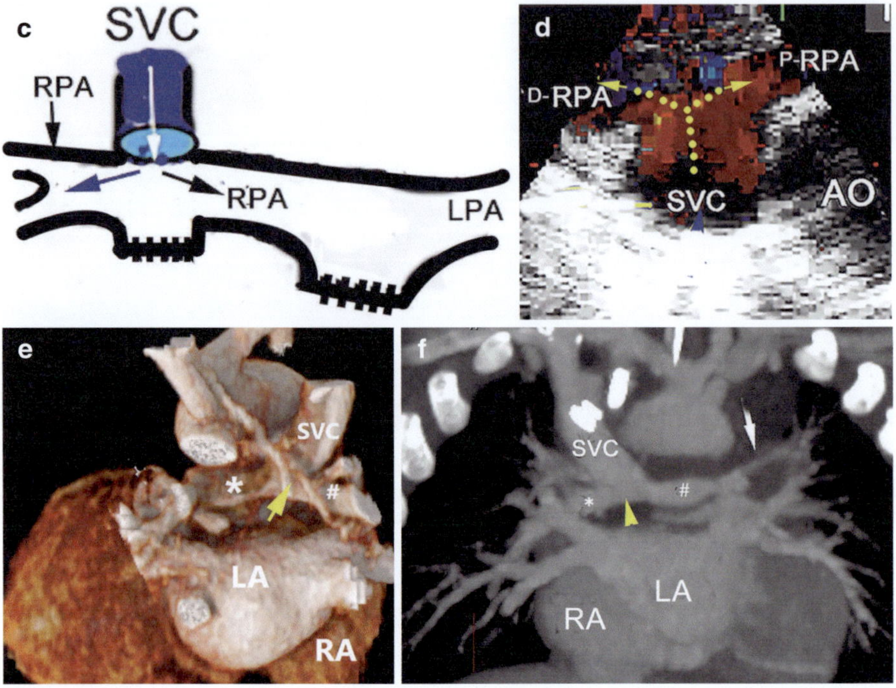

Fig. 5.35 (continued)

References

1. Leung MP, Mok C-K, Hui P-W. Echocardiographic assessment of neonates with pulmonary atresia and intact ventricular septum. J Am Coll Cardiol. 1988;12(3):719–25.
2. Yoshimura N, Yamaguchi M, Ohashi H. Pulmonary atresia with intact ventricular septum: strategy based on right ventricular morphology. J Thorac Cardiovasc Surg. 2003;126:1417–26.

5.2 (B). Vascular Abnormalities

5.2.1 Coarctation of the Aorta (CoA)

Coarctation of the aorta (CoA) is a congenital heart defect characterized by a narrowing or constriction in the aorta. This constriction can impede blood flow to the lower body and cause increased blood pressure in the upper body.

CoA is usually diagnosed in infancy or childhood, and diagnosis typically involves multiple imaging tests such as transesophageal echocardiography (TEE, Fig. 5.36c), magnetic resonance imaging (MRI) (refer to Fig. 5.36a) or 3D cardiac

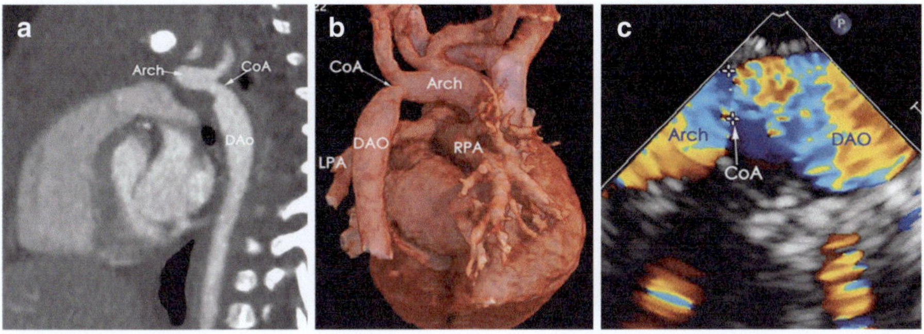

Fig. 5.36 Shows the case of a 7-day-old infant with a coarctation of the aorta (CoA) who presented with tachypnea and tachycardia, and underwent surgical repair. (**a**) The sagittal view of the computed tomographic (CT) scan shows a discrete narrowing (CoA) at the level of the aortic isthmus (arrow). (**b**) The 3D reconstruction of the CT angiography of the same patient, viewed from the right-dorsal aspect, clearly shows the site of the discrete narrowing (CoA). (**c**) During the surgery, intraoperative color TEE was performed, and the UE DAo view demonstrated turbulence at the site of coarctation (arrow). The postoperative TEE was not performed because it was considered that the insertion of the TEE probe might indirectly compress the surgical anastomosis

CT (refer to Fig. 5.36b). Surgical repair with TEE monitoring in the severe case is to remove the narrowed portion of the aorta and reconnect the remaining ends (refer to Fig. 5.36c).

5.2.2 Interrupted Aortic Arch (IAA)

Interrupted aortic arch (IAA) is a rare congenital heart defect that affects the aorta. In IAA (Interrupted Aortic Arch), a segment of the aorta is either missing or severely narrowed, resulting in a disruption of blood flow to the body. IAA typically manifests with symptoms shortly after birth or during the neonatal period.

Diagnosis of IAA is made through imaging tests including transesophageal echocardiography (TEE, Fig. 5.37c), and 3D cardiac CT (refer to Fig. 5.37b). Treatment usually involves surgery under TEE monitoring to reconstruct the aortic arch and restore normal blood flow. In some cases, multiple surgeries may be needed over time (refer to Fig. 5.37).

5.2.3 Double Aortic Arch (DAA)

A baby's aorta typically develops as one large vessel leaving the heart, but defects in aorta development can occur. Double aortic arch (DAA) is causing by failure of regression of both primitive arches and resulting in two transverse aortic arches over the trachea and bronchi. This creates a vascular ring (refer to Fig. 5.38c, d) that may lead to life-threatening airway blockages.

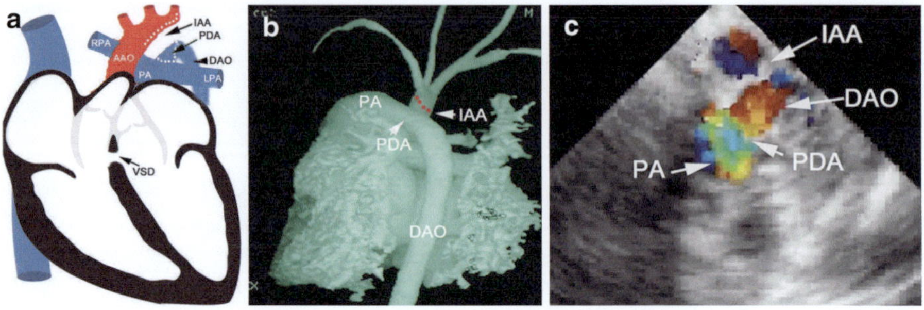

Fig. 5.37 Shows the case of a newborn with an interrupted aortic arch (IAA), who presented with tachycardia, gray skin color, and coldness over both legs. The patient underwent a surgical repair. (**a**) The diagram depicts an interrupted aortic arch (Type A), with the discontinuation occurring just past the left subclavian artery. To provide blood flow to the lower body, a patent ductus arteriosus (PDA) is present. The white dotted line indicates the surgical incisions for repairing the interrupted aortic arch. (**b**) The 3D reconstruction of the CT angiography in the left posterior oblique (LPO) view clearly shows the patent ductus arteriosus (PDA) directly arising from the pulmonary artery (PA) and connecting to the descending aorta (DAO). The red dotted line indicates the interrupted aortic arch (Type A). (**c**) During the surgery, the intraoperative color TEE revealed the direction of the PDA flow, which originated from the PA and drained toward the DAO. No postoperative TEE was performed because it was considered that inserting the TEE probe might potentially compress the reconstructed aortic anastomosis indirectly

A CT or 3D test is useful in detecting DAA and other heart defects. Surgical treatment of DAA usually involves dividing and ligating one of the aortic arches, typically the smaller one, to relieve pressure on the trachea and esophagus. This procedure is called aortoplasty (refer to Fig. 5.38).

5.2.4 The Aortapulmonary Window (APW)

The aortapulmonary window (APW) is a congenital heart defect characterized by a communication between the ascending aorta and the main pulmonary artery. Their symptoms and signs are shortness of breath, fatigue, and poor weight gain, especially in infants result from increasing blood flow and pressure in the lungs.

Diagnosis of APW is typically made through imaging tests including transesophageal echocardiography (TEE, Fig. 5.39e), or 3D cardiac CT (Fig. 5.39b, c). In some cases, surgery under TEE monitoring may be necessary to repair the APW and separate blood flow between the aorta and pulmonary artery (refer to Fig. 5.39).

5.2.5 Diverticulum of Kommerell (KD)

Diverticulum of Kommerell is a rare congenital abnormality of the aorta. There is an outpouching or sac-like dilation of the aorta, usually located in the distal aortic

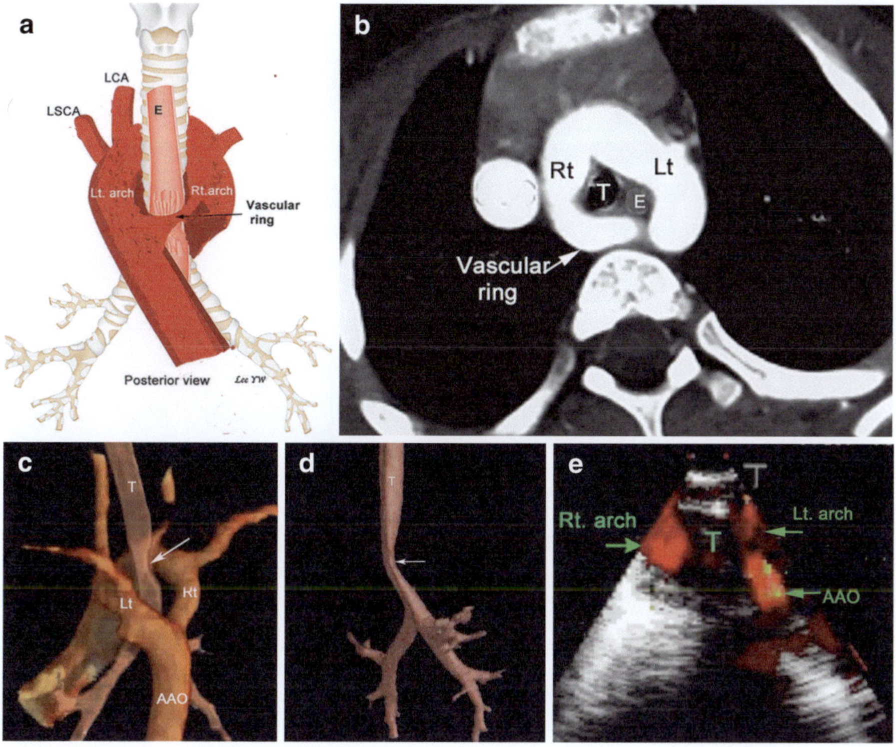

Fig. 5.38 Shows a case of double aortic arch in a 10-month-old boy who presented with chronic cough and choking while being fed. The patient underwent surgical correction. (**a**) This schematic representation shows the dorsal view of a double aortic arches, which causes a complete ring surrounding the esophagus and trachea, leading to compressive symptoms. (**b**) This axial CT scan illustrates a double aortic arch constricting the esophagus (E) and trachea (T) to form a complete vascular ring. (**c**) This 3D CT image of the ascending aorta depicts the vascular ring formed by the double aortic arch and extrinsic compression (indicated by a white arrow) at the lower third of the trachea by the right arch (Rt). (**d**) This 3D CT image of the trachea shows indentation at the lower part of the trachea (indicated by a white arrow). (**e**) This intraoperative TEE with color Doppler, in the UE AAO SAX view, demonstrates the ascending aorta (AAO) giving rise to right and left arches that encircle and compress the trachea (T)

arch where the left subclavian artery originates. Diverticulum of Kommerell can lead to compression of nearby structures, such as the trachea, esophagus, or nerves, causing symptoms such as difficulty breathing, coughing, or swallowing difficulties.

Diagnosis is typically made through imaging studies such as transesophageal echocardiography (TEE, Fig. 5.40d, e), and 3D cardiac CT scan (Fig. 5.40b, c). Surgery under TEE monitoring may also be recommended to repair any associated anomalies such as coarctation of the aorta and severe symptoms from compression by this diverticulum (refer to Fig. 5.40).

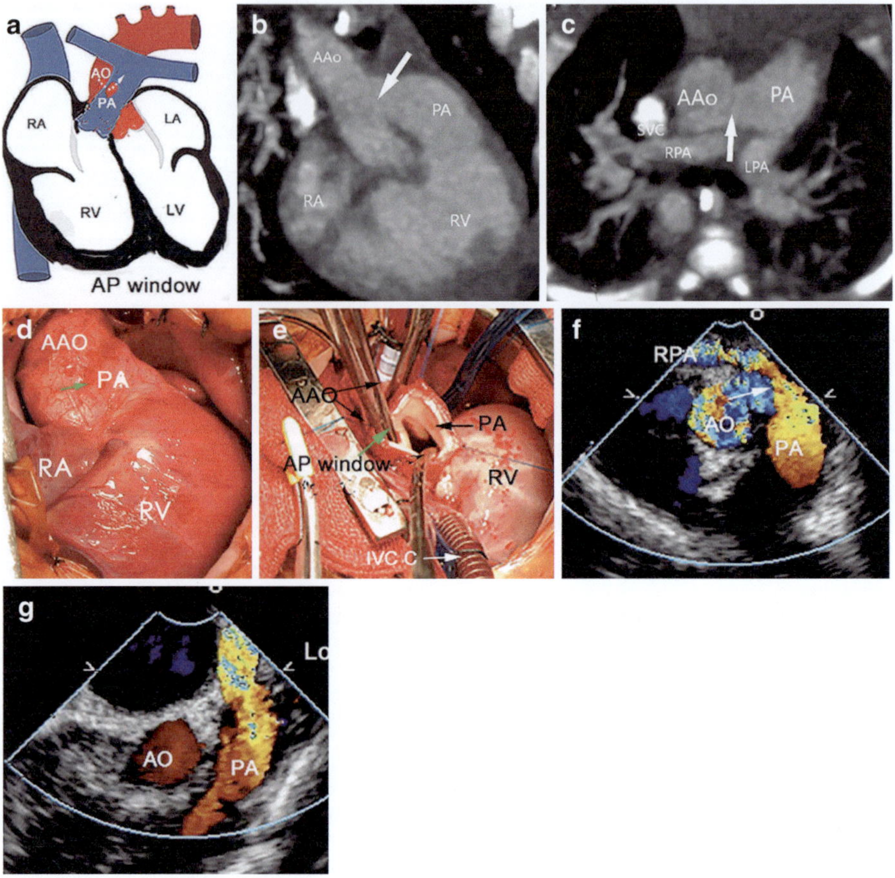

Fig. 5.39 Shows an aortopulmonary (AP) window in a 1-month-old infant who presented with recurrent chest infections, tachypnea, and cardiac murmur and underwent surgical correction. (**a**) The diagram shows an aortopulmonary (AP) window depicting communication between the aorta and pulmonary artery. (**b**, **c**) The maximal intensity projection images by thin-slab multiplanar reconstruction (MPR) in oblique coronal (**b**) and axial views (**c**) illustrate the aortopulmonary defect (indicated by the arrows) located before the pulmonary bifurcation. (**d**) The intraoperative photograph displays the external view of the AP window (indicated by the green arrow). (**e**) The intraoperative photograph, taken after pulmonary artery incision, illustrates a large oval-shaped defect (with a metal suction tube inserted, indicated by the green arrow) between the opened pulmonary artery and aorta. (**f**) The preoperative color TEE image, specifically the UE AAo SAX view demonstrates a big shunt between the aorta and pulmonary artery (arrow). (**g**) The postoperative color TEE image, specifically the UE AAo SAX view, demonstrates no more shunt between the aorta and pulmonary artery after patch closure of the aortopulmonary defect

5.2.6 Patent Ductus Arteriosus (PDA)

The ductus arteriosus is a blood vessel that connects the pulmonary artery and the aorta, allowing blood to bypass the nonfunctioning lungs of the fetus. In most

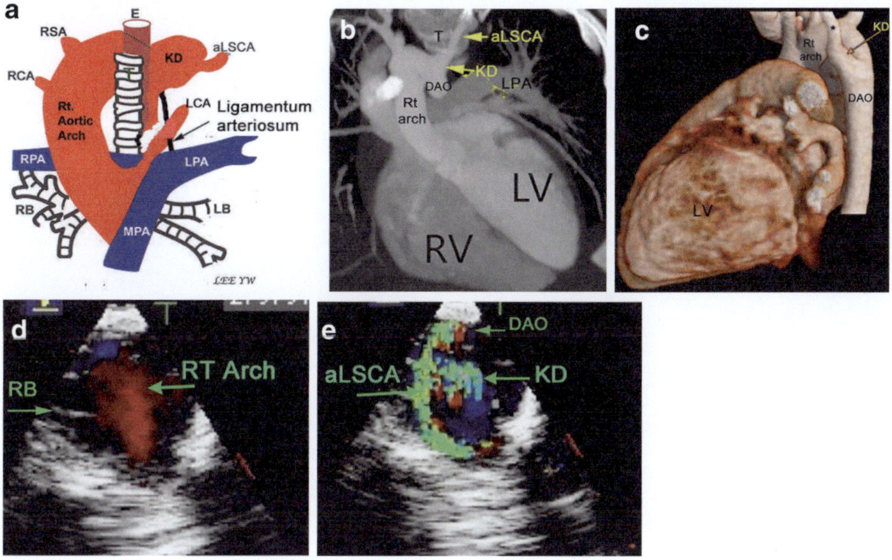

Fig. 5.40 Shows a case of right aortic arch with an associated aberrant left subclavian artery (aLSCA) and Kommerell's diverticulum (KD) in a 1-year-old boy weighing 7 kg. The patient presented with vomiting after feeding and coughing. (**a**) This diagram shows the anterior view of the descending aorta with a right-side aortic arch and Kommerell's diverticulum (KD), which is an aneurysmal dilatation of the descending aorta at the origin of the aberrant left subclavian artery (aLSCA). The presence of this aneurysm can cause external posterior compression of the esophagus and trachea due to vascular ring formation. (**b**, **c**) This reconstructed contrast-enhanced cardiac CT and 3D color volume rendering image in left lateral view show an aLSCA (*) originating from a KD. (**d**, **e**) This intraoperative color TEE image, in the UE AAO SAX view, shows the right-side (RT) aortic arch with a turbulent mosaic jet over the KD and aLSCA (RB indicating right bronchus)

infants, the ductus arteriosus closes spontaneously within a few days or weeks after birth. However, in some infants, the ductus arteriosus remains open, leading to patent ductus arteriosus (PDA). PDA is more common in premature infants and is more frequently found in females than in males.

If the PDA is large and causing symptoms in premature babies, medications such as indomethacin or ibuprofen may be used to facilitate the closure of the ductus arteriosus. If these medications are not effective, surgical PDA ligation or clipping may be necessary to close the ductus arteriosus. In cases where a PDA is high takeoff and large, it may be mistaken for the aortic arch, resulting in inadvertent ligation of the left pulmonary artery (LPA) (refer to Fig. 5.41), especially with the left thoracotomy approach. Therefore, to avoid this complication with certainty (refer to Fig. 5.42), TEE guidance should be used during surgical PDA ligation.

However, in premature or small infants, TEE-guided surgery may not be feasible. In such cases, a pediatric TEE transducer can be positioned at the parasternal area of the chest to facilitate continuous transthoracic echocardiographic (cTTE)

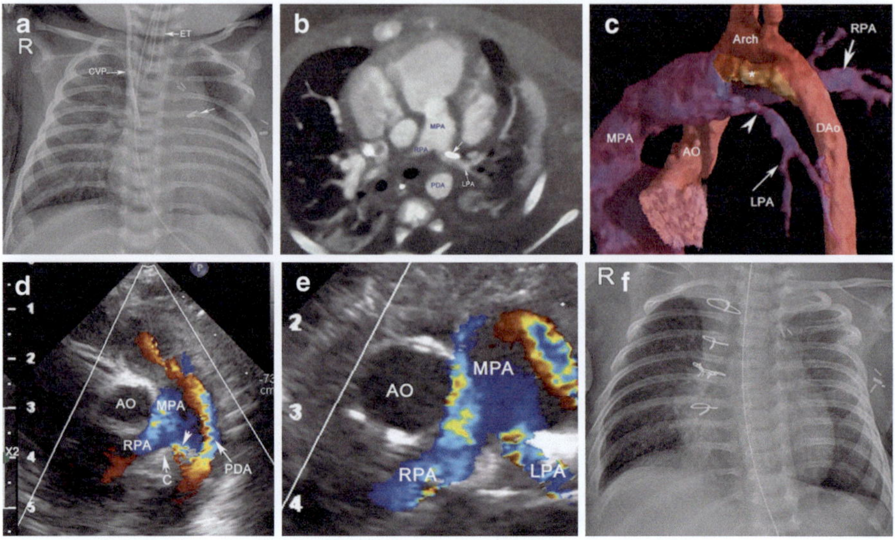

Fig. 5.41 Shows a female infant who was admitted to the hospital due to inadvertent ligation of the left pulmonary artery during surgical closure of a patent ductus arteriosus (PDA) performed 2 days prior at a different hospital. (**a**) The chest X-ray revealed cardiomegaly, oligemia of the left hemithorax, and increased pulmonary vasculature in the right hemithorax. Additionally, a dense opaque clip, indicated by an arrow, was seen superimposed over the left lung hilum. Furthermore, the infant was placed under mechanical ventilation due to respiratory failure, as indicated by the presence of an endotracheal tube (ET). (**b**) A dense opaque clip (indicated by a white arrow) was identified at the proximal left pulmonary artery on the cardiac CT scan. (**c**) A 3D volume rendering image obtained 48 h after the inadvertent ligation procedure showed the persistent presence of a large PDA (indicated by an asterisk and presented by a golden segment vessel). The left pulmonary artery (LPA) was clipped just distal to the main pulmonary artery bifurcation, which resulted in discrete and nearly interrupted proximal LPA stenosis (indicated by an arrowhead). (**d**) The transthoracic echocardiogram before redo surgery revealed the presence of a residual PDA, and a dense opaque clip (C) at the proximal site of the left pulmonary artery (LPA) causing near-total occlusion of LPA flow. (**e**) Immediately following the redo surgical removal of the clip and LPA reconstruction, a transthoracic echocardiogram revealed symmetric bilateral pulmonary flow. (**f**) A chest X-ray taken 7 days after the redo surgical reconstruction revealed symmetrical bilateral pulmonary vasculature. Moreover, there was no evidence of a dense opaque clip at the left lung hilum. Furthermore, there was no presence of an endotracheal tube for mechanical ventilation

monitoring during surgical ligation. This monitoring method is crucial in preventing inadvertent ligation. Please refer to Fig. 5.43.

References

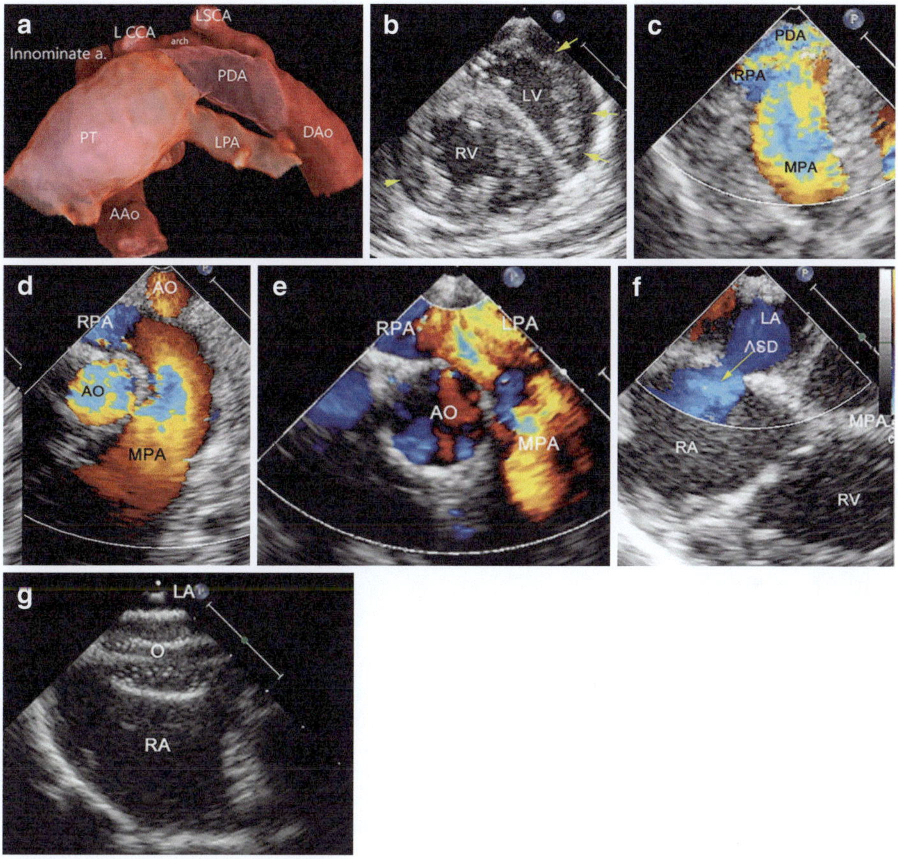

Fig. 5.42 Shows a case of a large patent ductus arteriosus (PDA) in an infant who presented with respiratory distress and congestive heart failure. The patient underwent surgical ligation to treat the condition. (**a**) A preoperative 3D CT image reveals a large PDA (lighten partially transparent segment) viewing from left lateral aspect. The real aortic arch can also be seen through this PDA. (**b**) This image, taken during intraoperative TEE and viewed from the transgastric angle, highlights the presence of pericardial effusion (indicated by the yellow arrows). (**c**) During the pretest PDA ligation, an intraoperative image was captured from the UE PA view, which showed a turbulent mosaic jet of PDA still present. These findings suggest that there may have been an incorrect ligation, possibly involving the descending aorta instead of the PDA. (**d**) Shows a continuous TEE image captured during the same time period as **c**. This image reveals that the LPA was not visible, indicating an incorrect PDA ligation on LPA. Consequently, the pretest LPA ligation was released, and the real one PDA was ligated instead. This TEE image confirmed the surgical findings. (**e**) After the PDA correction surgery, a color TEE image was taken and showed the absence of the PDA. The image also demonstrated normal blood flow from the MPA to the LPA and RPA, as shown in the left panel. (**f**) In addition, this infant was found to have an ASD with left-to-right shunting on a TEE in the ME four-chamber view. At the age of 3, transcatheter closure of the ASD was performed using an occluder, as shown in **g**. **Note**: If a PDA is high take-off level and large (as shown in **a**), it can be mistaken for the aortic arch, resulting in inadvertent ligation of the LPA especially at the left thoracotomy approach. Therefore, using TEE guidance during surgical PDA ligation can help to avoid this complication with certainty

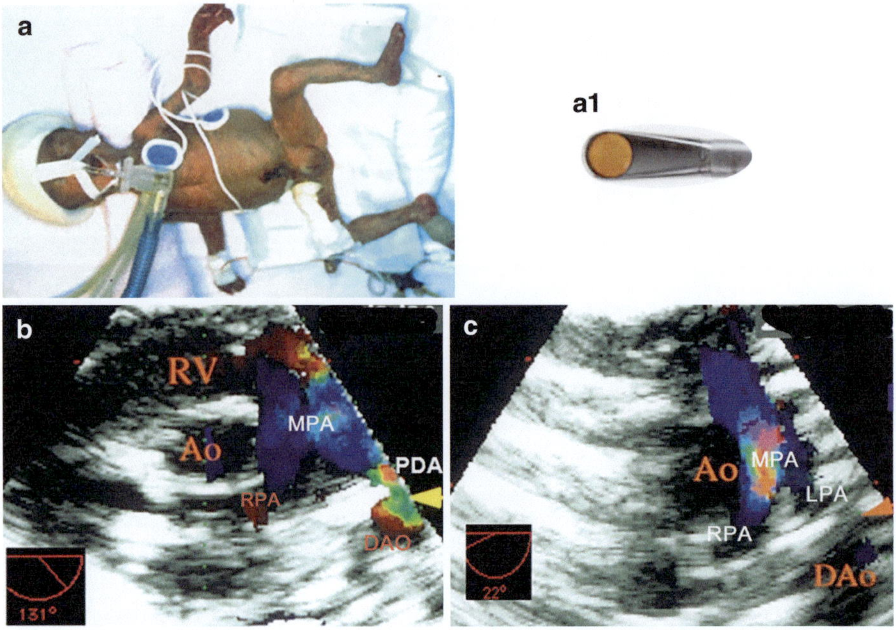

Fig. 5.43 Shows a PDA in a premature infant weighing 1500 g who presented with respiratory distress despite receiving the standard dose of pharmacological treatment. The infant underwent bedside PDA ligation. (**a**) A premature infant receiving mechanical ventilator therapy and medication for heart failure underwent bedside PDA ligation with a right lateral decubitus position. Throughout the procedure, a pediatric mini-multiplane transesophageal echocardiography (TEE) transducer (as shown in **a1**) was positioned and secured at the parasternal area of the chest. This transducer was utilized for continuous transthoracic echocardiographic (cTTE) monitoring. (**b**) The preoperative cTTE echocardiogram shows a large MPA and a turbulent jet across the PDA (indicated by the yellow arrow) from the DAo, resulting in a left-to-right shunt. (**c**) The postoperative cTTE echocardiogram after PDA ligation shows closure of the PDA (indicated by the brown arrow) and absence of blood flow from the DAo into the PA

1. Jaffe RB, Orsmond GS, Veasy LG. Inadvertent ligation of left pulmonary artery. Radiology. 1986;161:355–7.
2. Kilcoyne MF, Do-Nguyen CC, Stevens RM. A review of the surgical ligation of patent ductus arteriosus in a neonate. CTSNet, Inc Media; 2020.

5.2.7 Left Pulmonary Artery Sling (LPAS)

A left pulmonary artery sling (LPAS), also known as pulmonary artery sling, is a rare congenital heart defect in which the left pulmonary artery is abnormally posterior positioned and encircles the trachea, resulting in compression of the airway. In the case of LPAS, the left pulmonary artery arises from the right pulmonary artery and forms a sling around the trachea, which can cause respiratory problems. Symptoms can range from mild to severe and may include difficulty in breathing, wheezing, coughing, recurrent respiratory infections, and cyanosis.

Diagnosis of LPAS typically involves a combination of imaging tests, such as transesophageal echocardiography (TEE, Fig. 5.44d, e), and computed tomography (CT) (Fig. 5.44b). The treatment option for LPAS is surgery with TEE monitoring, which involves repositioning the left pulmonary artery to relieve airway compression. Please refer to Fig. 5.44.

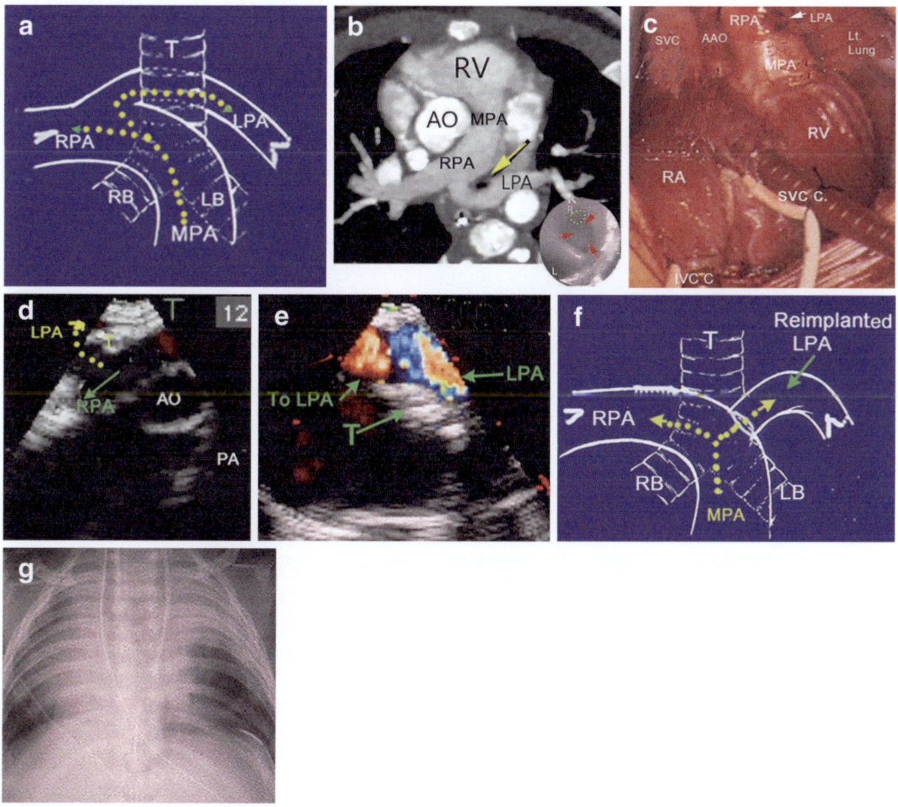

Fig. 5.44 Shows a case of left pulmonary artery (LPA) sling in a 6-month-old boy weighing 4 kg. The patient presented with respiratory distress and underwent LPA reimplantation. (**a**) This is a schematic representation of an LPA sling, where the LPA arises from the right pulmonary artery (RPA) and runs posteriorly between the trachea and esophagus to reach the left lung, forming a sling around the airway (RB indicating right bronchus, LB indicating left bronchus). (**b**) This CT scan demonstrates the LPA arising from the RPA and coursing posterior to the trachea, passing between the lower tracheal and esophagus (E), causing focal lower tracheal stenosis (indicated by a yellow arrow). The lower right circle diagram is an intraoperative bronchoscopy image which also shows a small opening of the main RB (indicated by a yellow dotted circle) and red arrows indicating stenosis of the lower trachea just proximal to the orifice of the main RB. (**c**) This intraoperative surgical photograph shows the LPA (arrow) arising from the RPA instead of the main pulmonary artery (MPA). (**d**) This preoperative TEE in the UE AAO SAX view shows a clear echo drop-out (indicated by a yellow dotted arrow line) of the LPA arising from the RPA. (**e**) This preoperative color TEE image shows the LPA arising from the RPA and running posteriorly to the trachea (T). (**f**) This diagram displays the transected LPA being anastomosed to the opening created in the MPA, while the opening of the RPA is closed. (**g**) This CXR after LPA reimplantation surgery shows the reexpansion of the right lung

5.2.8 Anomalous Origin of the Left Coronary Artery from the Pulmonary Artery (ALCAPA)

Anomalous origin of the left coronary artery from the pulmonary artery (ALCAPA) syndrome is a rare congenital heart defect where the left coronary artery, which normally arises from the aorta, instead originates from the pulmonary artery. This results in decreased oxygenated blood flow to the heart muscle, which can lead to heart failure, arrhythmias, and sudden cardiac death.

Diagnosis of ALCAPA in infants is typically made through imaging tests including transesophageal echocardiography (TEE, Fig. 5.45f) or 3D cardiac CT (Fig. 5.45b, c). The main treatment for ALCAPA syndrome is surgical repair by reimplantation of the left coronary artery into the aorta (refer to Fig. 5.45).

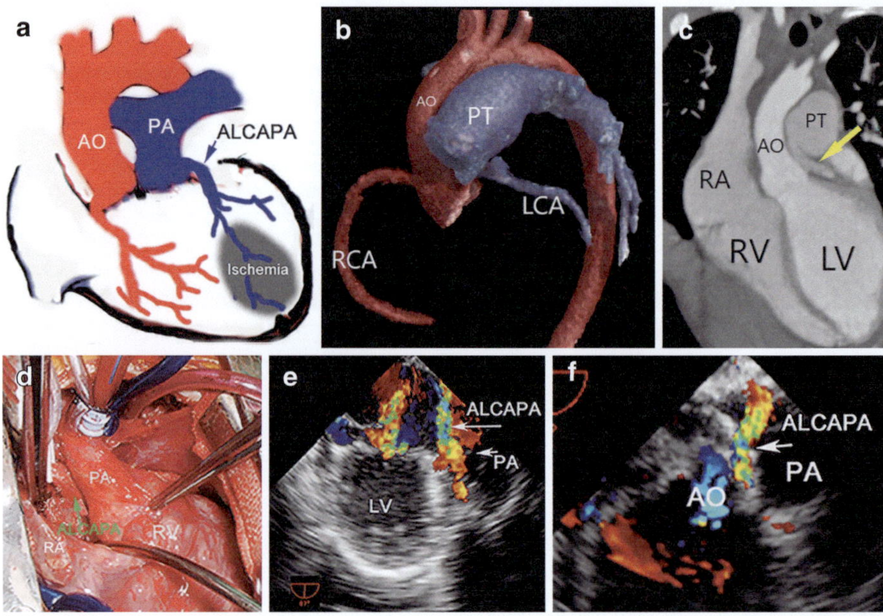

Fig. 5.45 Shows a case of ALCAPA (anomalous origin of the left coronary artery from the pulmonary artery) syndrome in an 8-year-old boy who presented with tachycardia and dyspnea, and underwent surgical repair. (**a**) The diagram shows an ALCAPA, where the left coronary artery (LCA) arises from the main pulmonary artery (PA). Due to the limited oxygenated blood supply to the left ventricular myocardium, there is a relatively chronic myocardial ischemia (gray zone) in the left ventricle, which can lead to heart failure. (**b, c**) The 3D volume rendering color mapping from cardiac CT image clearly distinguishes between the left coronary artery (LCA) originating from the pulmonary trunk (PT) and the right coronary artery (RCA) originating from the aorta. The axial multidetector CT angiogram (as depicted in **c**) displays the origin of the LCA (indicated by the yellow arrow) from the pulmonary trunk (PT). (**d**) The intraoperative photograph illustrates the origin of the LCA from the undersurface of the main pulmonary artery (indicated by the green arrow). (**e**) The preoperative color TEE image, specifically the ME four-chamber view, exhibits a dilated left ventricle with mitral regurgitation and the LCA opening from the main pulmonary artery (arrow). (**f**) The color TEE image, specifically the ME AV SAX view, displays the origin of the ALCAPA from the main pulmonary artery with turbulent flow

5.2.9 Total Anomalous Pulmonary Venous Connection (TAPVC)

Total anomalous pulmonary venous connection (TAPVC), also known as total anomalous pulmonary venous return, is an uncommon congenital heart defect that affects around 1–5% of individuals with congenital heart diseases [1]. This condition occurs when the four pulmonary veins, responsible for transporting oxygen-rich blood from the lungs to the left atrium of the heart, are improperly connected to the heart. In TAPVC, the pulmonary veins merge behind the heart to form the pulmonary venous confluence (PVC), which then drains into the right atrium or a nearby vein instead of the left atrium. This results in poorly oxygenated blood being circulated throughout the body.

Classifying TAPVC is crucial as the type of surgical repair varies depending on the location where the pulmonary veins drain. TAPVC can be categorized into four types based on this location:

Type 1 TAPVC, known as supracardiac type TAPVC [1, 2], occurs when the pulmonary veins merge behind the heart and drain upwards to an abnormal vertical vein that connects to the innominate vein, then to the superior vena cava (SVC), and finally, the right atrium (RA). This type of TAPVC is the most prevalent, making up around 50–60% of cases. Diagnosis imaging (such as TEE or CT) and management will be discussed in Fig. 5.46.

Type 2 TAPVC, also known as cardiac type TAPVC [1, 3], is characterized by the pulmonary veins draining directly into the RA or through the coronary sinus without any connection to the left atrium. The diagnosis imaging (such as TEE or CT) and management will be discussed in Fig. 5.47.

Type 3 TAPVC, also known as infracardiac type TAPVC [1, 4], is characterized by the pulmonary veins draining into a descending vertical vein that empties into the main portal vein most commonly or one of its tributaries, which then carries blood to the liver. The diagnosis imaging (such as TEE or CT) and management will be discussed in Fig. 5.48.

Type 4 TAPVC, or mixed type TAPVC, is a combination of the three previous types, with the pulmonary veins draining into more than one location.

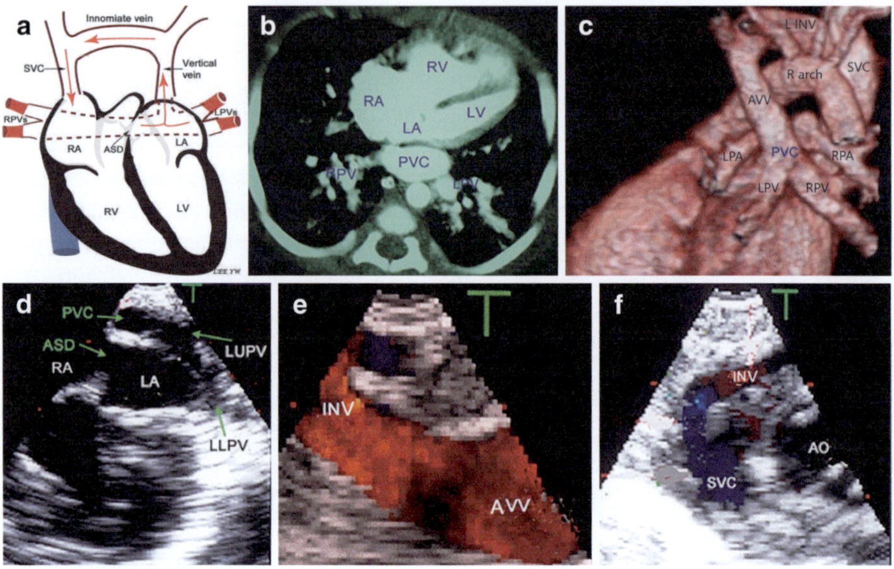

Fig. 5.46 Shows a case of total anomalous pulmonary venous connection (TAPVC) with the supracardiac type in a 2-day-old girl who weighed 3.3 kg. The patient presented with cyanotic respiratory distress and underwent surgical correction. (**a**) This diagram illustrates supracardiac TAPVC, in which all of the left- and right-side pulmonary veins drain into a confluence located behind the left atrium (LA). From the confluence, an ascending vertical vein connects to the left innominate vein, which then drains into the superior vena cava (SVC). The blood then flows from the SVC into the right atrium (RA). (**b**) This is a transverse sectional image of a contrast-enhanced cardiac CT, which shows the dilatation of the RA and a small LA with an ASD. The image also shows that the right pulmonary veins (RPV) and left pulmonary veins (LPV) merge together to form a pulmonary vein confluence (PVC) located behind the LA. (**c**) This is a 3D volume rendering image (dorsal view) generated from CT, which illustrates supracardiac TAPVC. The image shows that the LPVs and RPVs join together to form a PVC. From the PVC, the blood drains into the SVC and the RA through the ascending vertical vein (AVV) and the innominate vein (INV). (**d**) This is a preoperative TEE image in a four-chamber view, which shows that the left-sided pulmonary veins drain into the PVC chamber located behind the LA and the ASD. (**e**) This is a color TEE image, which shows the blood flow from the pulmonary vein confluence (PVC) connecting to the ascending vertical vein (AVV) and then flowing upward to drain into the innominate vein (INV). (**f**) This color TEE image is a continuation of the previous images (**d**, **e**) and shows the blood flow from the innominate vein (INV) draining into the superior vena cava (SVC)

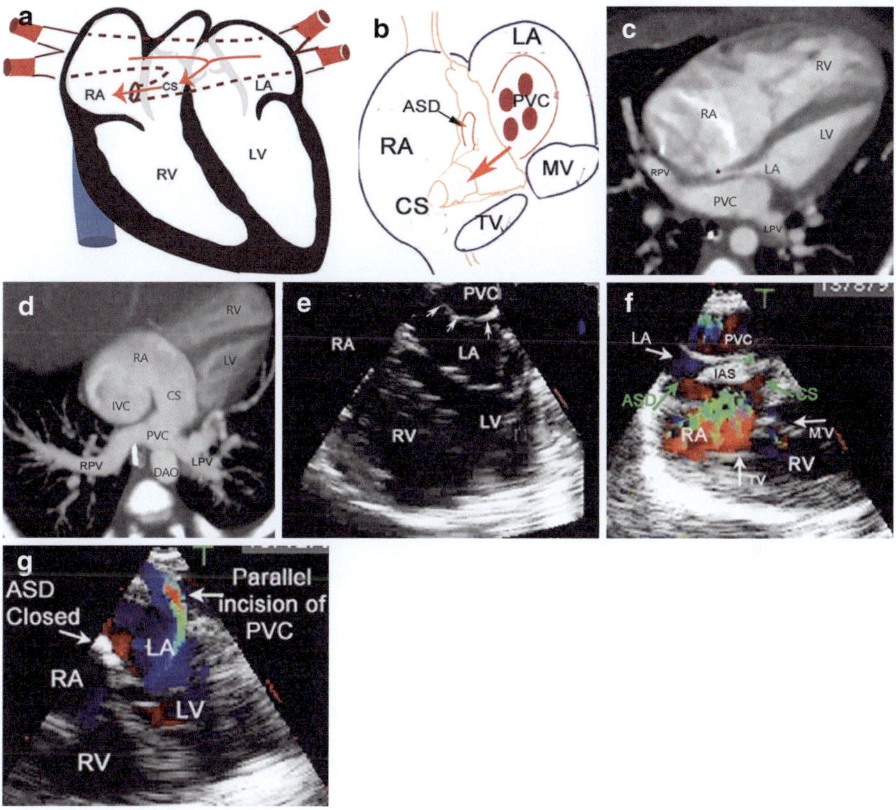

Fig. 5.47 Shows a case of total anomalous pulmonary venous connection (TAPVC) with intracardiac type in a 1-week-old male baby who presented with cyanosis, rapid breathing, and grunting. The baby underwent surgical treatment. (**a**) This schematic diagram depicts the direction of blood flow from the pulmonary veins, which drain into the coronary sinus and then flow into the right atrium (illustrated by the red curved arrow line). (**b**) Diagram of enface LA view illustrating four pulmonary veins (red dot) come together behind the LA into the pulmonary venous confluence (PVC) chamber connecting the CS (red arrow) and drain to RA. Part of this oxygen-rich blood drains to LA through the ASD (arrow). (**c**) Preoperative cardiac CT demonstrates a large PVC behind the LA. ASD (asterisk) between LA and RA. A small LA, LV, and dilated RA were noted. (**d**) This cardiac CT scan shows a pulmonary venous connection (PVC) draining into a dilated coronary sinus (CS), which then drains into the RA. This finding indicates a cardiac type of total anomalous pulmonary venous connection (TAPVC). (**e**) Preoperative TEE shows the PVC chamber (small white arrows) located behind the LA. (**f**) Preoperative TEE with color Doppler, in the ME four-chamber view, shows a large PVC located behind the LA draining into the RA via the coronary sinus (CS). A broad-mouthed opening with turbulent flow at the entrance is visible. Additionally, an atrial septal defect (ASD) with right-to-left shunt is noted. This TEE image confirmed the surgical finding. (**g**) This postoperative TEE with color Doppler shows the rerouting of the pulmonary vein confluence (PVC) into LA. The pulmonary venous return is now directed into the LA and then drains into the mitral valve. Additionally, the atrial septal defect (ASD) has been closed with a patch

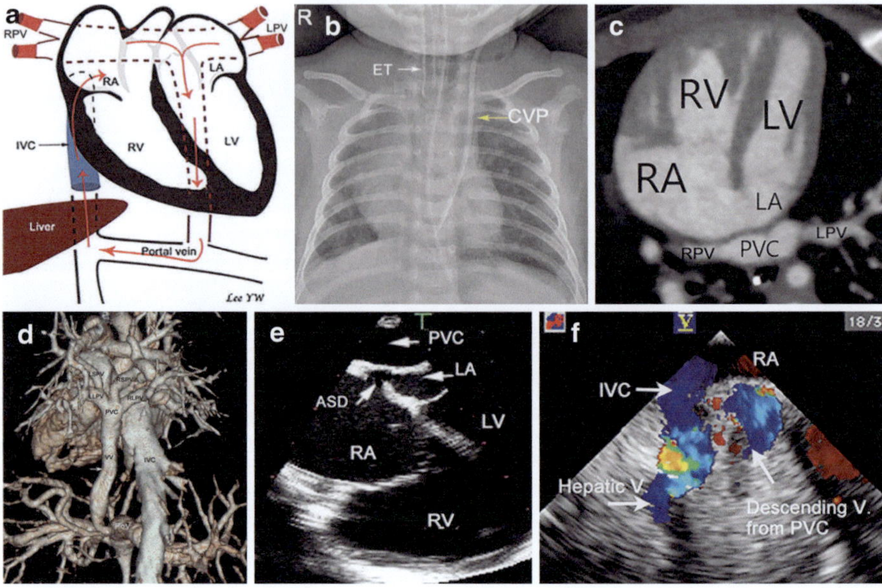

Fig. 5.48 Shows an infracardiac type of total anomalous pulmonary venous connection (TAPVC) with obstruction of the portal vein in a 14-day-old girl weighing 2.5 kg. The patient presented with cyanosis, respiratory failure, and required ventilatory support. She underwent a surgical rerouting operation to correct the condition. (**a**) The diagram shows an infracardiac type of TAPVC, in which the four pulmonary veins join together behind the heart and finally drain into the right atrium (RA) by a descending vertical vein (VV) downwards at the supraphrenic segment. After penetrating the diaphragm, this VV connects to the portal vein (PoV) and drains through the liver before upward entering the RA. (**b**) The chest X-ray showed cardiomegaly with an upturned cardiac apex, which is suggestive of right ventricular hypertrophy. There was also pulmonary congestion with diffuse prominence of the pulmonary interstitium. A trace of right pleural effusion was also observed, and an endotracheal tube was in place. Additionally, the CVP in the LSVC was noted. (**c**) The transverse section image of the contrast-enhanced cardiac CT shows dilatation of the right atrium (RA) and a small left atrium (LA). The right and left pulmonary veins (RPV and LPV) merge together behind the LA to form a pulmonary venous confluence (PVC). (**d**) The 3D volume-rendered cardiac CT image in a dorsal view demonstrates the bilateral pulmonary veins merging together to form a PVC that connects to the PoV via a descending vertical vein. The vertical vein is encased by the diaphragm (indicated by a white arrow) and is stenotic at its connection to the PoV (marked by an asterisk). (**e**) The preoperative TEE shows a ME four-chamber view with dilatation of the RA and RV. There is slight hypoplasia of the LA and an atrial septal defect (ASD). A PVC chamber is also visible behind the LA. (**f**) The color Doppler TEE in the transgastric view shows the descending vertical vein arising from the pulmonary venous confluence (PVC) and draining into the PoV. This blood into the hepatic sinusoid and further be collected by hepatic veins which then connects to the inferior vena cava (IVC) before entering the RA. (**g**) Color Doppler TEE in the transgastric view reveals dilation and engorgement of the hepatic vein, which indicates overflow by adding all pulmonary venous return combined with original portal venous flow into hepatic sinusoid. (**h**) The intraoperative surgical photograph displays engorgement of the RA. (**i**) The postoperative TEE in the ME four-chamber view displays the surgical incision of both the anterior wall of the PVC and the posterior wall of the LA with a side-to-side anastomosis. The atrial septal defect closure was performed but not shown in this image. However, the color TEE image showed turbulent flow in the rerouting site, indicating an inadequate anastomosis between the PVC and LA. As a result, the patient was immediately taken for reoperation to repair the anastomosis. However, due to a small LA in TAPVC, the anastomosis between the PVC and LA was challenging

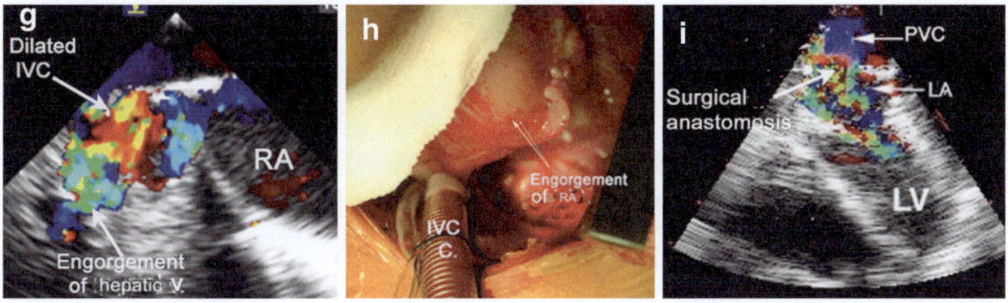

Fig. 5.48 (continued)

References

1. Karamlou T, Gurofsky R, Al SE, Coles JG, Williams WG, Caldarone CA. Factors associated with mortality and reoperation in 377 children with total anomalous pulmonary venous connection. Circulation. 2007;115:1591–8.
2. Wu FM, Emani SM, Landzberg MJ, Valente AM. Rare case of undiagnosed supracardiac total anomalous pulmonary venous return in an adult. Circulation. 2014;130:1205–7.
3. Sharma A, Fulwani M, Kulkarni V. Total anomalous pulmonary venous drainage into coronary sinus along with atrial septal defect and pulmonary stenosis—a rare congenital anomaly in an adult. Indian J Thorac Cardiovasc Surg. 2013;29(1):14–5.
4. Bhatia A, Sodhi KS, Saxena AK, Singhal M, Khandelwal N. Infracardiac total anomalous pulmonary venous return: an unusual cause of neonatal portal vein enlargement. World J Pediatr Congenit Heart Surg. 2014;5(1):131–2.

5.2.10 Complex Partial Anomalous Pulmonary Venous Connection (PAPVC)

Partial anomalous pulmonary venous connection (PAPVC) is a rare congenital heart defect that affects only on part of the pulmonary veins. With PAPVC, some pulmonary veins deviate from their normal path and do not connect to the left atrium of the heart. Instead, they may connect to different parts of the heart or even veins that lead to the heart. PAPVC is frequently linked with sinus venous type atrial septal defect (ASD). The abnormal blood flow can increase pressure in the right side of the heart, leading to the development of ASD-like hemodynamic effect by a right-to-left shunt through a patent foramen ovale. The typical form of PAPVC has been discussed in Figs. 3.2, 3.4, and 3.5.

However, complex PAPVC is a condition where there are multiple anomalous connections between the pulmonary veins and the heart, and the connections are often in unusual locations. This can make the diagnosis and treatment of complex PAPVC more challenging than the typical form of PAPVC [1]. The diagnosis imaging (such as TEE or CT) and surgical options will be discussed detail in Fig. 5.49.

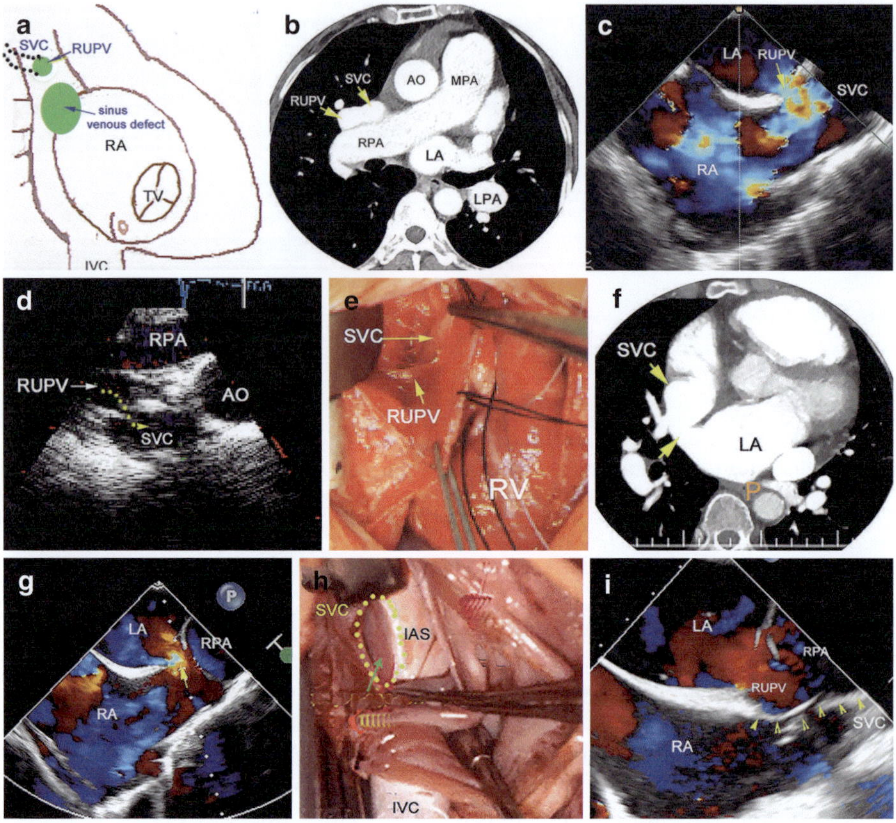

Fig. 5.49 Shows a case of complicated partial anomalous pulmonary venous connection (PAPVC) and superior sinus venosus atrial septal defect (SVASD) in a 16-year-old child who presented with an exertional dyspnea and underwent a surgical repair. (**a**) This is a schematic drawing that shows two defects: a sinus venosus defect of the superior vena cava (SVC) (large green circle) and an isolated right upper pulmonary vein (RUPV) draining into the SVC (small green circle), as viewed from the unroofed right atrium. These images (**b–e**) demonstrate the isolated right upper pulmonary vein (RUPV) draining into the superior vena cava (SVC). (**b**) This preoperative CT image demonstrates the isolated right upper pulmonary vein (RUPV) connecting to the superior vena cava (SVC). (**c**) This intraoperative TEE image in the bicaval view shows the isolated RUPV connecting to the SVC, as indicated by the yellow arrow. (**d**) This image taken from the (**e**) AAO SAX view demonstrates the RUPV connecting to the SVC, as indicated by the yellow curved dots line and arrow. (**e**) This intraoperative photograph also shows the RUPV connecting to the SVC. The following images (**f–h**) show superior sinus venosus atrial septal defect (SVASD). (**f**) This preoperative CT image shows the superior SVASD, as indicated by the yellow arrow, connecting to the LA. (**g**) This bicaval view image demonstrates the discontinuity of the SVC-interatrial septum (IAS) junction, as indicated by the yellow arrow, indicating a superior SVASD. (**h**) This intraoperative photograph also shows the discontinuity of the SVC-IAS junction, indicating a superior SVASD. (**i**) This postoperative TEE image in the ME bicaval view demonstrates the implementation of a large intra-atrial baffle with a patch repair to reroute both defects, as highlighted by the small arrowheads

Reference

1. Hatipoglu S, Almogheer B, Mahon C, et al. Clinical significance of partial anomalous pulmonary venous connections (isolated and atrial septal defect associated) determined by cardiovascular magnetic resonance. Circ Cardiovasc Imaging. 2021;14:e012371.

Cardiac Chamber Anomalies

6

6.1 Cor Triatriatum

Cor triatriatum is a rare congenital heart defect in which the left or right atrium of the heart is divided into two compartments by a membrane, resulting in a triatrial heart. Cor triatriatum sinister is a condition characterized by the presence of a membrane in the left atrium (LA). This membrane restricts the orifice, leading to an obstruction of pulmonary venous drainage. Consequently, pulmonary arterial and venous hypertension can occur, potentially resulting in congestive heart failure. In this condition, a membrane tissue divides the left atrium (LA) into two parts. The proximal chamber is located superoposteriorly, while the distal chamber, where the mitral valve and left atrial appendage are situated, is positioned anteroinferiorly [1].

Transesophageal echocardiography (TEE) and contrast CT scan, as shown in Fig. 6.1, revealed the presence of an obstructing membrane in the cor triatriatum sinister. The proximal chamber appeared dilated, while the distal chamber appeared relatively small. Additionally, an atrial septal defect (ASD) was identified. Surgical repair is the definitive treatment for removing the obstructing membrane and achieving favorable outcomes [2].

S.-K. Tsai et al., *Transesophageal Echocardiography in Pediatric Congenital Cardiac Surgery and Catheter Intervention*, https://doi.org/10.1007/978-981-99-6582-3_6

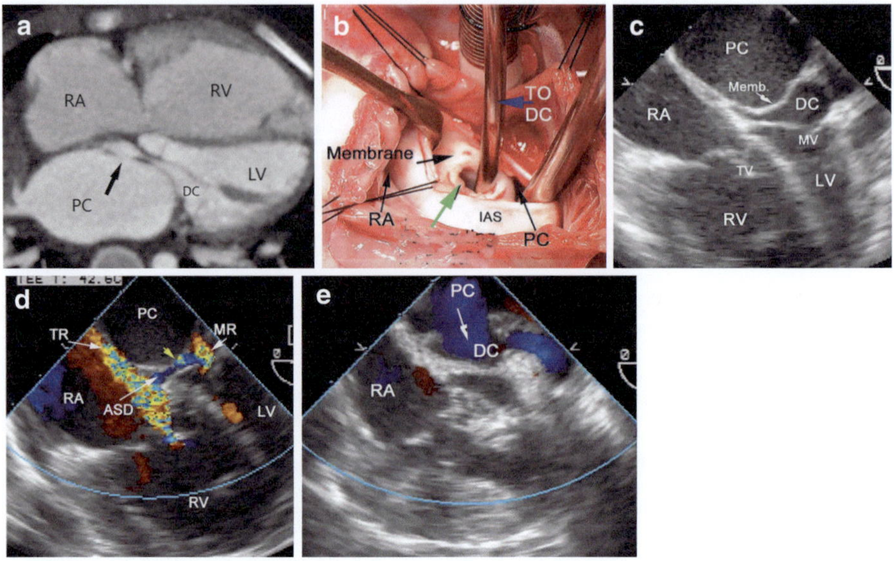

Fig. 6.1 A case of cor triatriatum sinistrum (CTS) and atrial septal defect (ASD) in a 3-year-old girl weighing 10 kg who presented with dyspnea and underwent surgical repair. (**a**) This girl has been diagnosed with cor triatriatum, which is characterized by a restrictive opening (indicated by the arrow) between the proximal chamber (PC) and the distal chamber (DC) in the left atrium (LA). A contrast-enhanced cardiac CT in a four-chamber view reveals that the septum between the PC and DC is bowing toward the DC, but an ASD not shown in this image. (**b**) This photograph during operation shows cor triatriatum sinistrum as seen through the septostomy after opening the RA. A membrane (black arrow) is visible between the PC and DC, with a small central fenestration (green arrow). The metal suction tube (indicated by the blue arrow) is extended through the fenestration and into the distal chamber. (**c**) Left atrium (LA) appears dilated and is divided by a membrane into two distinct chambers. The pulmonary veins drain into the posterosuperior PC, while the DC communicates with the left atrial appendage (LAA) and the mitral valve, as shown in the ME four-chamber view on this preoperative TEE. (**d**) This preoperative color TEE image shows a crescent-shaped membrane within the LA, with a fenestration (yellow arrow) between the PC and DC. Mitral regurgitation (MR) and tricuspid regurgitation (TR) are also visible, and an ASD is noted. (**e**) In the postoperative TEE image, it can be seen that most of the membrane has been excised, and there is a high signal intensity of normal blood flow across the residual membrane. Additionally, the ASD has been closed

References

1. Salomone G, Tiraboschi R, Bianchi T, et al. Cor triatriatum. Clinical presentation and operative results. J Thorac Cardiovasc Surg. 1991;101:1088–92.
2. Yaroglu Kazanci S, Emani S, et al. Outcome after repair of cor triatriatum. Am J Cardiol. 2012;109:412–6.

6.2 Right Atrial Isomerism (RAI)

Right atrial isomerism (RAI), also known as asplenia syndrome or right atrial appendage isomerism, is a rare and complex congenital disorder that affects the development of multiple organs in the body [1, 2], including the heart. This condition leads to intricate anatomical variations that can be challenging to diagnose due to their complexity. RAI is typically characterized by bilateral atria with similar right atrial morphology, along with right atrial appendages. This condition is often accompanied by anomalies in the ventricles and arteries. Patients with RAI commonly present with total anomalous pulmonary venous connection (TAPVC), a single ventricle, asplenia, and bilateral right-sided liver or horizontal liver.

The presence of bilateral right atria and atrial appendages, along with the absence of left-sided structures, is a key characteristic of RAI. A chest X-ray can reveal the abnormal positioning of the stomach and liver. Echocardiograms such as trans-esophageal echocardiography (TEE, Fig. 6.2d) demonstrated common atria, a single atrioventricular valve, and a large ventricular septal defect with TAPVC. Cardiac CT scan is particularly important in such syndromes as it can clearly delineate cardiovascular and extra-cardiac anatomies (as discussed in Fig. 6.2b, c).

RAI commonly presents with TAPVC, a common atrium, a single ventricle, and asplenia. The treatment approach varies depending on the severity of the heart condition and other associated organ abnormalities, and unfortunately, mortality rates are high [3]. The treatment for RAI with a single ventricle typically involves staged palliative surgeries, including a Blalock-Taussig shunt and bilateral Glenn shunts (as discussed in Fig. 4.2), followed by a Fontan procedure (as discussed in Fig. 4.10 and Fig. 4.11). Repairing TAPVC to alleviate pulmonary venous obstruction is crucial especial at the early stage (as discussed in Sect. 5.2.9). However, the management of extracardiac lesions is not addressed in this chapter.

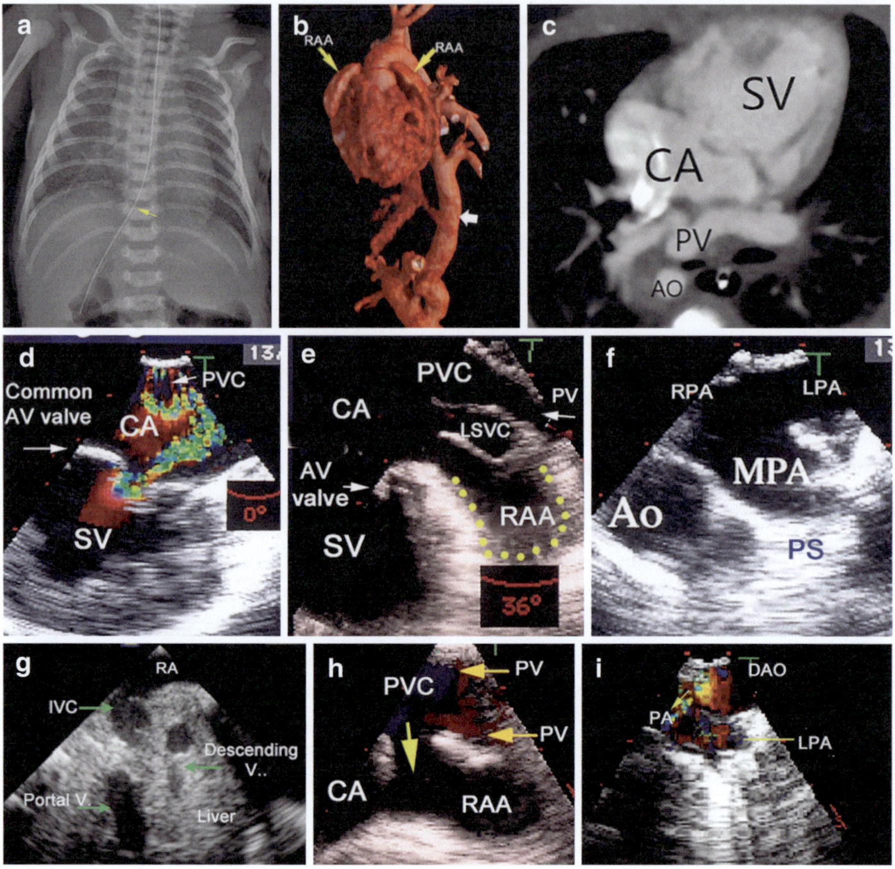

Fig. 6.2 A case of asplenia syndrome (right atrial isomerism) in a 1-month-old female baby who presented with cyanosis and heart failure. The patient underwent surgical rerouting of the infracardiac type of total anomalous pulmonary venous connection (TAPVC), with the creation of a Blalock-Taussig (BT) shunt and ligation of the patent ductus arteriosus. (**a**) Chest X-ray, including the upper abdomen, shows a horizontally positioned liver and a midline stomach position, which is confirmed by a nasogastric tube (indicated by the yellow arrow). (**b**) This 3D volume-rendered image, on the frontal view, displays symmetrical bilateral right atrial appendages (RAA), as indicated by the yellow arrows, in this baby. The patient exhibits a TAPVC to the portal vein through an engorged descending vertical vein, as pointed out by the white large arrow. Specifically, this TAPVC is of the infracardiac type. (**c**) Contrast-enhanced CT image in the transverse section shows a common atrium (CA) opening into a single ventricle (SV) via a common atrioventricular valve and connection. (**d**) This preoperative color TEE view shows the presence of a CA, a SV, and a common atrioventricular valve with regurgitation. A pulmonary vein confluence (PVC) of her TAPVC is visible behind the CA, with turbulent flow. (**e**) This preoperative TEE image in the ME four-chamber view shows the PVC of the TAPVC and a broad base of the RAA (dotted yellow line). (**f**) This preoperative TEE image in the ME four-chamber view shows that the aorta (Ao) is anterior left to the main pulmonary artery (MPA). Infundibular pulmonary stenosis (PS) is also visible. (**g**) This TEE image with a transgastric view shows a descending vertical vein connecting to the portal vein, indicating the presence of the infracardiac type of TAPVC. (**h**) This postoperative TEE image shows the excision and anastomosis of the common wall between the PVC and the CA (indicated by a clear echo drop-out and the yellow arrow). The pulmonary venous (PV) return is diverted into the CA. (**i**) This postoperative color TEE image of the BT shunt shows the blood flow traveling through the shunt (indicated by the yellow arrow) into the pulmonary artery (PA), increasing pulmonary circulation

References

1. McLaughli JF, Anderson, RH. Right atrial isomerism: clinical and anatomic features. J Am Coll Cardiol. 1990;15(3):655–61.
2. Jehle MK, Tchervenkov, CI. The clinical spectrum of the heterotaxy syndrome with right atrial isomerism. Cardiol Young 2012;22(4):385–98.
3. Hashmi A, Abu-Sulaiman R, McCrindle BW, et al. Management and outcomes of right atrial isomerism: a 26-year experience. J Am Coll Cardiol. 1998;31(5):1120–6.

6.3 Double-Chambered Right Ventricle (DCRV)

Double-chambered right ventricle (DCRV) is a rare congenital heart defect. In this condition, the right ventricle is divided into two chambers by muscular ridges, which can partially obstruct blood flow from the right ventricle to the pulmonary artery [1]. DCRV is commonly associated with other congenital anomalies, such as a large ventricular septal defect (VSD), in approximately 80% to 90% of patients [2]. Echocardiography such as TEE can show RV hypertrophy and severe obstruction of the outflow tract, while cardiac CT also can confirm the presence of DCRV.

Echocardiography (TEE) showed RV hypertrophy, severe obstruction of the outflow tract, and cardiac CT, which can confirm the presence of DCRV.

DCRV can be classified into two types [1–4], based on the location and extent of the obstruction:

Type I DCRV: In this type, the obstruction is caused by anomalous fibromuscular bundles that separates the right ventricle (RV) into proximal high-pressure part and distal low-pressure part. These bundles are thick and partially obstructive at the middle RV (as illustrated in Fig. 6.3).

Type II DCRV is characterized by obstruction caused by marked hypertrophy of the parietal and septal muscles of the RV. A large VSD can cause increased blood volume to be shunted from the left to the RV, which can result in the enlargement of the RV and the development of the hypertrophied muscle band that causes the obstruction. This band separates the proximal and distal chambers of the RV. Therefore, it is crucial to evaluate the presence of any residual obstruction resulting from inadequate hypertrophied muscle resection immediately after DCRV surgery, as illustrated in Fig. 6.4. The treatment for both types of DCRV involves surgery to remove the obstructing ridges or hypertrophied muscles to relieve the middle right ventricle obstruction [5, 6].

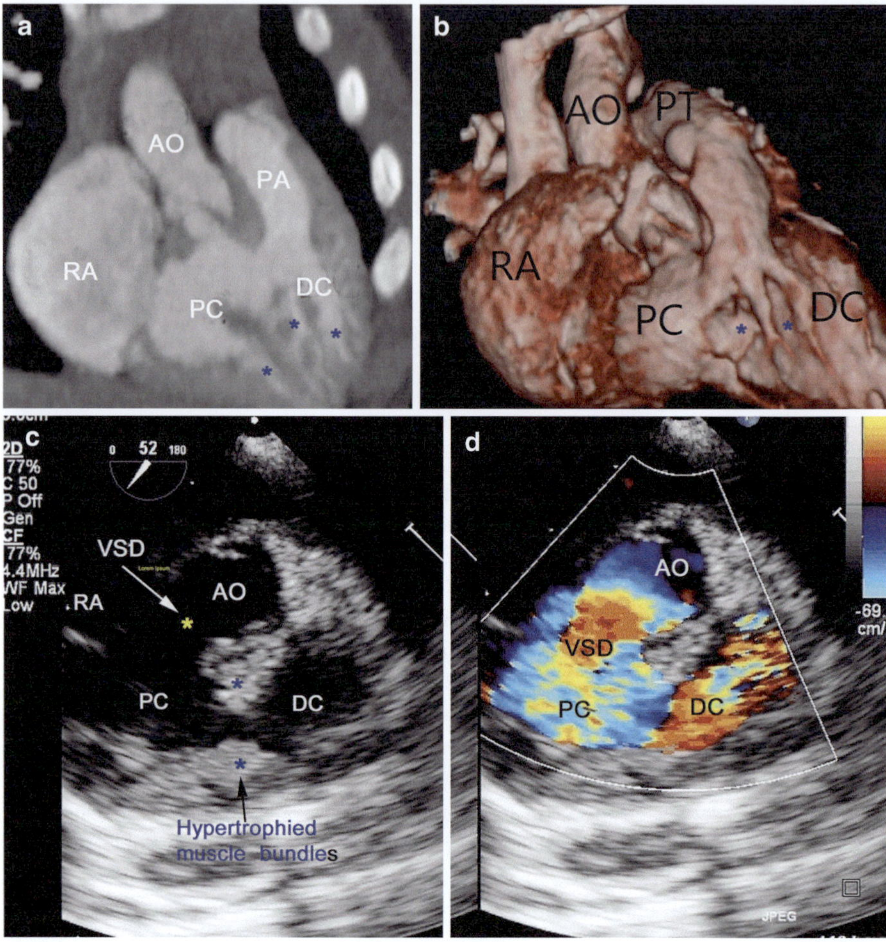

Fig. 6.3 A case of double-chambered right ventricle (DCRV type I) in a 12-year-old child who presented with mild exercise intolerance and underwent surgical correction. (**a**) This oblique-coronal thin-slab maximum intensity projection (MIP) reconstruction of the contrast-enhanced cardiovascular computed tomography (CT) image shows the separating of the proximal chamber (PC) and distal chamber (DC) by the hypertrophied muscle bundles (indicated by the blue asterisks) in the right ventricle (RV). (**b**) This 3D reconstruction image by contrast-pooling volume rendering shows the separation of the PC and DC by the hypertrophied muscle bundles (indicated by the blue asterisks) in the RV. (**c**) This preoperative TEE image in the ME AV SAX view shows the division of the RV into a high-pressure (PC) and a lower-pressure (DC) by anomalous RV muscle bundles with insertion at the interventricular septum and right ventricular free wall (indicated by the blue asterisks), causing mid-cavitary obstruction. A large malalignment ventricular septal defect (VSD) is also visible (indicated by the yellow asterisk). (**d**) This color TEE image shows a turbulent Doppler color flow velocity pattern, suggesting a middle RV obstruction, along with a large malalignment VSD with a left-to-right shunt

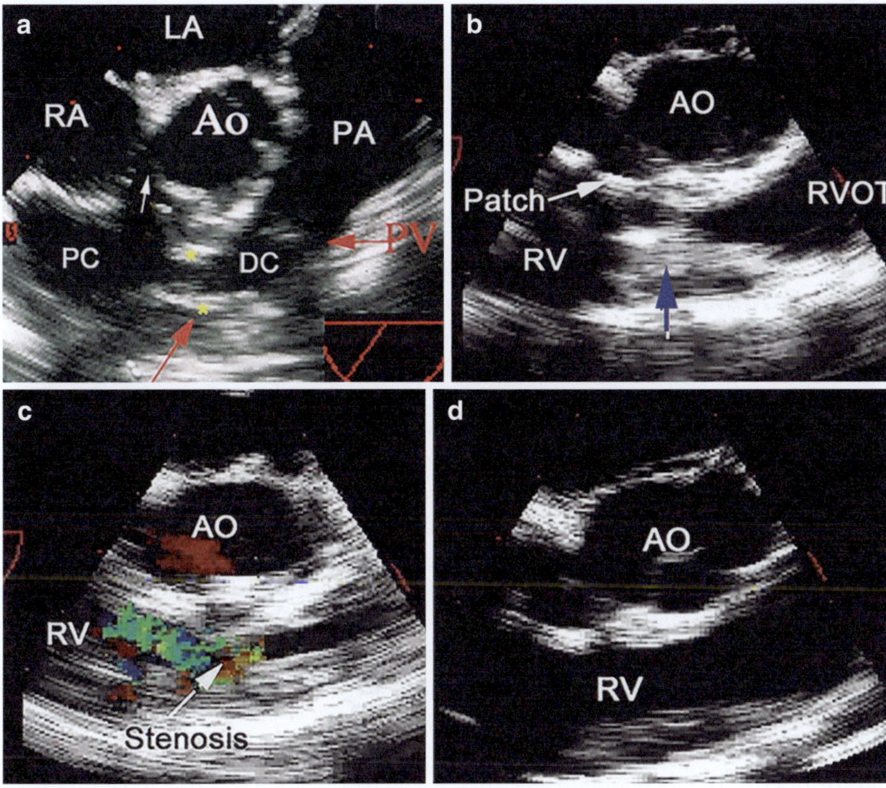

Fig. 6.4 A double-chambered right ventricle (DCRV type II) in a 9-year-old child with tetralogy of Fallot, who underwent surgical correction. (**a**) Preoperative TEE, ME AV SAX view, shows significant obstruction of the middle right ventricular outflow tract by hypertrophied parietal and septal muscles (yellow stars) and a ventricular septal defect (white arrow). (**b**) Postoperative TEE, ME AV SAX view, shows a patch used for repairing the VSD (white arrow), but residual middle RV stenosis due to inadequate removal of hypertrophied muscle tissue (blue arrow) in the subinfundibular region of the RV. (**c**) Postoperative color Doppler TEE, ME AV SAX view, also shows the presence of middle RV stenosis with a turbulent flow pattern. Its pressure gradient is >40 mmHg. (**d**) Therefore, the patient was immediately reoperated to excise residual hypertrophied muscles. A TEE image after this immediate reoperation shows a patent middle RV with no any more residual structural narrowing detected

References

1. Alva C, Ho SY, Lincoln CR, et al. The nature of the obstructive muscular bundles in double-chambered right ventricle. J Thorac Cardiovasc Surg. 1999;117(6):1180–9.
2. Restivo A, Cameron AH, Anderson RH, et al. Divided right ventricle: a review of its anatomical varieties. Pediatr Cardiol. 1984;5(3):197–204.
3. Galiuto L, O'Leary PW, Seward JB. Double-chambered right ventricle: echocardiographic features. J Am So Echocardiogr. 1996;9(3):300–5.

4. Loukas M, Housman B, Blask C et al. Double-chambered right ventricle: a review. Cardiovasc Pathol. 2013;22:417–23.
5. Kottayil BP, Dharan BS, Pillai VV, et al. Surgical repair of double-chambered right ventricle in adulthood. Asian Cardiovasc Thorac Ann. 2011;19(1):57–60.
6. Penkoske PA, Duncan N, Collins-Nakai RL. Surgical repair of double-chambered right ventricle with or without ventriculotomy. J Thorac Cardiovasc Surg. 1987;93(3):385–93.

6.4 Double Outlet Right Ventricle (DORV)

Double outlet right ventricle (DORV) is a rare congenital heart defect where both the aorta and pulmonary artery arise from the right ventricle. A child with DORV may also have other heart problems, including pulmonary stenosis, pulmonary atresia, coarctation of the aorta, and mitral valve abnormalities [1–3].

The symptoms of DORV depend on the location and size of the ventricular septal defect (VSD), which is a common accompanying defect characterized by an opening in the wall separating the two ventricles of the heart. Therefore, DORV is classified based on the location of the VSD and the position of the great arteries in relation to the ventricular septum [1–5]. There are four types of DORV that can be identified through a 3D cardiac CT scan (as shown in Fig. 6.5).

DORV with a Subaortic VSD: In this type of DORV, the VSD is located just beneath the aortic valve, as illustrated in Fig. 6.6.

DORV with a Subpulmonary VSD (also known as Taussig-Bing Syndrome): This form of DORV is distinguished by a VSD positioned just below the pulmonary valve, with the aorta typically arising right lateral and a little anteriorly to the pulmonary artery, as depicted in Fig. 6.7.

DORV with a Noncommitted (or remote) VSD [3]: The VSD is situated neither near the aorta nor the pulmonary artery, typically in the muscular or inlet portion, as depicted in Fig. 6.8.

DORV with a Doubly Committed VSD: In this type of DORV, there is a large VSD located under each of the great arteries, with both the aorta and pulmonary artery arising above the VSDs, as shown in Fig. 6.10.

Imaging studies such as echocardiography, magnetic resonance imaging (MRI), or computed tomography (CT) scans can provide detailed images of the heart, which can help identify DORV and the specific type of VSD. However, the utilization of Three-dimensional volume-rendered cardiac CT (as depicted in Fig. 6.5) can specifically highlight the infundibular morphology, encompassing the size and orientation of the outlet septum in relation to the ventricular septal defect margin. Additionally, it provides valuable information regarding the extent of the muscular infundibulum, which serves as an important additional estimation of the distance between the ventricular septal defect margin and the arterial valve or valves for the feasibility of intracardiac reouting if needed [4, 5].

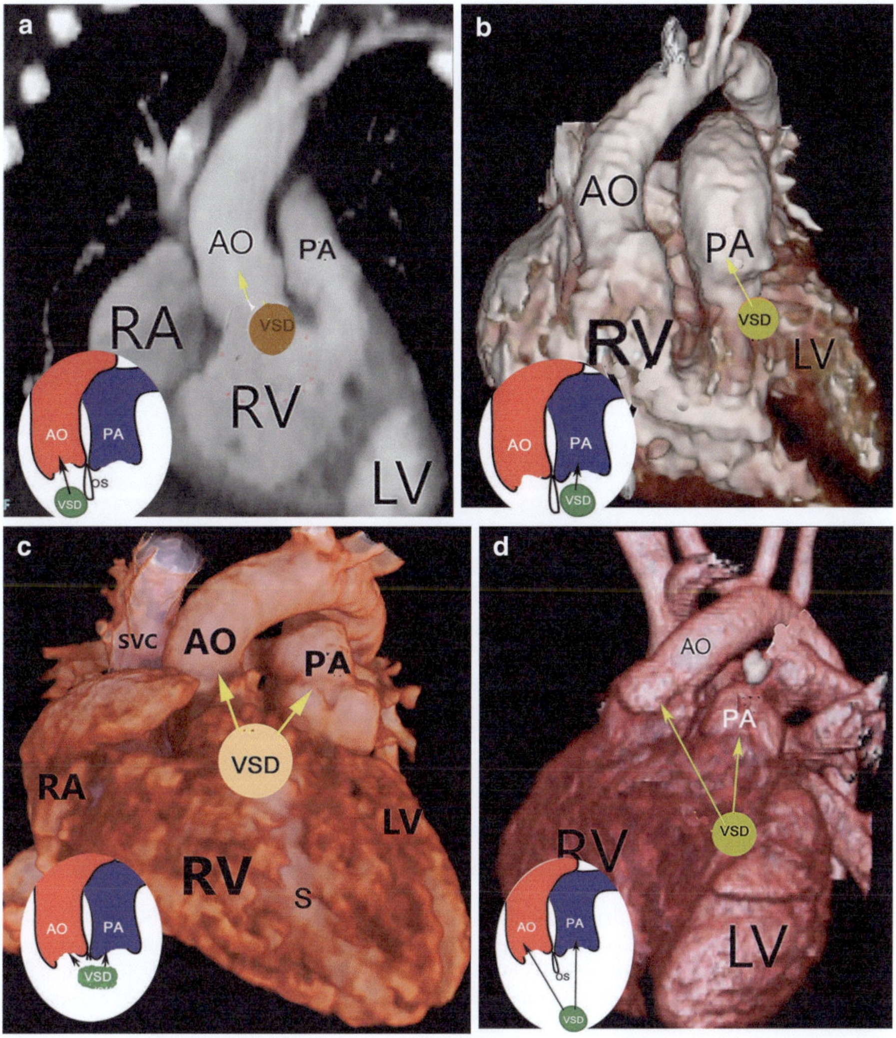

Fig. 6.5 Overview of double outlet right ventricle (DORV). Three-dimensional volume-rendered cardiac images present the different locations of four types of ventricular septal defects (VSDs) in DORV (from fig. **a**–**d**). The left lower circle diagrams show the relationship of the outlet septum (OS) to the VSD. (**a**) Subaortic Type VSD: The defect is located just under the aortic valve. The left lower circle diagram shows that the OS is fused to the left margin of the VSD. (**b**) Subpulmonary Type VSD: The defect is located just under the pulmonary valve. The left lower circle diagram shows that the OS is fused to the right margin of the VSD. (**c**) Doubly Committed Type VSD: The defect is adjacent to the semilunar valves of the great arteries. The left lower circle diagram shows that the OS is parallel to the plane of the VSD. (**d**) Remote type of DORV: The VSD is not located near the aorta (AO) or pulmonary trunk (PT). The left lower circle diagram shows that the OS is not fused to either side of the VSD

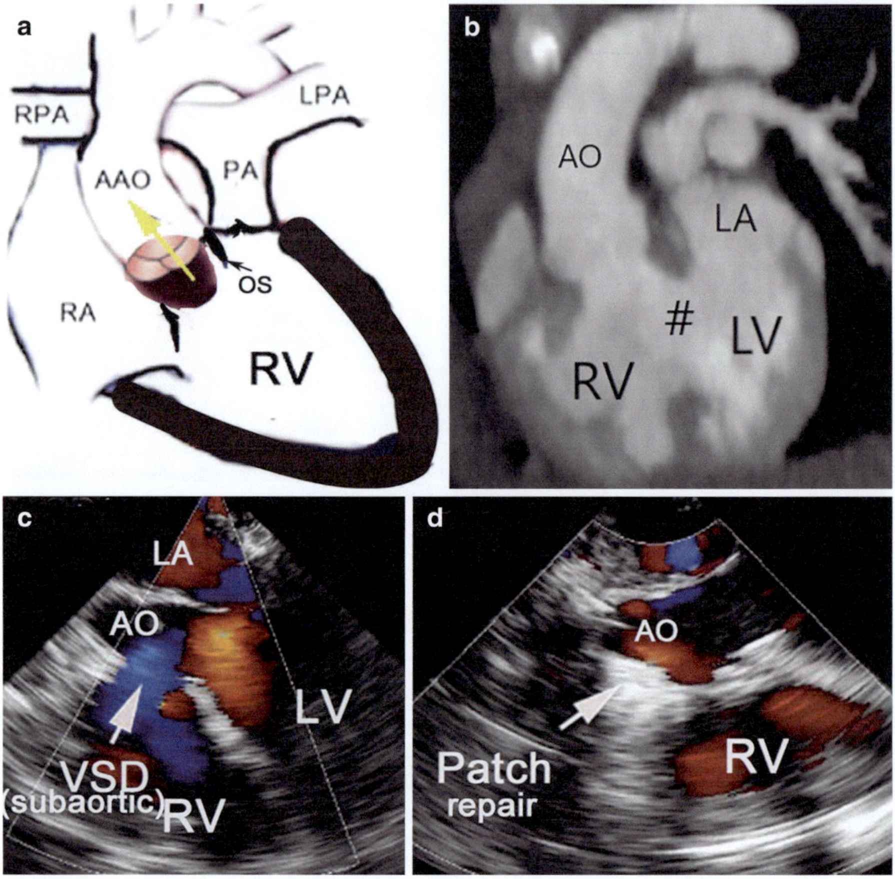

Fig. 6.6 A case of double outlet right ventricle (DORV) with a subaortic ventricular septal defect (VSD) in a 10-month-old boy who presented with impending heart failure and underwent surgical treatment. (**a**) This is a diagram of DORV with a subaortic VSD, which shows the VSD located just below the aortic valve. The outlet septum (OS) is anteriorly and leftward deviated, causing the aorta to override the VSD and resulting in the narrowing of the subpulmonary region. (**b**) This is a contrast-enhanced cardiovascular CT image that shows a nonrestrictive subaortic VSD (#) on an oblique-sagittal view. (**c**) This is a preoperative color TEE image, showing a large subaortic VSD (white arrow) with a left-to-right shunt in the ME four-chamber view. (**d**) This is a postoperative color TEE image that shows successful intraventricular VSD repair by a rerouting tunnel patch, without any residual shunting, in the ME four-chamber view

The specific type of DORV determines the symptoms and treatment options associated with it. Treatment options may involve surgery to repair the VSD and redirect blood flow. In certain cases, treatment may also involve addressing single ventricle physiology or considering a heart transplant. The intraventricular tunnel repair is the most common surgical procedure for DORV with a subaortic VSD. This procedure involves creating a tunnel that connects the left ventricle to the aorta, using a patch to redirect blood flow.

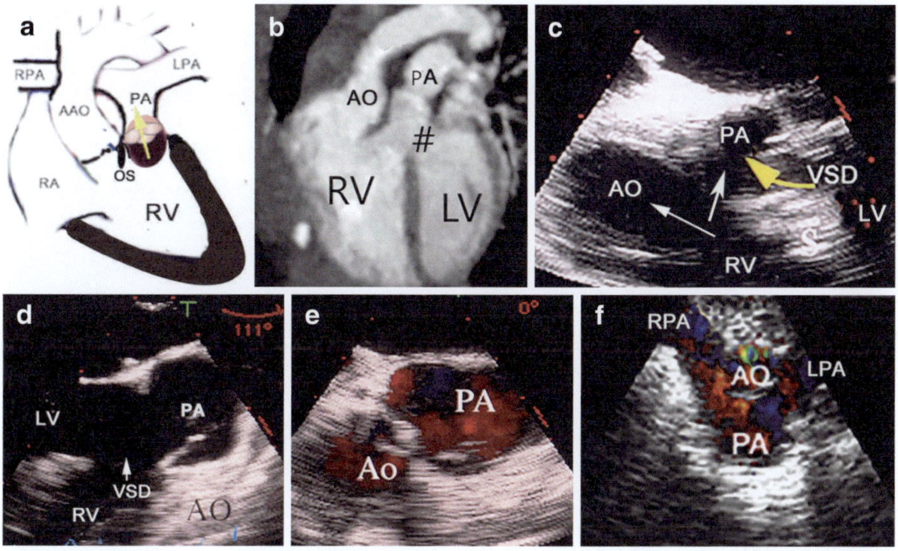

Fig. 6.7 A case of double outlet right ventricle (DORV) with a subpulmonary ventricular septal defect (VSD), which is also known as the Taussig-Bing anomaly. The image is of a 3-day-old male baby who presented with tachypnea and underwent surgical correction. (**a**) This diagram illustrates DORV with a subpulmonary VSD, showing a nonrestrictive subpulmonary VSD. The conal septum (CS) is posteriorly and rightwardly deviated, which may cause the pulmonary artery to override the VSD. (**b**) This image is a thin-slab maximal intensity projection reconstruction of the cardiovascular CT, which displays a VSD (#) located just below the pulmonary valve. Both the aorta (AO) and pulmonary artery (PA) are seen originating from the right ventricle (RV). Additionally, in this image, the aorta is positioned anterior and right to the PA. (**c**) This preoperative TEE image, taken from the ME AV SAX view, shows a VSD (indicated by the yellow arrow) located below the pulmonary valve. The transseptal flow is directed from the left ventricle (LV) to the PA, which results in the dilation of the pulmonary trunk. The aorta AO is positioned anterior and to the right of the pulmonary artery. Additionally, in this image, the right ventricular flow is draining toward both the aorta and pulmonary artery. (**d**) This image, specifically the ME AV LAX view, shows the PA overriding the VSD (indicated by the white arrow). Furthermore, the aortic trunk is positioned anterior to the dilated pulmonary trunk. (**e**) This image is taken from the UE AAO SAX view and displays the aorta positioned anterior and to the right of the PA, which results in mimics D-transposition of the great arteries. (**f**) This postoperative image shows Jatene's arterial switch operation (ASO) with the LeCompte maneuver, demonstrating the successful switching of both great arteries and reattaching them to their anatomically correct ventricle. Additionally, the PA has been repositioned anterior to the aorta. It is worth noting that the VSD closure by a patch is not visible in this image

An arterial switch operation is required when the aorta and pulmonary artery are reversed in DORV, particularly in cases where it mimics the hemodynamics of transposition of the great arteries (TGA). In more complex cases, a univentricular repair such as the Fontan operation may be recommended. Surgical complications may arise, including residual pulmonary stenosis or right ventricular obstruction, as demonstrated in Fig. 6.9.

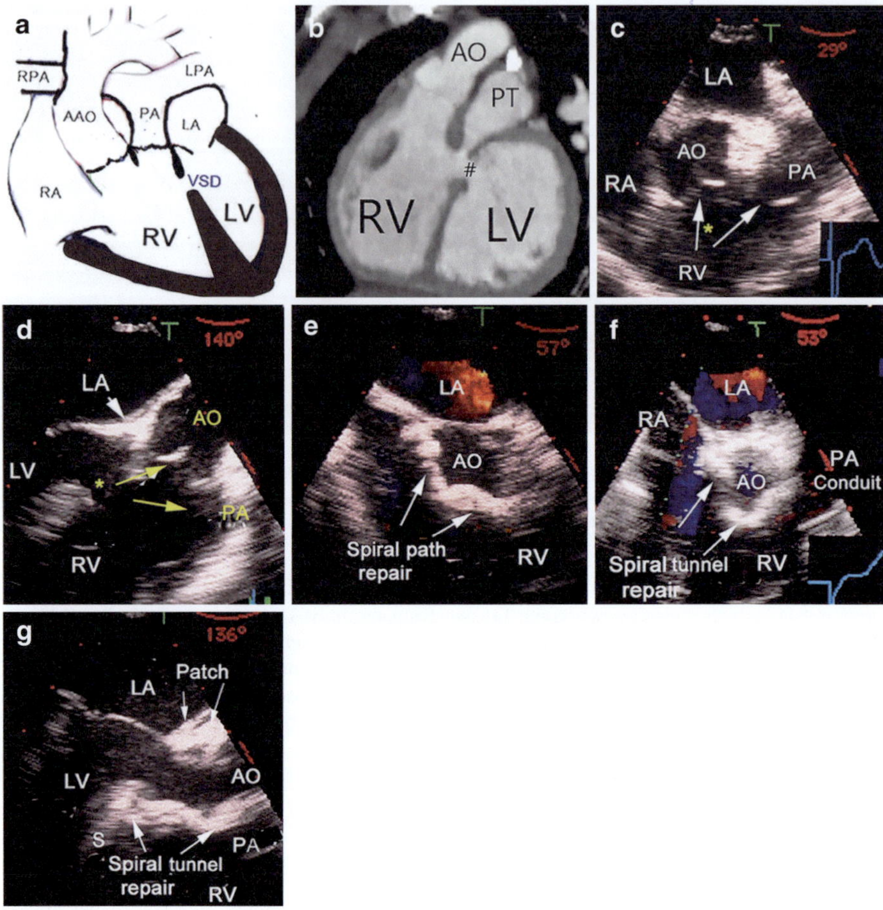

Fig. 6.8 A case of DORV (double outlet right ventricle) with a noncommitted VSD (ventricular septal defect) (also known as remote type of DORV) in a 1-year-old girl who underwent surgical repair of the defect. (**a**) This illustration depicts DORV with a noncommitted VSD, where the VSD is located far away from the great arteries. Both the aorta (AO) and pulmonary artery (PA) arise from the right ventricle (RV), and the VSD is covered by a double conus. (**b**) A CT image reconstructed using thin-slab maximal intensity projection shows a noncommitted ventricular septal defect (VSD) (#), with both great vessels arising entirely from the right ventricle (RV). (**c**) Preoperative TEE in a ME AV SAX view reveals a noncommitted ventricular septal defect (VSD) (*) positioned at a considerable distance from both arterial valves. Additionally, both great vessels originate exclusively from the right ventricle (RV). (**d**) Preoperative TEE in a ME AV LAX view displays a noncommitted VSD (*) located far away from the parallel great arteries, with the great arteries spiraling around each other in a normal position without pulmonary outlet tract obstruction. A large conal tissue results in aorto-mitral discontinuity (short white arrow). (**e**) Postoperative image after VSD repair with intraventricular baffle rerouting. TEE in a ME four-chamber view shows a spiral path for the VSD repair without any shunt. (**f**) Postoperative image following intraventricular baffle and Rastelli pulmonary artery (PA) conduit repairs is shown in the image. A TEE in the ME AV SAX view reveals a spiral tunnel patch (indicated by white arrows) surrounding the aorta and Rastelli PA conduit for right ventricular outflow tract (RVOT) repair. No evidence of RVOT or LVOT obstruction is observed. (**g**) Postoperative TEE in a ME AV LAX view displays a long tunnel with a spiral patch repair connecting the left ventricle to the aorta, without any residual shunt. No left ventricular outflow tract or right ventricular outflow tract obstruction is observed

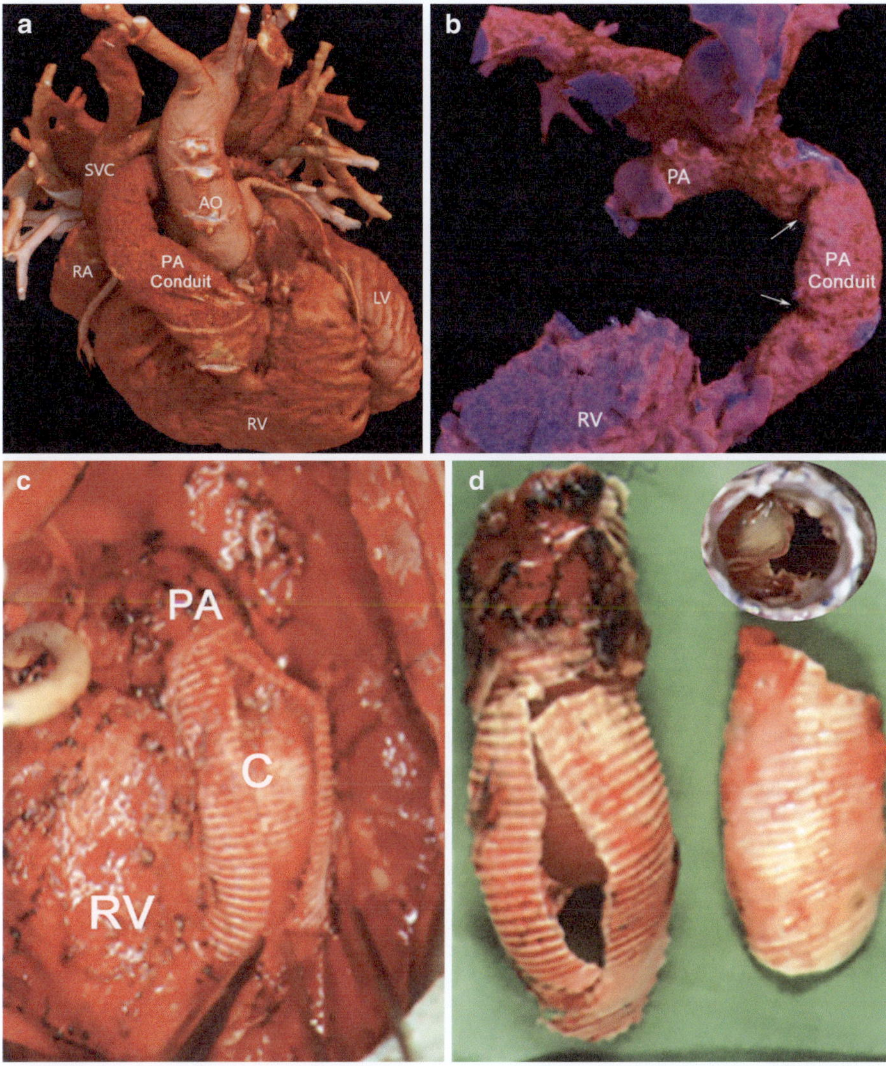

Fig. 6.9 Patient's condition 23 years after the initial operation presented in Fig. 6.8. Unfortunately, the patient's Rastelli conduit has developed segmental stenosis and has become infected, necessitating an exchanged new conduit. (**a**) A 3D image of the heart viewed from the front view shows a Rastelli PA conduit that is tortuous and originates from the ventral-cephalic wall of the right ventricle. (**b**) A right lateral view of the outlet portion of the right ventricle, along with the deformed Rastelli PA conduit, shows deep ventral folding (indicated by arrows) on the dorsal side of the conduit. The native pulmonary artery and the bilateral arteries are preserved. (**c**) This intraoperative surgical photograph shows a folded and tortuous Rastelli PA conduit (C) that is consistent with the findings seen in the 3D images. (**d**) Rastelli PA conduit was excised and revealing evidence of endocarditis and valvular degeneration

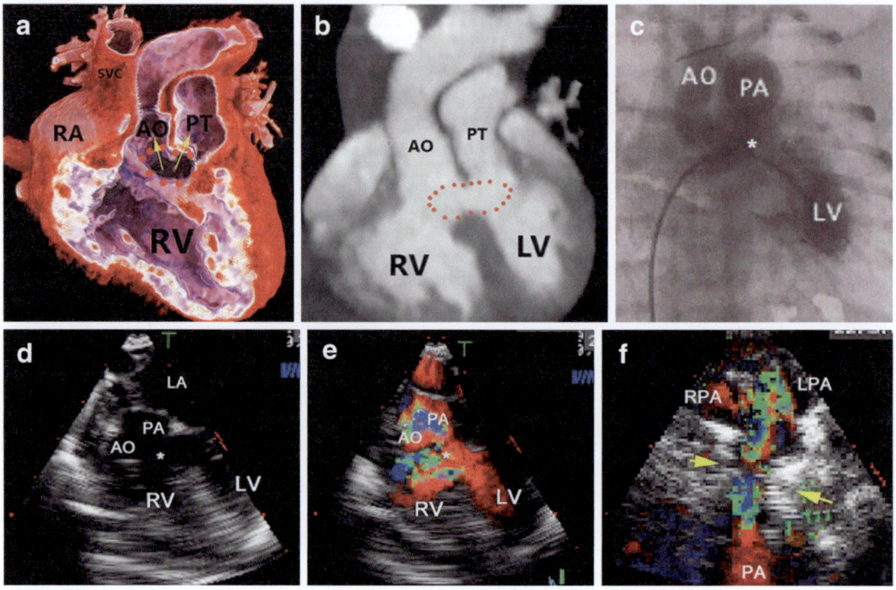

Fig. 6.10 A 3-month-old girl with DORV and a doubly committed VSD who presented with respiratory distress. The patient underwent PA banding. (**a**) A virtual image of a solid cardiac model in a right anterior oblique view reveals a large VSD (red dotted circle) located just below the annuli of both great arteries. The VSD is large and roofed by the great arterial valves in fibrous continuity due to the absence of the conal septum. (**b**) A thin-slab maximal intensity projection image in a double oblique-coronal view displays a large doubly committed VSD (red dotted circle) located just below the parallel great arteries. (**c**) Left ventricular angiography shows a VSD (*) located just under the arterial valves. (**d**) Preoperative TEE with ME AV SAX view shows a doubly committed VSD) (*) that is not suited to either of the two arterial valves, with the aorta anterior and to the right of the PA. (**e**) Color TEE image shows blood flow from the RV directed toward both the aorta (AO) and pulmonary artery (PA) through a doubly committed ventricular septal defect (VSD) (indicated by a white star). Additionally, aortic regurgitation is visible with turbulent mosaic flow. (**f**) Color TEE image taken after pulmonary artery banding (PAB) shows the banding site (indicated by two yellow arrows) on the main pulmonary artery, with turbulent mosaic flow pattern and a velocity of 3.6 m/s

References

1. Ebadi A, Spicer DE, Backer CL, et al. Double-outlet right ventricle revisited. J Thorac Cardiovasc Surg. 2017;154:598–604.
2. Tynan MJ, Becker AE, Macartney FJ, Jiménez MQ, Shinebourne EA, Anderson RH. Nomenclature and classification of congenital heart disease. Br Heart J. 1979;41:544–53.
3. Belli E, Serraf A, Lacour-Gayet F, et al. Double-outlet right ventricle with non-committed ventricular septal defect. Eur J Cardiothorac Surg. 1999;15:747–52.
4. Mazzucco A, Faggian G, Stellin G, Bortolotti U, Livi U, Rizzoli G, Gallucci V. Surgical management of double-outlet right ventricle. J Thorac Cardiovasc Surg. 1985;90:29–34.
5. Udson JP, Danielson GK, Puga FJ, Mair DD, McGoon DC. Double-outlet right ventricle. Surgical results, 1970-1980. J Thorac Cardiovasc Surg. 1983;85:32–40.

6.5 Univentricular Heart (Single Ventricle, SV)

Single ventricle (SV) physiology refers to a condition where there is only one functional pumping chamber in the circulation. There are various types of single ventricle defects, which can be classified based on the missing or abnormal structures within the heart. In other words, SV physiology can indicate the presence of a true anatomical isolated left or right ventricle, or it may suggest a bilateral atrioventricular connections with only one functioning ventricle, even though both ventricles are present. Anatomically, single ventricles account for less than 2% of congenital heart defects (CHD), while functionally, SV cases comprise approximately 1.5–3%.

There are a variety of anatomical variations of functional SV, such as tricuspid atresia (Fig. 6.11b1) and hypoplastic left heart syndrome (Fig. 6.11b2). In both tri cuspid atresia (as discussed in Chap. 4) and HLHS (as discussed in Sect. 4.3), the surgical procedures used to treat these conditions are complex and often require multiple stages [1].

Two unique types of anatomical single ventricle defects that are related to each other are double inlet of the right ventricle (DIRV, Fig. 6.11a2) and double inlet of the left ventricle (DILV, Fig. 6.11a1). In DIRV, both the left and right atria are connected to the right ventricle, while the left ventricle is either absent or very small. In contrast, DILV is a type of single ventricle anomaly where both the left and right atria are connected to a single left ventricle, while the right ventricle is either absent or very small, as seen in conditions such as pulmonary atresia. DIRV is considered rare. Among hearts with a univentricular atrioventricular (AV) connection, the morphologically left ventricular type is the most commonly observed. As for treatment, establishing Fontan circulation is a justifiable approach for patients with single ventricle physiology [2].

The following is some examples of complex SV anomalies:

DILV with Normally Related Great Arteries (also Known as a Holmes Heart, Fig. 6.11a): Both atrioventricular valves are connected to the left ventricle (LV). The right ventricle (RV) lacks an inlet and body portion; only the outflow part (infundibulum) remains. This rudimentary RV serves as a pathway from the LV to the pulmonary artery (PA) and is connected to the LV through a ventricular septal defect (VSD), also known as the bulboventricular foramen, and an outflow chamber. The size of the PA depends on the size of the bulboventricular foramen. The aorta arises from the LV and is well-developed (similar to the anatomy seen in tricuspid atresia), which will be further discussed in Fig. 6.14.

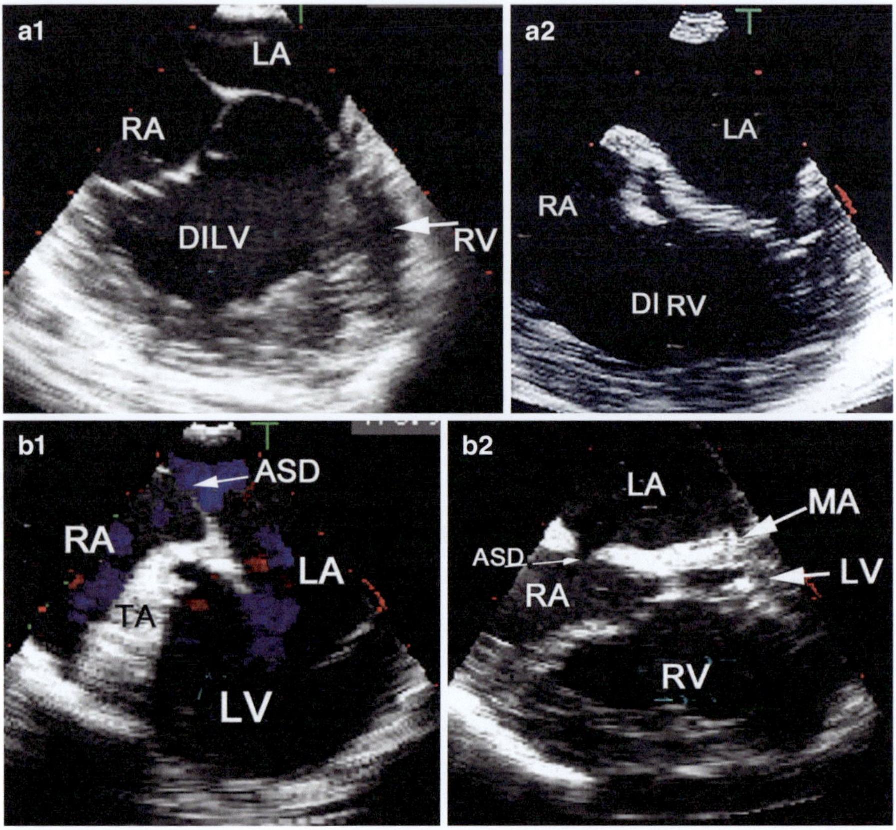

Fig. 6.11 Case of functionally univentricular (UV) heart, which is a rare and complex congenital heart defect (CHD) where both atria mainly drain into one ventricle. This cardiac malformation may have a dominant ventricle of either left or right ventricular morphology. Chronic volume overload and persistent hypoxia can lead to atrioventricular incompetence. Based on the TEE images, two subtypes of UV heart can be described as follows: (1) **Subtype A (a1,a2)**: The ventricular septum is totally absent, and both atria empty into a dominant morphological ventricle, as seen in patients with double inlet of the left ventricle (DILV) (a1 also, see Sect. 6.6.1) and double inlet of the right ventricle (DIRV) (a2 also, see Sect. 6.7). However, DILV is the most frequent type and will be discussed in Sect. 6.5. DIRV is rare [1] with a greater prevalence of right atrial isomerism (RAI) that is usually associated with DIRV in Chinese patients [2] (see Sect. 6.7). (2) **Subtype (b1,b2):** The absence or severe stenosis of either the right or left atrioventricular valve connection is associated with hypoplasia of the corresponding ventricle, as seen in patients with: (b1) Tricuspid Atresia: See Sect. 4.1. (b2) Mitral Atresia with Hypoplastic Left Heart Syndrome (HLHS): See Sects. 4.3.1 and 4.3.2

References

1. Van Praagh R. Van Praagh S. Blad P, et al. Diagnosis of the anatomic types of single or common ventricle Am J Cardiol. 1965;15:345.
2. Kawahira Y, Uemura H, Yoshikawa Y et al. Double inlet right ventricle versus other types of double or common inlet ventricle: its clinical characteristics with reference to the Fontan procedure. Eur J Cardio-thorac Surg. 2001;20:228–32.

6.6 Double Inlet of Left Ventricle (DILV)

6.6.1 L-TGA, Hypoplastic Left-Sided Morphological Right Ventricle (RV), Atrial Septal Defect (ASD), and Ventricular Septal Defect (VSD)

The diagnosis by using an echocardiogram (TEE) and cardiac CT or 3D CT scan is illustrated in Fig. 6.12b, c, e, f. This condition requires complex surgical interventions, typically in the form of staged procedures, but single-stage ventricular septation [1] as shown in Fig. 6.12g, h, i.

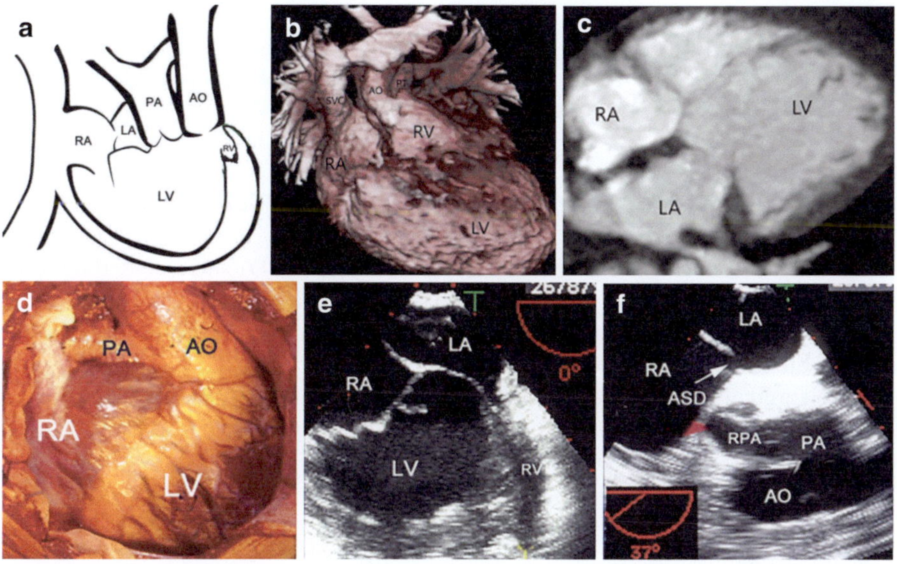

Fig 6.12 A 2-month-old boy was diagnosed with double inlet of the left ventricle (DILV) with transposition of the great arteries (TGA), hypoplastic left-sided right ventricle (RV), atrial septal defect ASD, and ventricular septal defect (VSD) underwent surgical correction. (**a**) This diagram shows a DILV with TGA. Both atria are connected to the left ventricle (LV), while a small hypoplastic right ventricle (RV) is located on the opposite side of the heart (l-loop). The aorta (AO) arises from the RV, and the pulmonary artery (PA) arises from the LV. (**b**, **c**). CT and 3D images reveal a DILV with a rudimentary RV located at the left frontal cephalic aspect adjacent to the dominant LV. The ventriculoarterial connection is discordant with the AO arising from the rudimentary RV and the pulmonary trunk (PT) originating from the dominant LV. The AO is situated right anterior to the pulmonary trunk (PT). (**d**) This intraoperative photograph shows a large right atrium (RA) and LV, an anteriorly positioned AO, and a small PA. (**e**) This preoperative TEE ME four-chamber view shows a large RA and LV, a hypoplastic RV, and both atria draining into the LV. (**f**) This preoperative TEE ME AV SAX view shows an atrial septal defect (ASD) and an anteriorly positioned AO relative to the PA. (**g**) This postoperative TEE ME four-chamber view shows successful surgical repair with ventricular septation and no residual defect in both the atrial and neo ventricular septa. (**h**) Postoperative TEE four-chamber view shows that blood flow from the RA now drains to the LV and then to the PA after the biventricular repair. (**i**) Postoperative TEE AV LAX view shows that blood flow from the LA now drains to the neo RV and then to the AO after the ventricular septation procedure. A turbulent mosaic flow over the RVOT was observed, indicating a focal stenosis

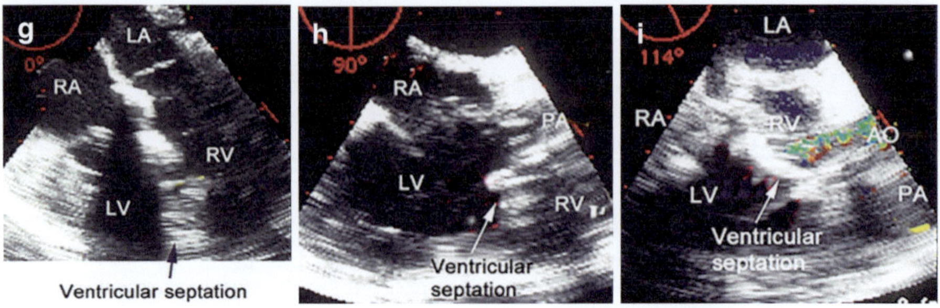

Fig. 6.12 (continued)

Reference

1. Margossian RE, Apray TL, Kugler RD, et al. Septation of the single ventricle: revised. J Thorac Cardiovasc Surg. 2002;124:442–7.

6.6.2 L-TGA with Pulmonary Atresia/VSD (PA/VSD) and ASD

Pulmonary atresia (PA) with ventricular septal defect (VSD) and congenitally corrected transposition of the great arteries (L-TGA) is a complex congenital heart defect that requires complex surgical intervention to correct the defect and restore normal blood flow to the body. Treatment options for PA/VSD and L-TGA may include surgical repair [1, 2] or a series of staged surgeries to gradually correct the defect. Figure 6.13 discusses the use of the Senning operation, ventricular septation, and Rastelli procedure for total surgical repair.

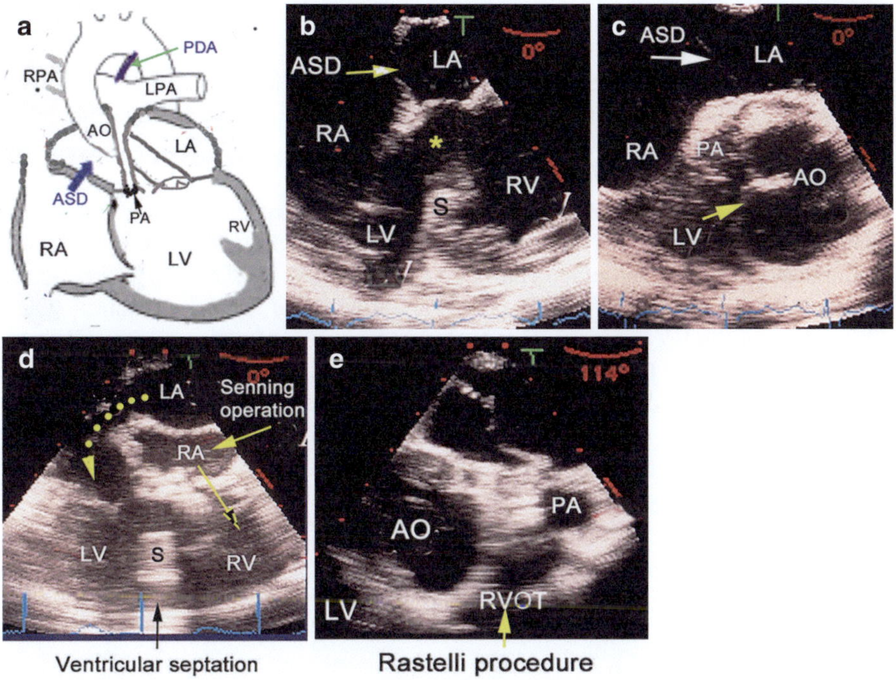

Fig. 6.13 A 5-year-old male patient with double inlet of left ventricle (DILV), transposition of the great arteries (TGAs), atrial septal defect (ASD), ventricular septal defect (VSD), and pulmonary atresia who underwent surgical repair. (**a**) Diagram depicts a case of DILV, TGA, and pulmonary atresia, with a dominant left ventricle (LV) and hypoplastic right ventricle (RV) containing a large VSD and an ASD. A small RV on the opposite side of the heart. The ventriculoarterial connection is discordant. (**b**) This preoperative TEE shows the four-chamber view of the heart. The morphologically LV is on the right, and the RV is on the left. There is a large VSD (*) and ASD. (**c**) This preoperative TEE in the ME AV SAX view reveals a large ASD, with the anterior positioning of the aorta and hypoplasia of the posteriorly located PA. (**d**) This postoperative TEE was taken after the Senning operation, ventricular separation, and Rastelli procedure. The ME four-chamber view shows the intra-atrial baffle used in the Senning operation to redirect systemic venous return to the RV. The dotted curve line represents the pulmonary venous return, which flows directly to the LV. The image also shows the closure of a large VSD and ventricular septation. (**e**) This postoperative TEE in the ME AV SAX reveals the reconstruction of the right ventricular outflow tract (RVOT) using a valved conduit, which was part of the Rastelli procedure performed to connect the RV to the PA

References

1. Kumar TKS. Congenitally corrected transposition of the great arteries. J Thorac Dis. 2020;12:1213–18.
2. Hiramatsu T, Matsumura G, Konuma T, et al. Long-term prognosis of double-switch operation for congenitally corrected transposition of the great arteries. Eur J Cardiothorac Surg. 2012;42:1004–8.

6.6.3 Holmes Heart

Double inlet of the left ventricle (DILV) is a congenital heart defect characterized by the normal positioning of the great arteries, but with a rudimentary right ventricle (RV) and ventriculoarterial concordance. It is also known as a "Holmes Heart." In this condition, the pulmonary artery arises from a small infundibular outlet chamber of the RV, while the aorta arises from the single left ventricle. The rudimentary RV functions as a pathway from the left ventricle (LV) to the pulmonary artery (PA) and is connected to the LV through a ventricular septal defect (VSD), also known as the bulboventricular foramen (BVF), and an infundibular outlet chamber (OC). Obstruction of the BVF can complicate the management of patients with a Holmes heart. The size of the BVF can be measured using color two-dimensional echocardiography, as depicted in Fig. 6.14d (transesophageal echocardiography image). Additionally, surgical biventricular repair, discussed in Fig. 6.14e, f, may also be considered as an option.

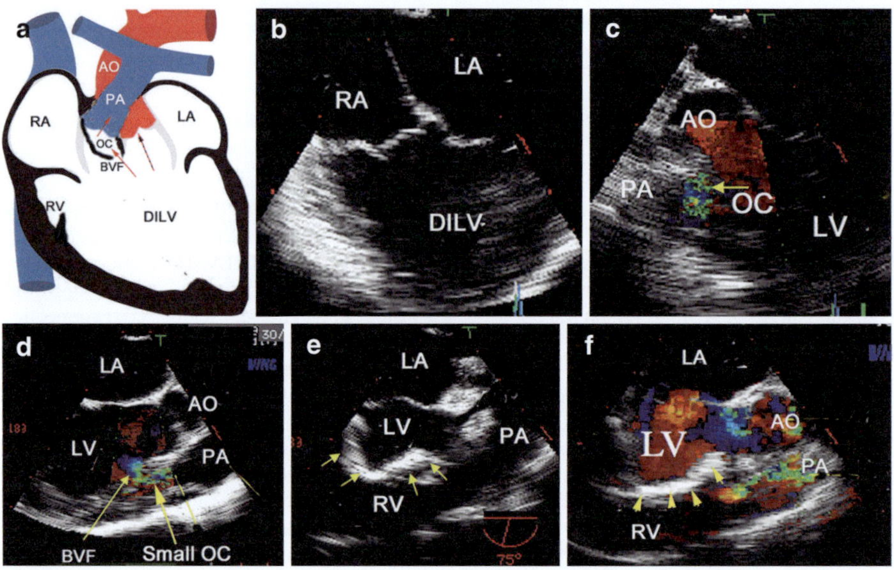

Fig. 6.14 A 5-year-old boy who received surgical correction for his Holmes heart condition. (**a**) Diagram of a Holmes heart, a rare congenital heart defect characterized by DILV (double inlet of the left ventricle) and the absence of the inflow tract of the morphologically RV. This condition is associated with a dominant morphological left ventricle (LV) and normally related great arteries. In a Holmes heart, the pulmonary artery (PA) arises from the infundibular outlet chamber (OC) of the RV, while the aorta arises from the dominant morphological LV. (**b**) Preoperative TEE. In the ME four-chamber view, this dominant LV has both atrioventricular orifices. (**c**) Preoperative color TEE. In the ME five-chamber view, the PA is seen arising from a small OC with a small turbulent flow. (**d**) Preoperative color TEE. In the ME AV LAX view, a small bulboventricular foramen (BVF) is visible with a small turbulent flow between the LV and infundibular OC. (**e**) Postoperative TEE after a biventricular repair. In the ME AV SAX view, ventricular septation with a patch (indicated by yellow arrows) is visible between the RV and LV. (**f**) Postoperative color TEE. In the ME AV LAX view, successful ventricular septation without residual shunt is confirmed, but a minor turbulent flow over the right ventricular outflow tract (RVOT) can be seen

References

1. Dobell AR, Van Praagh R. The Holmes heart: historic associations and pathologic anatomy. Am Heart J. 1996;132:437–45.
2. Bharucha T, Agarwal R, Siddiqui S. Double inlet left ventricle (DILV) with normally related great arteries (NRGA): our experience and review of literature. Ann Pediatr Cardiol. 2019:12:263–9.

6.7 Double Inlet of Right Ventricle (DIRV)

6.7.1 With Systemic Outflow Obstruction

DIRV is a rare cardiac malformation. In patients with DIRV and systemic outflow obstruction, the hemodynamics can present similarly to hypoplastic left heart syndrome. In such cases, a variation of the Norwood stage operation leading to a Fontan-type circulation is often recommended. Figure 6.15 discusses a case of DIRV with severe systemic outflow obstruction, resembling hypoplastic left heart syndrome.

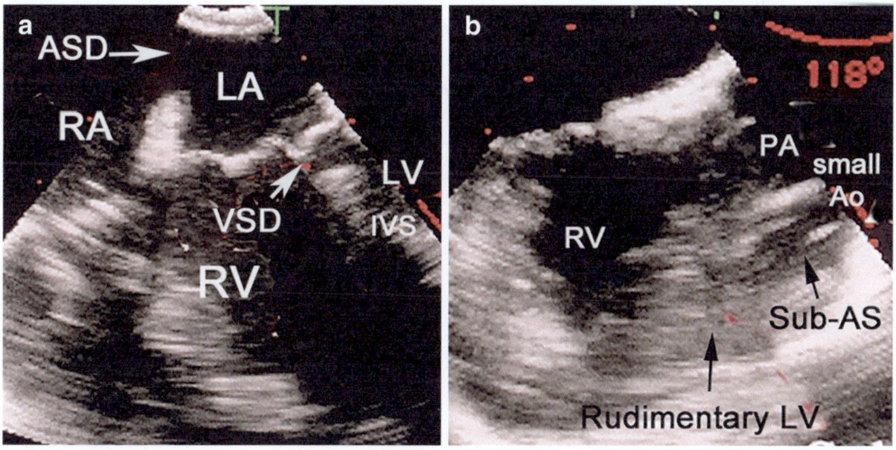

Fig. 6.15 Case of a newborn who underwent the Norwood operation and modified Blalock-Taussig shunt for very complex congenital heart defects, including double inlet right ventricle (DIRV), double outlet right ventricle (DORV), atrial septal defect (ASD), ventricular septal defect (VSD), and subaortic stenosis (Sub-AS). (**a**) Preoperative TEE. The ME four-chamber view shows that the patient has a DIRV, with both atria connected to the dominant right ventricle (RV) and a rudimentary left ventricle (LV). ASD and VSD were also observed. (**b**) Preoperative TEE. The ME AV LAX view shows a rudimentary LV, a small aorta with Sub-AS, located anterior to the pulmonary artery (PA). (**c**) Postoperative TEE image of the Norwood procedure (for detailed information, see Fig. 4.8). The UE AAO SAX view shows a neoaorta (Neo-AO) arising from the RV without focal stenosis. (**d**) Postoperative TEE image of the Blalock-Taussig (BT) shunt used to create pulmonary circulation, as seen in the UE PA SAX view, shows a successful shunt with turbulent blood flow from the descending aorta (not visible in this view) drains into the PA

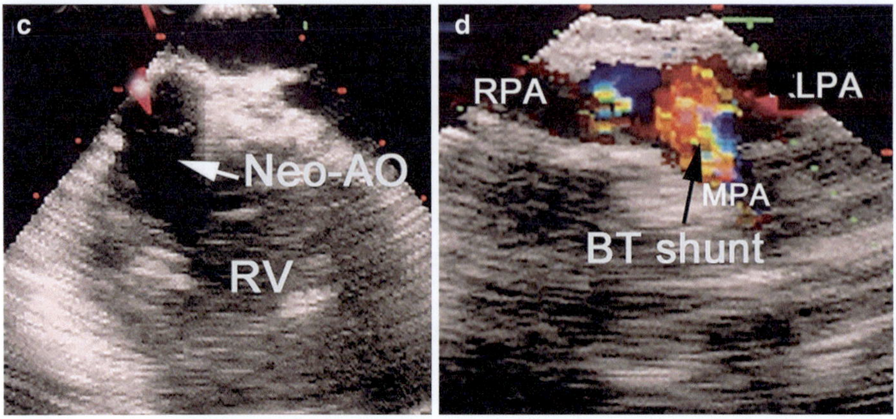

Fig. 6.15 (continued)

References

1. Shiraishi H, Silverma NH. Echocardiographic spectrum of double inlet ventricle: evaluation of the interventricular communication. J Am Coll Cardiol. 1990;15:1401–8.
2. Norwood WI. Hypoplastic left heart syndrome. Cardiol Clin. 1989;7:377–85.

Miscellaneous Congenital Heart Diseases

7

7.1 Primary Neonatal Cardiac Tumors

The most common primary cardiac tumors are mostly benign, including rhabdomyoma, teratoma, and fibroma [1, 2]. Symptoms of a cardiac tumor in postnatal life depend on its size and location. A large tumor can compress cardiac chambers or vital structures, obstruct cardiac valves, and disrupt blood flow. This can lead to symptoms such as bluish skin, breathing problems, feeding difficulties, or heart failure. Surgical resection is the most common treatment, and echocardiography is preferred for diagnosis and determining the size and location of the tumor.

Rhabdomyomas, which originate from striated muscle cells within the ventricles, are a rare form of cardiac tumor that typically develops during neonatal stages. Although they are usually benign, a significant large tumor or blockage of blood flow can lead to symptoms of heart failure.

Diagnostic imaging modalities such as transesophageal echocardiography (TEE) can confirm the diagnosis, and management strategies are outlined in Fig. 7.1.

Rhabdomyosarcoma is a rare type of cancer that arises from skeletal muscle cells and typically has a poor prognosis in neonates. Figure 7.2 outlines diagnostic imaging modalities, such as TEE or CT, as well as management strategies for this condition.

S.-K. Tsai et al., *Transesophageal Echocardiography in Pediatric Congenital Cardiac Surgery and Catheter Intervention*, https://doi.org/10.1007/978-981-99-6582-3_7

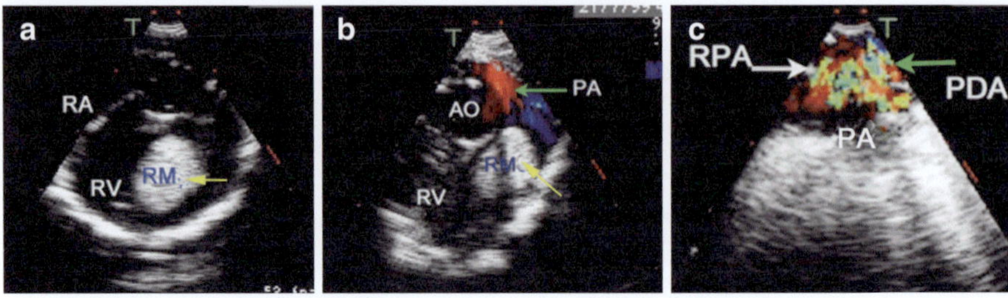

Fig. 7.1 A newborn with a cardiac rhabdomyoma (RM) underwent surgical intervention. (**a**) Preoperative TEE, modified four-chamber view, illustrates a distinct hyperechoic mass with clearly defined borders in the right ventricle (RV), measuring 1.8 × 1.4 cm. This mass was verified as a cardiac rhabdomyoma (RM) through pathology study, indicated by the yellow arrow. (**b**) TEE-In the short-axis view demonstrates the cardiac rhabdomyoma (indicated by yellow arrow) located in the right ventricular outflow tract (RVOT) during systole, causing total RVOT obstruction. (**c**) TEE in the UE AAO SAX with color flow view reveals the presence of a turbulent flow in the patent ductus arteriosus (PDA), which flows into the pulmonary artery (PA) to enhance blood oxygenation, and it is aggravated by the obstruction caused by this tumor

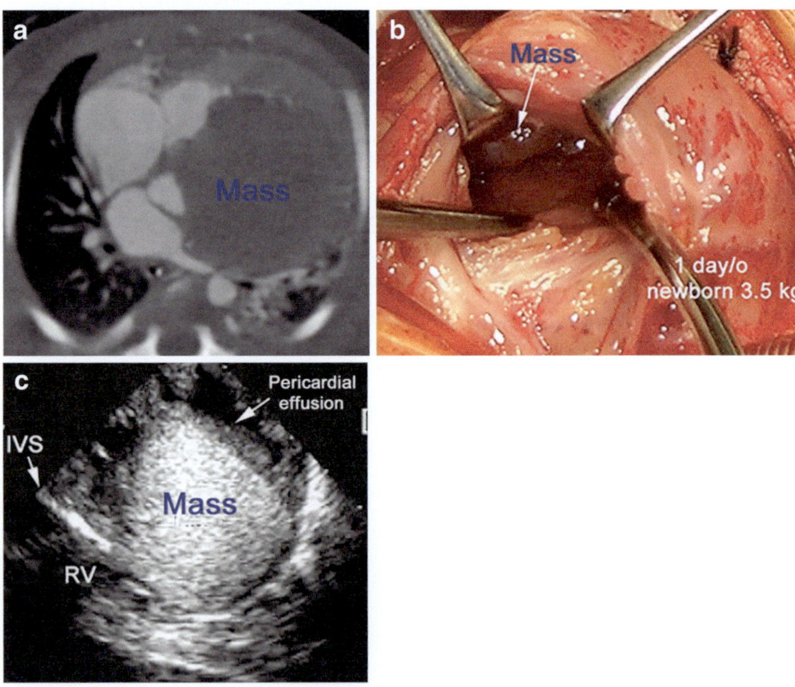

Fig. 7.2 A 1-day-old newborn presenting with heart failure due to cardiac tamponade. (**a**) Preoperative cardiac computed tomography in axial view demonstrates the presence of a large mass occupying the entire cavity and anterior-lateral wall of left ventricle, which is obstructing the LV outflow tract. (**b**) Intraoperative image of the cardiac tumor. The extent of local tumor infiltration made it inoperable. A biopsy and immunohistochemistry analysis were conducted. (**c**) 2D TEE image in the modified four-chamber view displays a solid mass occupying the entire outlet portion of the left ventricle. Additionally, pericardial effusion is evident

References

1. Isaacs H Jr. Fetal and neonatal cardiac tumors. Pediatr Cardiol. 2004;25:252–73.
2. Gazit AZ, Gandhi SK. Pediatric primary cardiac tumors: diagnosis and treatment. Curr Treat Options Cardiovasc Med. 2007;9:399–406.

7.2 Congenital Right Coronary Artery Aneurysm with a Fistula to the Right Heart Chamber

A right coronary artery (RCA) aneurysm fistula draining into the right atrium (RA) or right ventricle (RV) is a rare cardiac condition. This condition occurs when an aneurysm, which is a bulging and weakened section, develops in the RCA, and a fistula, an abnormal connection, forms between the aneurysm and either the RA or RV.

The diagnosis of RCA aneurysm fistula draining into RA or RV is usually made through imaging tests such as echocardiography, CT, or MRI. Treatment depends on the severity and symptoms of the condition. Options may include medication, surgery to repair the aneurysm, and fistula.

Cardiac CT and transesophageal echocardiography (TEE) can confirm the diagnosis of RCA aneurysm fistula to the RA, and Fig. 7.3 outlines management strategies for this condition. Similarly, Fig. 7.4 outlines diagnostic imaging modalities such as TEE or CT, as well as management strategies, for RCA aneurysm fistula to the RV in a child.

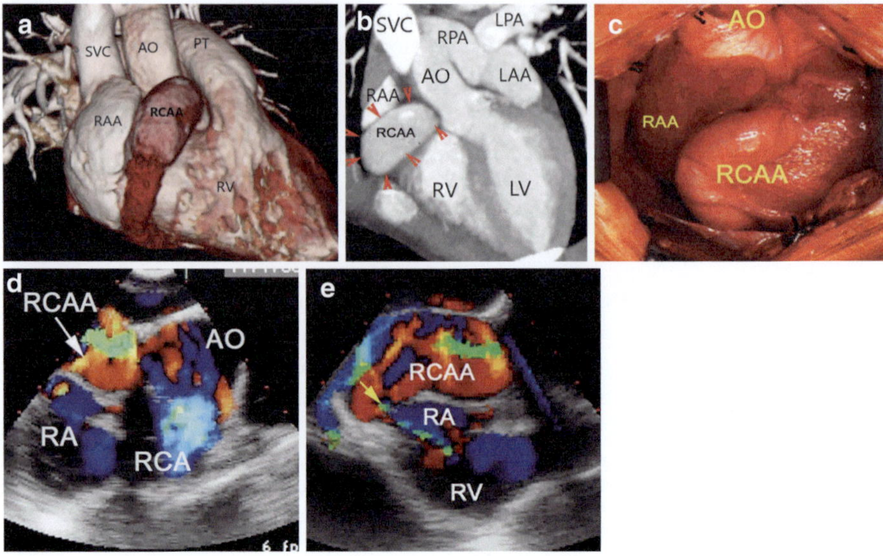

Fig. 7.3 A giant isolated aneurysm in the right coronary artery (RCA) in a 10-year-old girl who presented with chest tightness after physical activity and underwent surgical intervention. (**a**) Preoperative 3D volume-rendered image shows a large proximal aneurysm in the right coronary artery (RCA) with significant dilation of the remaining right coronary artery. (**b**) Enhanced CT image in an oblique-coronal view shows a large RCAA (indicated by red arrowheads) separating apart of the RAA and RV. (**c**) Intraoperative photograph revealed marked dilation of the right coronary artery (RCA), including a giant RCA aneurysm (RCAA) that was compressing the right atrium (RA) and right ventricle (RV). (**d**) During the intraoperative TEE, a marked dilation of the right coronary artery (RCA) was observed, including the presence of a giant RCA aneurysm (RCAA), which was compressing the right atrium (RA). (**e**) Color TEE image displayed the right coronary artery aneurysm (RCAA) and a small fistula (indicated by the yellow arrow) connecting it to the right atrium (RA) and draining into the right ventricle (RV)

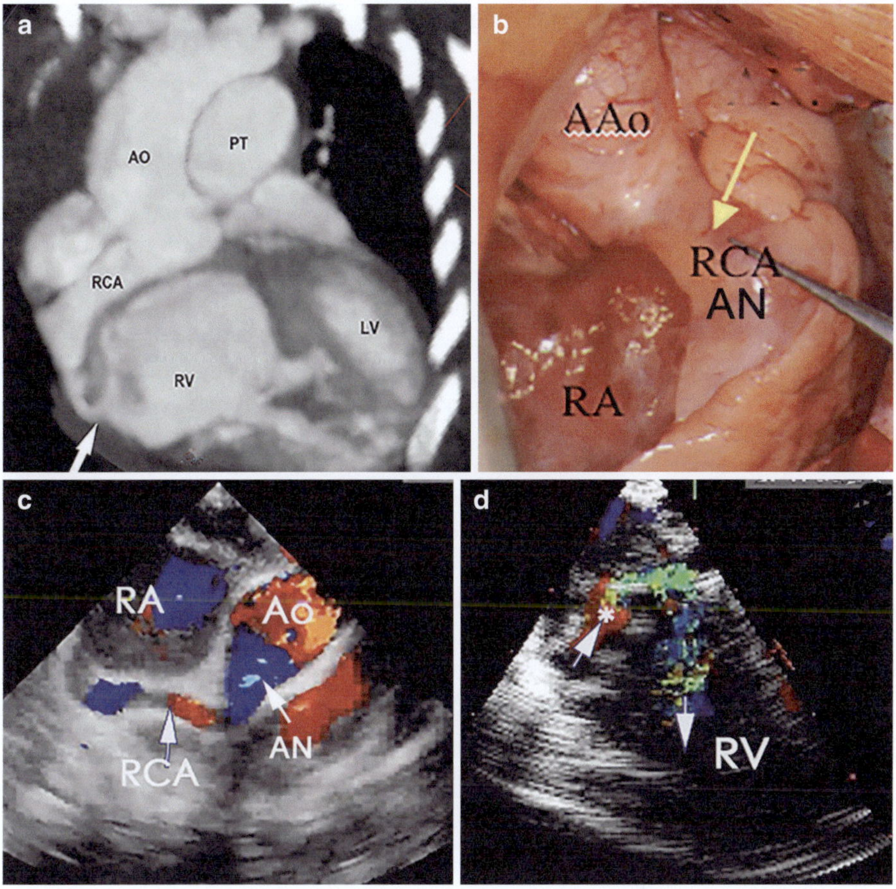

Fig. 7.4 A right coronary artery (RCA) aneurysm in a 12-year-old boy with a history of Kawasaki disease, who presented with exertional chest pain. Despite failed attempts at device closure, the aneurysm and fistula were successfully resected through surgical intervention. (**a**) Preoperative cardiac CT scan revealed the presence of an RCA aneurysm. The aneurysm was found to be fistulizing into the lateral wall of the subvalvular inlet of the right ventricle (arrow). (**b**) Intraoperative surgical photograph shows an external view of the tortuous and aneurysmal dilation of the RCA (indicated by an arrow) and a fistula leading to the right ventricle (not shown). (**c**) Preoperative color TEE, ME four-chamber view shows the aneurysm dilation (AN) of the right coronary artery and its long fistulous tract extending laterally along the atrioventricular groove. (**d**) Preoperative color TEE, ME four-chamber view shows the folded-back fistulous trajectory of the RCA (*) from the lateral side and its drainage into the basal portion of the RV (indicated by an arrow) along the atrioventricular groove with a turbulent mosaic jet

References

1. Choi JH, Kim J Y, Cho JY, et al. Aneurysm of the right coronary artery with fistula to the right atrium. Korean Circ J. 2006:36:619–21.
2. Balasubramanian S, Jothi M, Shanmugam Ml. Right coronary artery aneurysm with fistula to the right ventricle. Heart Lung Circ. 2009;18:153–4.

7.3 Pediatric Heart Transplant

Pediatric heart transplantation is the recommended treatment for children with end-stage heart failure caused by complex congenital heart defects, cardiomyopathy, or other heart diseases that cannot be treated effectively with medications or other surgical options [1, 2]. Recent data show favorable outcomes, with a median survival of 22.3 years for children receiving heart transplant under one year of age, 18.4 years for those between 1 and 5 years of age, and 14.4 years for those between 6 and 10 years of age. However, the mortality rate remains high [3].

Pediatric heart transplantation is complex and requires careful evaluation and planning. The size of a donor depends on various factors, including weight, height, and age. For infants and young children [4, 5], it is recommended to have a weight ratio of 1:1 to 1.2:1. When selecting a donor heart, it is important to consider factors such as the size of the heart, any structural abnormalities and the urgency of the transplant. In certain circumstances, there may be a need to accept an oversized donor heart if an appropriately sized donor heart is not available for a small child, or if waiting for a suitably sized donor heart presents greater risks than accepting a larger one [6]. Figures 7.5 and 7.6 show the management of a 6-month-old boy weighing 5 kg with heart failure who received a heart transplant for cardiomyopathy.

Great vessels stenosis occurred in 13.6% of the study population after heart transplantation [7] and was associated with a higher risk of mortality and retransplantation. Infants with congenital heart diseases, especially those with a single ventricle and related abnormalities in the great vessels, had a higher likelihood of residual great vessels stenosis and requiring extracorporeal membrane oxygenation (ECMO) support before reoperation, as outlined in Fig. 7.7.

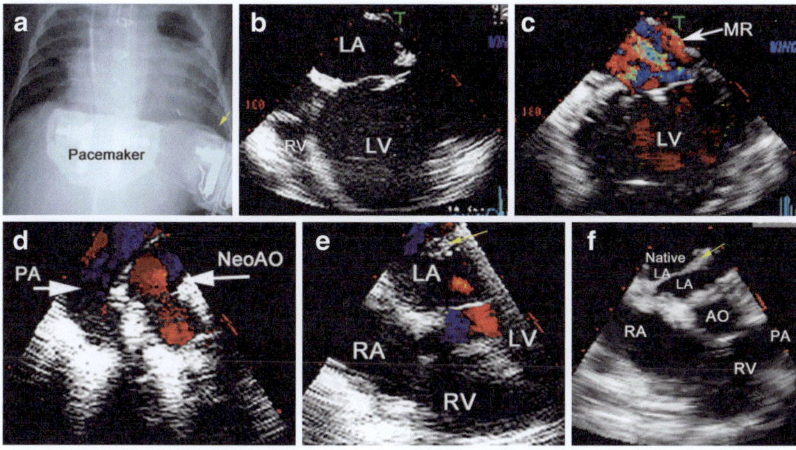

Fig. 7.5 Orthotopic heart transplantation in a 6-month-old boy with heart failure caused by tricuspid atresia and severe pulmonary stenosis who received the a Blalock-Taussig shunt and a pacemaker in Infancy. (**a**) Chest X-ray upon admission shows cardiomegaly, pulmonary congestion, and heart failure with pleural effusion (indicated by arrow). Pacemaker implantation is visible. (**b**) Preoperative TEE, with the four-chamber view showing a small right ventricle and marked left ventricular dilation. (**c**) Color TEE image in a similar view reveals dilated cardiomyopathy with severe mitral valve regurgitation, as indicated by the arrow. (**d**) Color Doppler TEE image post-heart transplantation, with a donor heart weighing 10 kg, demonstrates a successful anastomosis of the aorta (NeoAO) and pulmonary artery. (**e**) Postoperative TEE image, taken from a five-chamber view (including the unmarked native LA near the probe and the donor LA), displays a normal donor left atrium (LA) with an echodense suture line visible in between, as indicated by the yellow line. (**f**) Postoperative TEE image with orthotopic heart transplantation in the ME AV SAX view shows the left atrial suture line and residual native left atrium

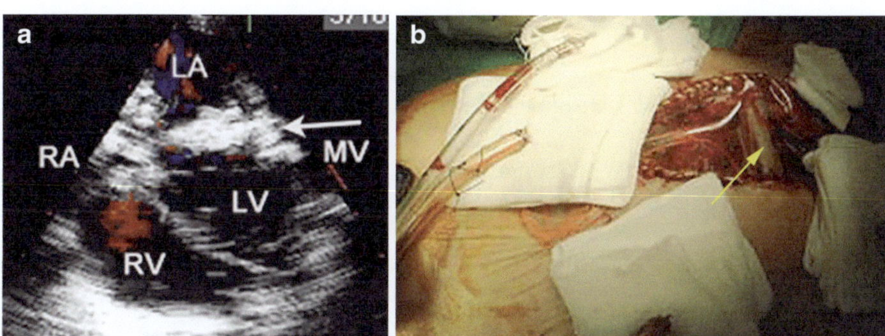

Fig. 7.6 Delayed sternal closure due to impaired cardiac function following heart transplantation in a baby, as shown in Fig. 7.5. (**a**) A 6-month-old boy underwent a successful heart transplantation procedure but experienced a sudden drop in blood pressure during sternal closure. The TEE image reveals that the mitral valve (MV) is being compressed by pressure from the sternal closure due to the larger size of the donor heart relative to the thoracic cavity. (**b**) Postoperative photograph depicts a delayed sternal closure utilizing the hand-cut syringes technique, as indicated by the arrow, and covered with a sterile, occlusive dressing following the surgery

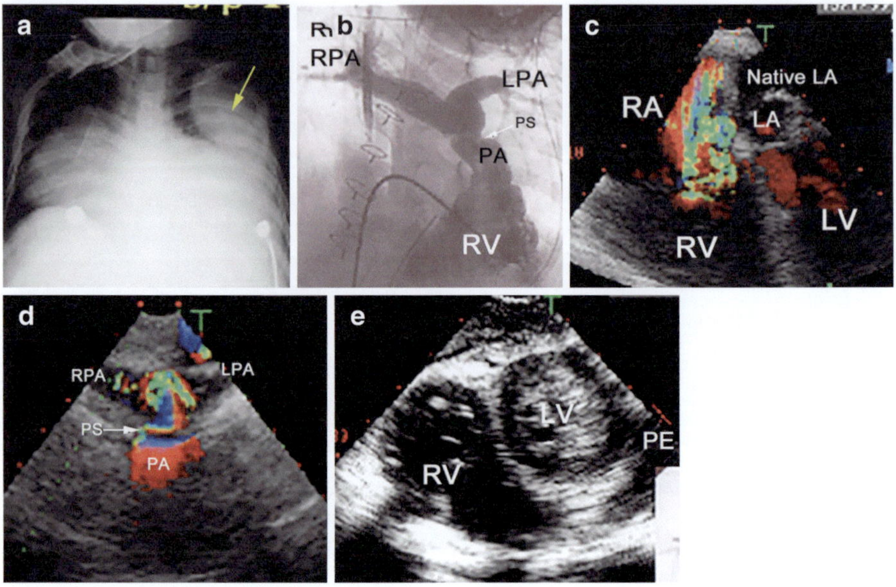

Fig. 7.7 Use of ECMO (extracorporeal membrane oxygenation) support for right ventricular failure in a 2-year-old boy after orthotopic heart transplantation. (**a**) Chest X-ray taken 5 days after orthotopic heart transplantation displays extreme cardiomegaly with prominent bilateral heart borders nearly attached on both chest wall that occupies the whole lower thorax. A lobulated pleural effusion is also seen, indicated by the yellow arrow. (**b**) Right ventricle angiography reveals an anastomotic pulmonary stenosis (PS) at the pulmonary trunk (white thin arrow). (**c**) 2D Color TEE image in the four-chamber view displays dilation of the right ventricle and severe tricuspid regurgitation. (**d**) TEE image of the pulmonary trunk in the UE AAO SAX view depicts a turbulent mosaic flow pattern, strongly suggesting an anastomotic pulmonary stenosis (PS) (white thin arrow). (**e**) Transgastric view image captured by TEE reveals a dilated right ventricle (RV), a collapsed left ventricle (LV), and the presence of pericardial effusion (PE), indicating right ventricular failure and the need for an emergency ECMO support

References

1. Dipchand AI. Current state of pediatric cardiac transplantation. Ann Cardiothorac Surg. 2018;7:31–55.
2. Dipchand AI, Mahle WT, Tresler M, et al. Extracorporeal membrane oxygenation as a bridge to pediatric heart transplantation: effect on post-listing and post-transplantation outcomes. Circ Heart Fail. 2015;8:960–9.
3. Pietra BA, Kantor PF, Bartlett HL, et al. Early predictors of survival to and after heart transplantation in children with dilated cardiomyopathy. Circulation. 2012;126:1079–86.
4. Dipchand AI, Kirk R, Edwards LB, et al. The International Society for Heart and Lung Transplantation Guidelines for the management of pediatric heart transplantation: executive summary—2014. J Heart Lung Transplant. 2014;33(9):888–909.

5. Zafar F, Castleberry C, Khan MS. Donor heart size and pediatric heart transplantation. Pediatr Cardiol. 2017;38(2):295–301.
6. Schueler S, Kuehne T, Grothoff M, et al. Successful use of an oversized donor heart in a small child with dilated cardiomyopathy. J Heart Lung Transplant. 2014;33:1318–20.
7. Berman DP, Willis BC, Sisk MA, et al. Great vessel stenosis after pediatric heart transplantation: incidence, management, and impact on outcomes. J Am Heart Assoc. 2017;6(3):e004739.

7.4 Situs Inversus, DIRV with VSD

When a patient has VSD with situs inversus, it usually presents with dextrocardia and dextroposition, which means the heart is located on the right side of the chest (Fig. 7.8). The incidence of VSD with dextrocardia is relatively low and occurs in about 0.2–0.5% of all congenital heart defects [1].

The treatment of VSD with dextrocardia is similar to that of VSD in patients with normal situs. However, the surgical approach for VSD with dextrocardia may be more challenging [2] due to the reversed position of the heart and the associated vascular anomalies that can occur in situs inversus. Figure 7.8 will provide information on the diagnosis and management of VSD in patients with situs inversus.

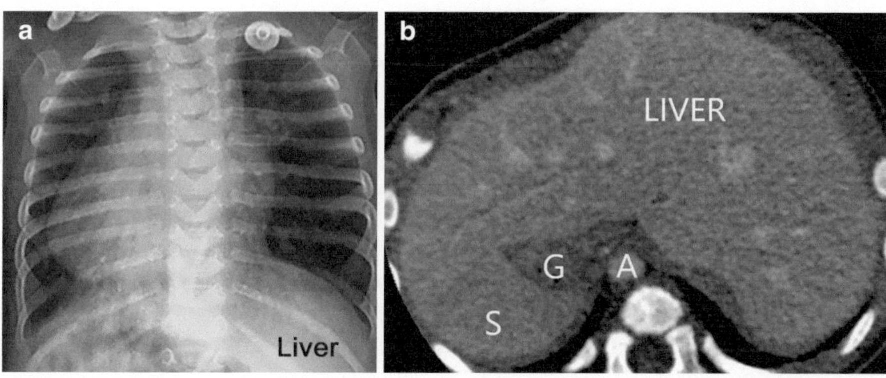

Fig. 7.8 Case of a 4-year-old boy with situs inversus and ventricular septal defect (VSD) who underwent surgical repair. (**a**) Chest X-ray shows a dextrocardia, a right-sided aortic knuckle, and gastric air bubble, but a left-sided liver. (**b**) Upper abdomen CT in the venous phase of contrast enhancement reveals situs inversus with the spleen (S), stomach (G), and descending aorta (A) all located on the right side. (**c**) Preoperative TEE. The ME four-chamber view shows a rightward cardiac apex and a VSD. Both atria opening into the morphologically right ventricle (RV) indicates he has a double inlet of the right ventricle (DIRV). (**d**) Preoperative TEE. The ME AV SAX view of the aortic valve and pulmonary artery (PA) shows the PA located anterior to the aorta (AO) on the right side

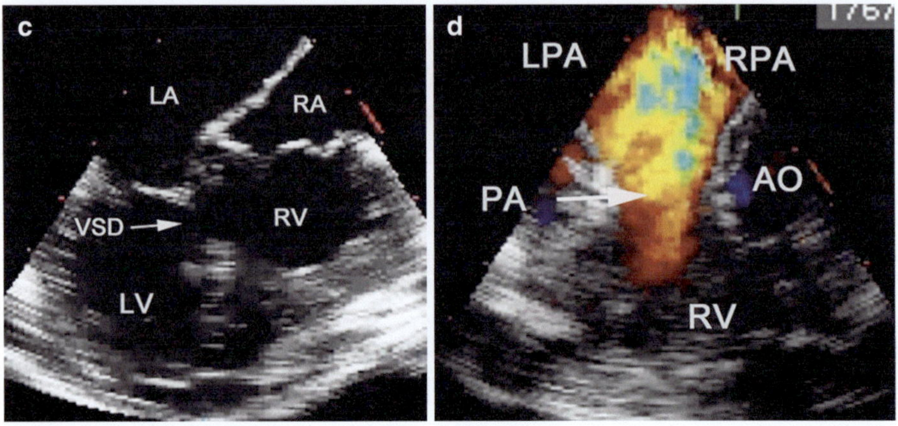

Fig. 7.8 (continued)

References

1. Aggarwal V, Natarajan P, Gupta SK, et al. Ventricular septal defect with situs inversus: a rare association. Ann Pediatr Cardiol. 2012;5(2):180–2.
2. Verma S, Gupta A, Abrol S, et al. Ventricular septal defect with dextrocardia and situs inversus: surgical challenges and management strategies. J Card Surg. 2015;30(7):587–9.

7.5 Congenital Giant Left Atrial Appendage Aneurysm

A giant left atrial appendage (LAA) aneurysm is a rare condition where the LAA is abnormally enlarged and exceeds 4 cm in diameter. LAA aneurysms are often asymptomatic and may be discovered incidentally during imaging tests such as echocardiography [1–3].

LAA aneurysm carries a risk of life-threatening complications, including atrial tachyarrhythmia, systemic embolism, myocardial dysfunction, and heart failure. Early surgical intervention in giant LAA aneurysm is generally recommended, even in asymptomatic cases [2].

The majority of cases of congenital LAA aneurysms are asymptomatic and are often discovered incidentally. The treatment approach depends on the severity of symptoms and the risk of complications. In the case of giant LAA aneurysms, aneurysmectomy is typically performed, even when the patient does not exhibit any symptoms. Figure 7.9 provides further details on diagnosis, management, and outcomes.

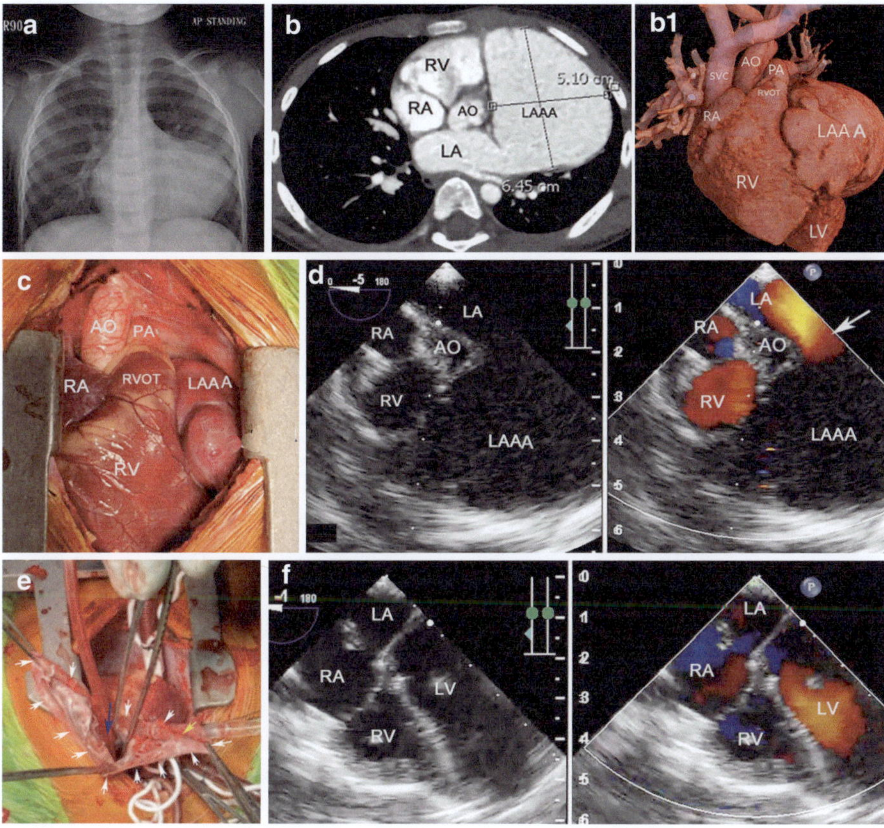

Fig. 7.9 A case of a 1.5-year-old boy with the incidental diagnosis of a giant congenital left atrial appendage (LAA) aneurysm (LAAA) and underwent an aneurysmectomy. (**a**) Posteroanterior chest X-ray demonstrates abnormal lateral protruding of the left heart border with upward lifting cardiac apex, which may mimic a right ventricular dilation. (**b**, **b**1) Contrast-enhanced CT (**b**) and 3D volume rendering CT (**b**1) images reveal a markedly enlarged LAAA (6.45 × 5.10 cm) causing mass effect on the basal anterior walls and downward displacement of the left ventricle. (**c**) Intraoperative photograph shows a large LAAA protruding out after opening the pericardium. (**d**) Preoperative 2D color TEE in the ME four-chamber view demonstrates a large LAA with an aneurysm and an annulus (neck) (indicated by arrow in the right diagram), which is direct communication with the left atrial cavity. Additionally, there is a small right atrium (RA) and ventricle (RV). (**e**) Photograph taken during the surgical incision of the LAAA shows a giant LAA aneurysm (as indicated by multiple arrows) with a fibrous annulus (neck) measuring 2 cm (large blue arrow) that was excised just above its attachment to the left atrium. An annuloplasty ring was sutured in place during the aneurysmectomy procedure. (**f**) Postoperative 2D color TEE image in the ME four-chamber view reveals the results of the surgery. The LAAA is no longer present, and the normal size and relationship of all four chambers were noted. (**g**) Postoperative 2D color TEE image visualizes the flow (right diagram) from the left lower pulmonary vein (LLPV). (**h**) Normal left pulmonary flow pattern was obtained by pulsed Doppler after resection of the LAAA

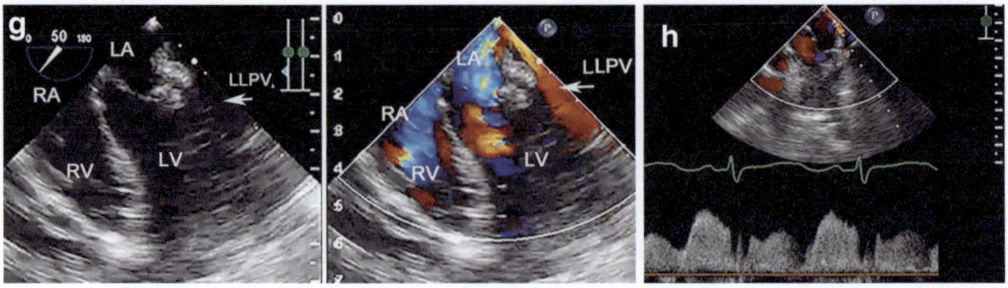

Fig. 7.9 (continued)

References

1. Ulucam M, Muderrisoglu H, Sezgin A. Giant left atrial appendage aneurysm: the third ventricle! Int J Cardiovasc Imaging. 2005;21(2-3):225–30.
2. Chowdhury UK, Seth S, Govindappa R, Jagia P, Malhotra P. Congenital left atrial appendage aneurysm: a case report and brief review of literature. Heart Lung Circ. 2009;18(6):412–6.
3. Morales JM, Patel SG, Jackson JH, Duff JA, Simpson JW. Left atrial aneurysm. Ann Thorac Surg. 2001;71(2):719–22.

Part III

TEE Guidance of Pediatric Catheter Intervention

The chapters of this part delve into the utilization of transesophageal echocardiography (TEE) to guide cardiac catheter interventions in pediatric patients who have congenital heart disease.

Septal Defects

8

8.1 Imaging Modality Monitoring During Transcatheter Intervention Procedure for Septal Defects

Traditionally, septal defects were repaired through open-heart surgery. However, advancements in interventional cardiology have led to the development of transcatheter techniques as an alternative option. The procedure involves inserting a thin, flexible tube called a catheter into a large blood vessel, usually through the groin vessels, and guiding it to the heart using imaging techniques. The continuous improvement of cardiac interventions has been accompanied by advancements in cardiac imaging. Fluoroscopy and transesophageal echocardiography (TEE) are utilized for procedural guidance. TEE [1–4] plays a crucial role in various aspects, including diagnosis, detailed anatomical assessment, device sizing and selection, periprocedure guidance, and post-device deployment surveillance (as depicted in Fig. 8.1).

Two-dimensional (2D) transesophageal echocardiography (TEE) cannot provide a comprehensive image of the defect and ventricular septum. However, three-dimensional (3D) TEE offers the advantage of projecting an enface view of the defect, which allows for better visualization of the entire defect, especially in cases of ventricular septal defect (VSD). These defects often have unusual or irregular shapes, and 3D TEE can accurately display such morphology, aiding in the selection of the appropriate occluder device (as depicted in Figs. 8.2, 8.3 and 8.4). The assessment of the morphology of atrial septal defects (ASDs) guided by 3D TEE will be discussed in Figs. 8.10 and 8.12. Four-dimensional (4D) [6] TEE is an innovative technique that utilizes dynamic 3D echocardiography to obtain a more comprehensive illustration of abnormalities and their relationship with other cardiac structures. It enhances our understanding of spatial relations and motion, providing a clearer

---

Supplementary Information The online version contains supplementary material available at https://doi.org/10.1007/978-981-99-6582-3_8.

S.-K. Tsai et al., *Transesophageal Echocardiography in Pediatric Congenital Cardiac Surgery and Catheter Intervention*, https://doi.org/10.1007/978-981-99-6582-3_8

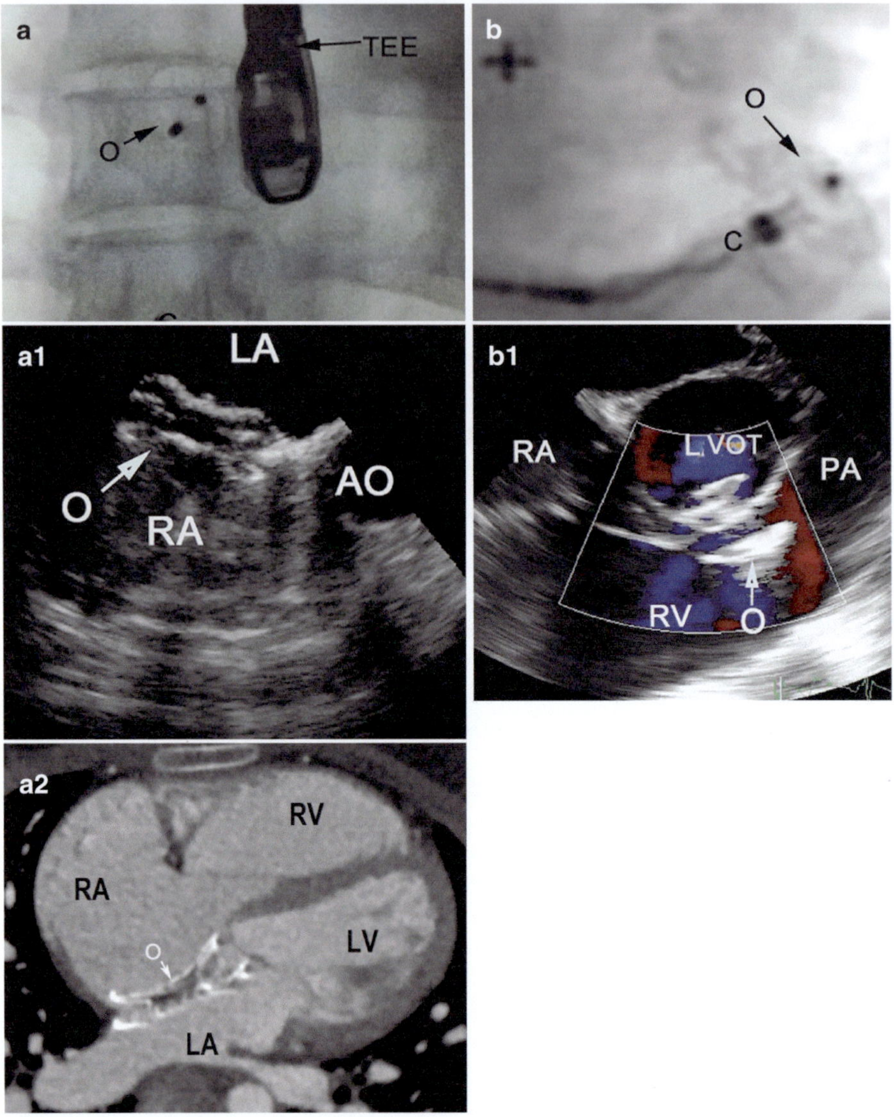

Fig. 8.1 Primary images of transcatheter closure using TEE and fluoroscopy for ASD or VSD. Combining TEE-guided and fluoroscopic techniques for transcatheter closure of ASD or VSD can enhance efficiency by minimizing fluoroscopic time and reducing radiation exposure. (**a**) and (**b**) Fluoroscopy images during device closure of an ASD and a VSD, respectively. (**a1**) and (**b1**) TEE images corresponding to the transcatheter closure of an ASD or a VSD offer vital information, including the relative position of the defect and occluders and confirmation of proper occluders positioning. (**a2**) Corresponding cardiac CT image on 4-chamber view shows dilated RA and RV with a large Amplatzer occluder (O) in between RA and LA for a large secundum type ASD

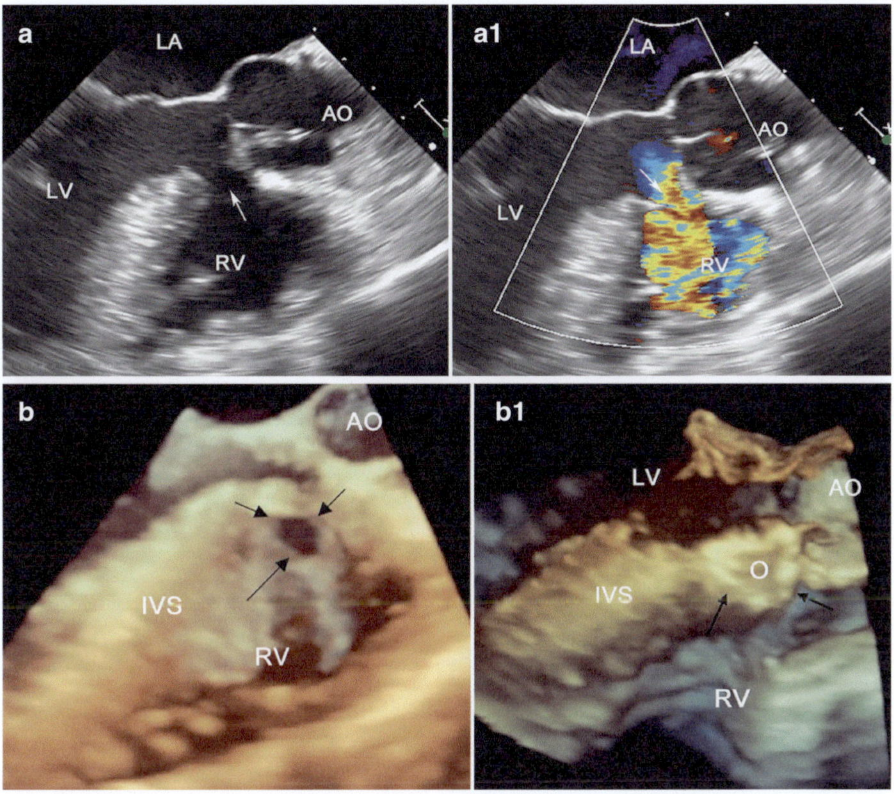

Fig. 8.2 Three-dimensional (3D) transesophageal echocardiography (TEE) versus 2D TEE for guiding the transcatheter closure of VSD. (**a**) 2D TEE image taken from the ME AV LAX view reveals a perimembranous ventricular septal defect (VSD) indicated by the arrow. Additionally, color Doppler imaging in (**a1**) displays a flow of blood, indicated by shunt flow, from the left ventricle (LV) to the right ventricle (RV). (**b**) In the 3D TEE image of the perimembranous VSD from the right ventricular (RV) enface view, the morphology of the VSD is clearly depicted. It appears as an irregular ovoid shape, indicated by three black arrows, with accurate sizing on the RV side of the septum. In (**b1**), after the deployment of the occluder (O), shown by two black arrows, the image demonstrates that the waist of the occluder effectively seals on the ventricular septum

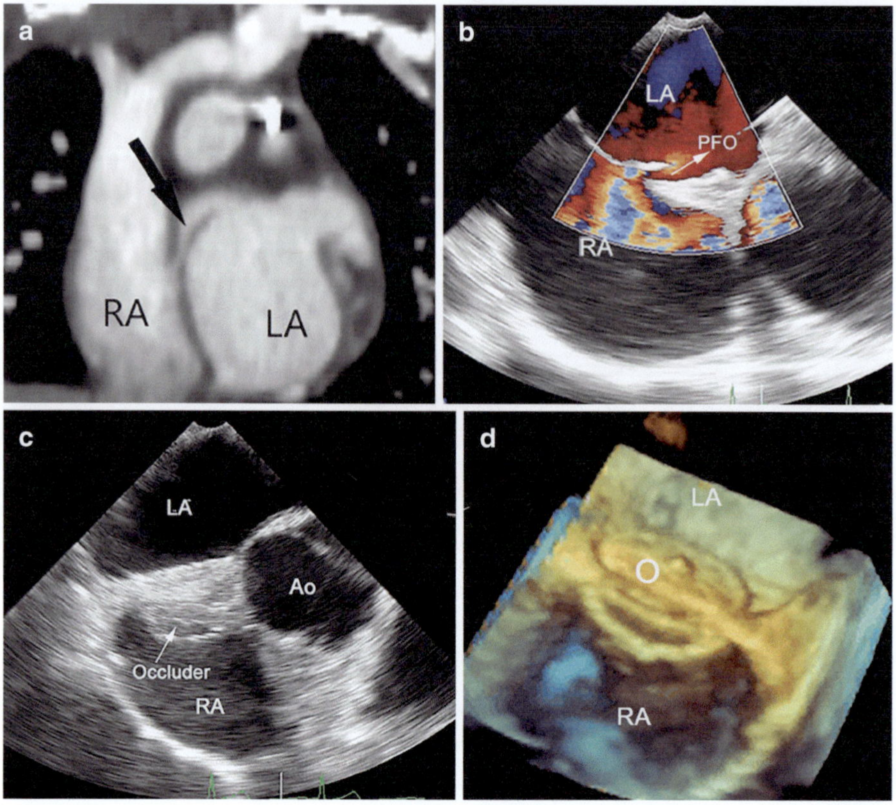

Fig. 8.3 A TEE-guided PFO closure procedure in a child using a catheter. (**a**) Contrast-enhanced cardiac CT, viewed in the coronal view, illustrates a small flaplike opening (indicated by the arrow) in the wall that separates the right atrium (RA) from the left atrium (LA) in a case of PFO. (**b**) Pre-procedural TEE, ME four-chamber view shows a small flaplike opening (arrow) at the atrial wall with turbulent flow from right-to-left atrium. (**c**) Post-procedural TEE and ME AV SAX view displays the Amplatzer occluder properly positioned on both the septum primum and secundum. (**d**) 3D TEE demonstrates proper placement of the occluder (O) with adequate coverage of all edges of the interatrial septum in the oblique enface atrial view

perspective. Additionally, it effectively demonstrates the abnormal shape and direction of blood flow, as discussed in Figs. 8.3 and 8.4.

Fluoroscopy employs X-rays to deliver continuous, real-time imaging. However, prolonged exposure to X-rays can potentially harm patients and personnel in the catheter room. On the other hand, TEE uses ultrasound (high-frequency sound waves) to provide detailed, continuous, real-time imaging of the heart's structures without posing potential radiation harm to the patient. In certain case reports, TEE can serve as the sole guidance for transcatheter intervention procedures, eliminating the need for fluoroscopy [7].

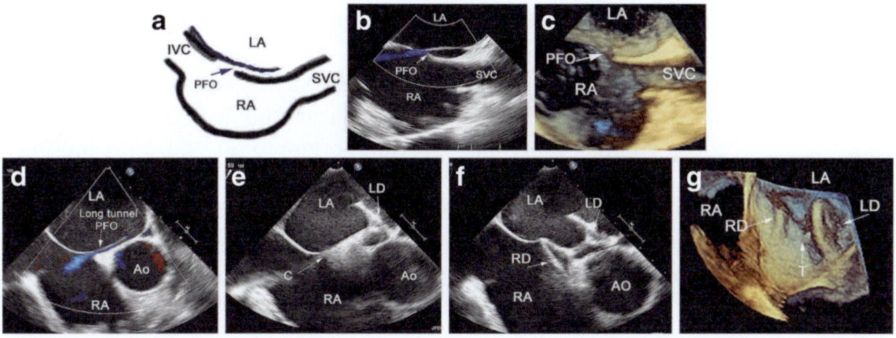

Fig. 8.4 Device closure of a long-tunnel patent foramen ovale (PFO) in a 16-year-old female who presented with migraines. (**a**) Diagram of a PFO displays a significant overlap between the septum primum and septum secundum. (**b**) Pre-procedural TEE with the bicaval view depicts a long-tunnel PFO located in the superior part of the fossa ovalis, and the color Doppler highlights left-to-right shunting. (**c**) 3D TEE image displays the fossa ovalis and a long tunnel between the septum primum (flap) and septum secundum. (**d**) Pre-procedural TEE in the ME AV SAX view shows a 15-mm long-tunnel PFO. (**e**) Intraprocedural TEE image used to guide the closure of a PFO shows the delivery catheter (C) advancing through the tunnel defect and deploying the left disk (LD) of the Amplatzer ASD occluder. (**f**) TEE imaging displays the occluder after complete deployment with a clear right disk (RD) tightly impinges on the right-side septum secundum. (**g**) Three-dimensional TEE image taken after the procedure illustrates the final placement of the device in the long tunnel (T). Tenting of the interatrial septum by margin of the RD toward the LA side is clearly demonstrated

References

1. Taniguchi M, Akagi T. Real-time imaging for transcatheter closure of atrial septal defects. Interv Cardiol. 2011;3.
2. Rana BS. Echocardiography guidance of atrial septal defect closure. J Thorac Dis. 2018;24:s2899–s2908.
3. Mendel B, Laurentius A, Ulfiarakhma D, et al. Safety and feasibility of transesophageal echocardiography in comparison to transthoracic echocardiography-guided ventricular septal defect percutaneous closure: an evidence-based case report. World Heart J. 2020;12(3):199–207.
4. Siagian SN, Prakoso R, Putra BE, et al. Echocardiography-guided percutaneous patent ductus arteriosus closure: 1-year single center experience in Indonesia. Front Cardiovasc Med. 2022;9:2–7.
5. Charakida M, Qureshi S, Simpson. 3D Echocardiography for planning and guidance of interventional closure of VSD. J Am Coll Img. 2013;6:120–23.
6. Wang XF, Li ZA, Cheng TO. Four-dimensional echocardiography methods and clinical application. Am Heart J. 1996;672–84.
7. Bu H, Yang Y, Wu Q, et al. Echocardiography-guided percutaneous closure of perimembranous ventricular septal defects without arterial access and fluoroscopy. BMC Pediatr. 2019;19:302.

8.2 Transcatheter Closure of Patent Foramen Ovale (PFO)

In the majority of individuals, the foramen ovale naturally closes after birth. PFO is present in 20% individuals. However, when paradoxical embolism or transient ischemic attacks occur in younger individuals, it is important to assess for the presence of a right-to-left shunt across the patent foramen ovale (PFO). The majority of PFO can be safely closed using the transcatheter technique, unless in rare situations such as complex heart conditions or when transcatheter closure is not feasible, surgical closure may be recommended.

There are several different types of PFOs that can occur:

1. Simple PFO: This is the most common type of PFO. The opening may vary in size and shape but does not involve any additional structures (as shown in Fig. 8.3).
2. Tunnel-type PFO: In this type, the PFO is characterized by a longer and more distinct tunnel or channel connecting the atria. The length of the tunnel can vary, and it may be associated with a higher risk of paradoxical embolism (as shown in Figs. 8.4 and 8.5).
3. Aneurysmal PFO: An aneurysmal PFO is characterized by a bulging or pouch-like formation on one side of the atrial septum (as shown in Fig. 8.6).

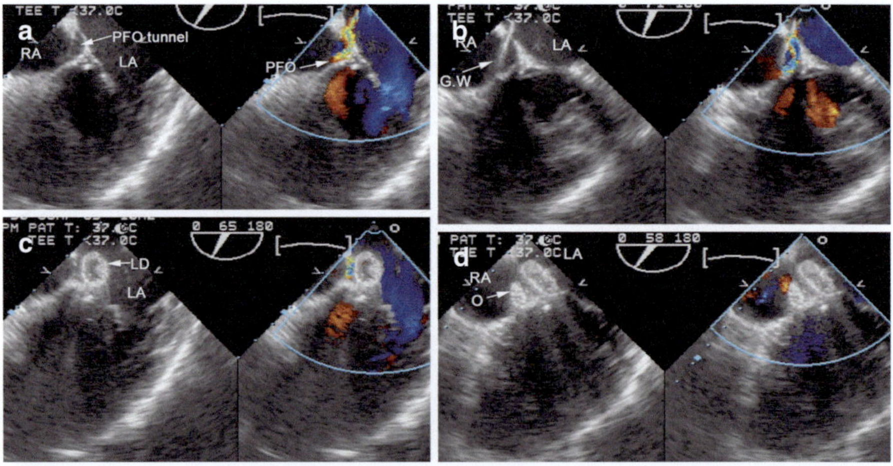

Fig. 8.5 A 12-year-old man underwent device closure for a patent foramen ovale (PFO) with an unusual tunnel and right-to-left shunting. (**a**) A pre-procedural TEE was performed in the ME four-chamber view, which revealed a PFO with an atrial septal aneurysm measuring 4 mm in diameter, along with a right-to-left shunt as seen in the color Doppler image on the right plane. (**b**) TEE image showing the guide wire (GW) pass through the PFO unusual tunnel into the LA (left atrium). (**c**) TEE image displaying the deployment of the 4-mm Amplatzer PFO occluder's left disk (LD) in the left atrium (LA). (**d**) TEE image demonstrating the correct positioning of the PFO occluder, with no evidence of residual shunting

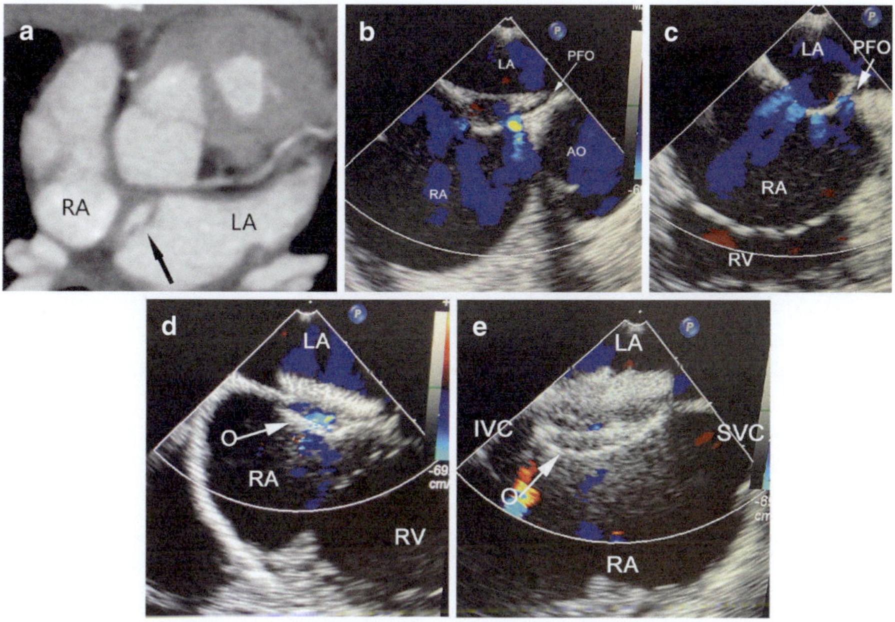

Fig. 8.6 A 10-year-old girl with a history of migraines and a PFO with an atrial septal aneurysm (ASA) underwent device closure. (**a**) Contrast-enhanced cardiac CT in axial view shows a PFO with an atrial septal aneurysm (black arrow). (**b**) Pre-procedural TEE in the ME AV SAX view demonstrating a PFO (14.5 mm) with an atrial septal aneurysm and several fenestrations resulting in significant left-to-right shunting. (**c**) TEE in the bicaval view demonstrates a PFO and a mobile atrial septal aneurysm, with several fenestrated shunts visible. (**d**) Post-procedural TEE in the ME four-chamber view displays complete splinting of the PFO and atrial septal aneurysm with a 25-mm Amplatzer cribriform multi-fenestrated septal occluder (O). (**e**) TEE in the bicaval view demonstrates the final, proper positioning of the occluder (O) with no evidence of residual shunting

References

1. Rigatelli G, Dell'Avvocata F, Ronco F, et al. Transcatheter closure of patent foramen ovale in pediatric patients: single center experience. Catheter Cardiovasc Interv. 2017;89(5):901–5.
2. Tzifa A, Moschovakou G, Zaqout M, et al. Transcatheter closure of patent foramen ovale in children: midterm follow-up results. J Interv Cardiol. 2016;29(6):639–45.

8.3 Transcatheter Closure of Atrial Septal Defect (ASD)

The first report showing transcatheter closure of an atrial septal defect was presented by King TD et al. in 1976 (JAMA). This procedure is now well-established and is advocated as an alternative to surgical repair. Transcatheter closure can close most secundum type ASDs.

1. Feasibility for Transcatheter Closure of ASD.
   (a) ASD device closure is suitable for most patients with secundum type ASDs, which are the most common type of ASDs. The size, location, and anatomy of the defect are evaluated to determine if device closure is appropriate [1, 2].
   (b) Other types of ASDs, such as primum-type or sinus venosus-type defects, or unroofed coronary sinus defects may require surgical intervention instead of transcatheter closure (as discussed in Sect. 3.1).
2. There are various types of devices utilized for transcatheter closure of atrial septal defects (ASDs). The following are some commonly employed devices:
   (a) Amplatzer Septal Occluder [2]: This widely used device is commonly employed for closing ASDs. It comprises two self-expandable disks made of a nitinol wire mesh connected by a waist. For further information, refer to Figs. 8.7 and 8.10.
   (b) Cera (Lifetech) Septal Occluder [3]: The Cera is a newer, cost-effective double-disk ASD occluder. It features as a self-expandable nitinol frame

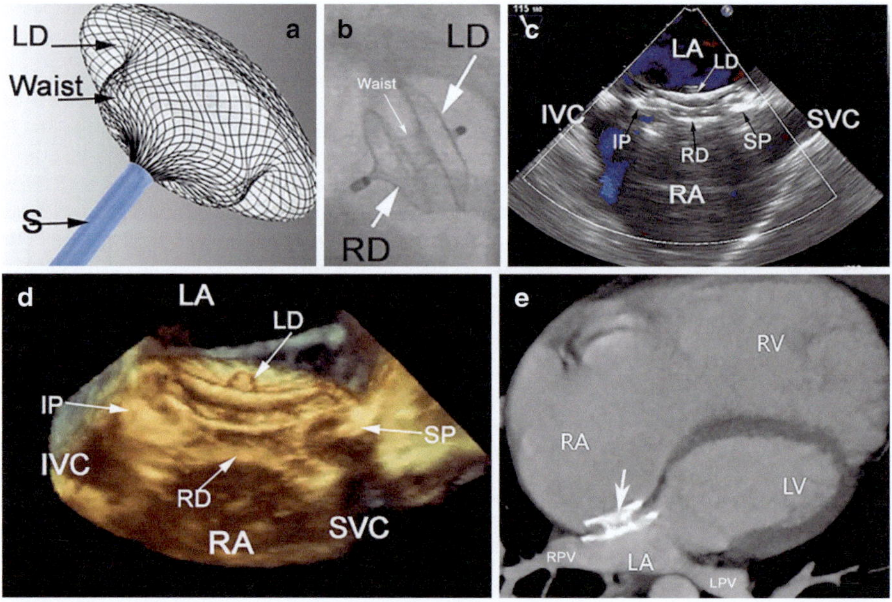

Fig. 8.7 Amplatzer atrial septal occluder deployment for closure of atrial septal defect (ASD). (**a**) Photograph of the Amplatzer septal occluder, including the delivery catheter (S), left disk (LD), and waist, with the right disk (RD) still contained within the delivery catheter. (**b**) Fluoroscopy image of the deployed Amplatzer septal occluder, displaying a clear separation of the two disks in the posterior-anterior view. (**c**) Post-procedural TEE image in the bicaval view showing the Amplatzer septal occluder properly positioned in the ASD with no residual shunting. (**d**) 3D TEE image demonstrating the Amplatzer septal occluder fully anchored at the superior (SP) and inferior (IP) posterior rims. (**e**) Contrast-enhanced cardiac CT in 4-chamber view shows the ASD occluder (arrow) in good position

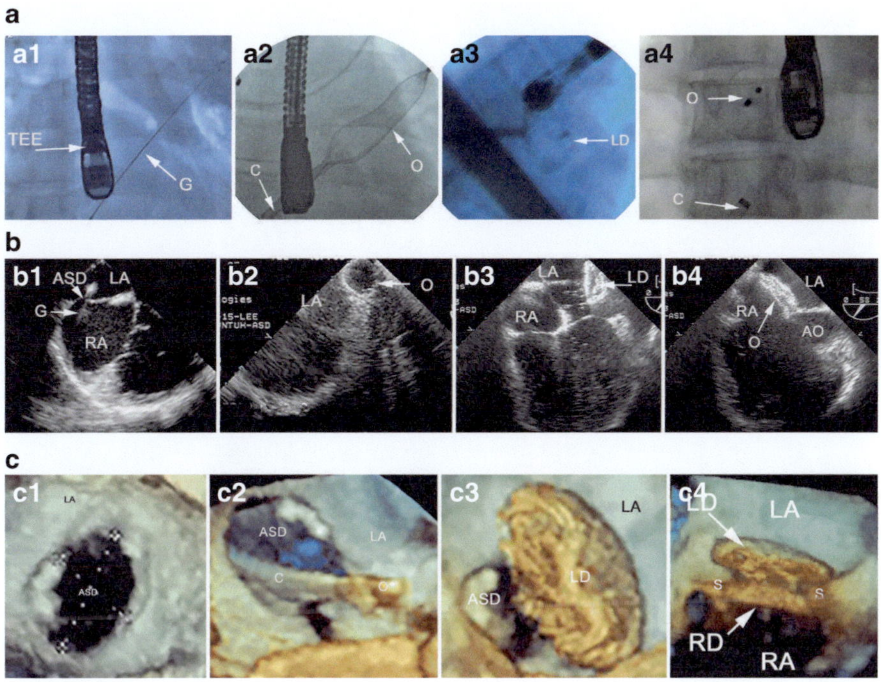

Fig. 8.8 Angiographic, 2D TEE, and 3D TEE images, respectively, depicting the procedure of closing an atrial septal defect (ASD) with an Amplatzer septal occluder. (**a**) Peri-procedural angiographic imaging during the device closure procedure is shown. Images **a1**, **a2**, **a3**, and **a4** depict the deployment of the device. The guideline (G) passes through the ASD from the right atrium (RA) to the left atrium (LA) (as shown in **a1**). The delivery-sheathed device (O) is inserted into the LA in **a2**. The left disk (LD) is deployed at the LA in **a3**. The device (O) is released from the delivery cable in **a4**. (**b**) Corresponding 2D TEE imaging during the device closure procedure is shown in **b1**, **b2**, **b3**, and **b4**. In **b1**, the guidewire is seen passing from the IVC to the LA across the atrial septal defect. The LD of the occluder (O) is deployed at the LA appendage in **b2**. The correct alignment of the LA disk on the atrial septum is seen in **b3**, and in **b4**, both disks are deployed ensuring that the atrial septum is captured between them. (**c**) Corresponding 3D TEE images are displayed in **c1**, **c2**, **c3**, and **c4**. **c1** shows an enface RA view of an oval-shaped ASD. **c2** shows the catheter passing through the ASD from the RA to the LA. **c3** shows the LD deployed in the LA. **c4** shows the right disk (RD) deployed and the device (O) capturing the atrial septum (S)

coated with bio-ceramic titanium nitride (TiN). The left disk is larger than the right disk and connected by a short 4 mm waist. The TiN coating on the Cera aims to reduce thrombosis, release nickel ion, and promote endothelial tissue growth. For additional details, see Fig. 8.8.

(c) CardioSEAL/STARFlex [4]: These devices consist of two self-expanding discs covered with polyester fabric, connected by a flexible center. They have demonstrated early safety and efficacy in percutaneous ASD closure. For more information, consult Fig. 8.9.

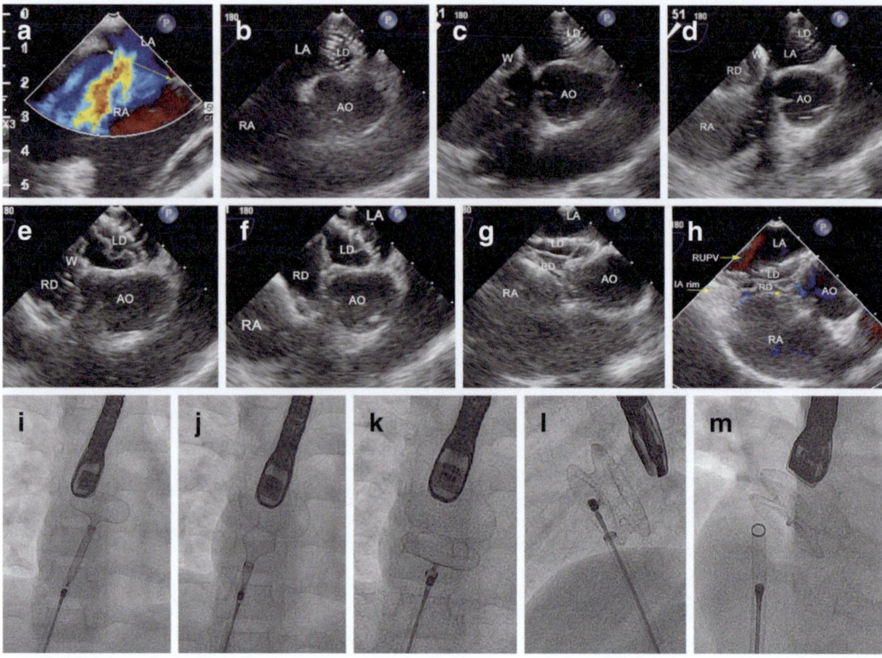

Fig. 8.9 A 2-year-old boy with an atrial septal defect (ASD) underwent device closure using the Cera (Lifetech) ASD occluder. (**a**) Pre-procedural TEE with color Doppler image shows a large ASD measuring 25 mm in diameter, with left-to-right shunting visible in the bicaval view. Intraprocedural TEE image of the device closure procedure using a 32 mm Cera ASD occluder. The sequence is shown from (**b**) to (**h**) as follows: (**b**) left disk (LD) deployed in the LA; (**c**) waist of occluder released; (**d**) right disk (RD) deployed in the RA; (**e**) both disks deployed; (**f**) device wiggling; (**g**) device released; (**h**) final position of the device anchored at the superior and inferior anterior septal rim. Accompanying angiogram depicting the device closure progression, from (**i**) to (**m**). The LD is shown and deployed in (**i**), the waist of the occluder is released in (**j**), both disks are shown deployed in (**k**), the device is completely deployed and ready to be released in (**l**), and the final position of the device in (**m**)

3. Morphology of ASD.

   ASDs can have different morphologies [5], which describe their specific characteristics and how they relate to the surrounding heart structures. In the case of a secundum type ASD, the rims refer to the border or edge that surrounds the defect. Assessing the presence and adequacy of these rims is crucial in determining the suitability of transcatheter closure and evaluating the risk of residual shunting or complications. For further details, refer to Figs. 8.11 and 8.12.

4. Balloon Sizing.

   Balloon sizing is a standard technique used to select the appropriate closure device size for transcatheter ASD closure [6]. It ensures choosing appropriate device for proper positioning, secure closure, and matching dimensions with the

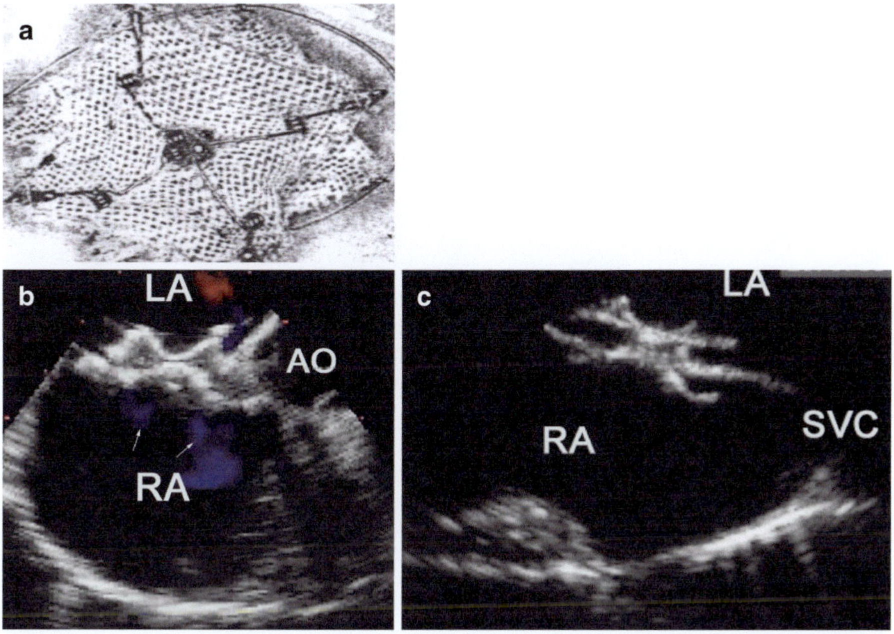

Fig. 8.10 A 15-year-old boy underwent device closure for an atrial septal defect (ASD) using the CardioSEAL/StarFlex septal occluder. (**a**) Photograph of the CardioSEAL/StarFlex atrial septal occluder (manufactured by NMT Medical, Boston, MA, USA) showcasing a spring-loaded dacron double-umbrella design and a framework with minimal fractures due to the flexibility of the metal hinge points. (**b**) Post-procedural TEE image in the ME AV SAX view of an ASD with a deficient superior-anterior rim depicts the square-shaped disks of the CardioSEAL/StarFlex septal occluder applied to both the left and right sides of the septum with a minimal residual shunt (indicated by arrow). (**c**) Post-procedural TEE image in the bicaval view displaying the four arms of the occluder securely positioned on both sides of the septum

defect. However, accidentally oversizing the closure device during balloon sizing may damage or tear the atrial septum, especially in cases with thin and flexible septal rims, as discussed in Fig. 8.14. Alternatively, the diameter measurement of an ASD can be determined without balloon sizing using three-dimensional (as shown in Figs. 8.11 and 8.12) or two-dimensional transesophageal echocardiography imaging techniques [7–9] as described in Fig. 8.13.

5. Transcatheter closure of an ASD with an attenuated anterior-superior (SA) septal subaortic rim poses additional challenges compared to cases with a fully developed rim [10, 11].

   Here are some potential complications (as discussed in Fig. 8.15) that may occur during or after the procedure: residual shunting, device-related complications such as cardiac erosion and perforation, arrhythmias (including heart block), and device instability resulting in device malposition or embolization (as discussed in Fig. 8.16).

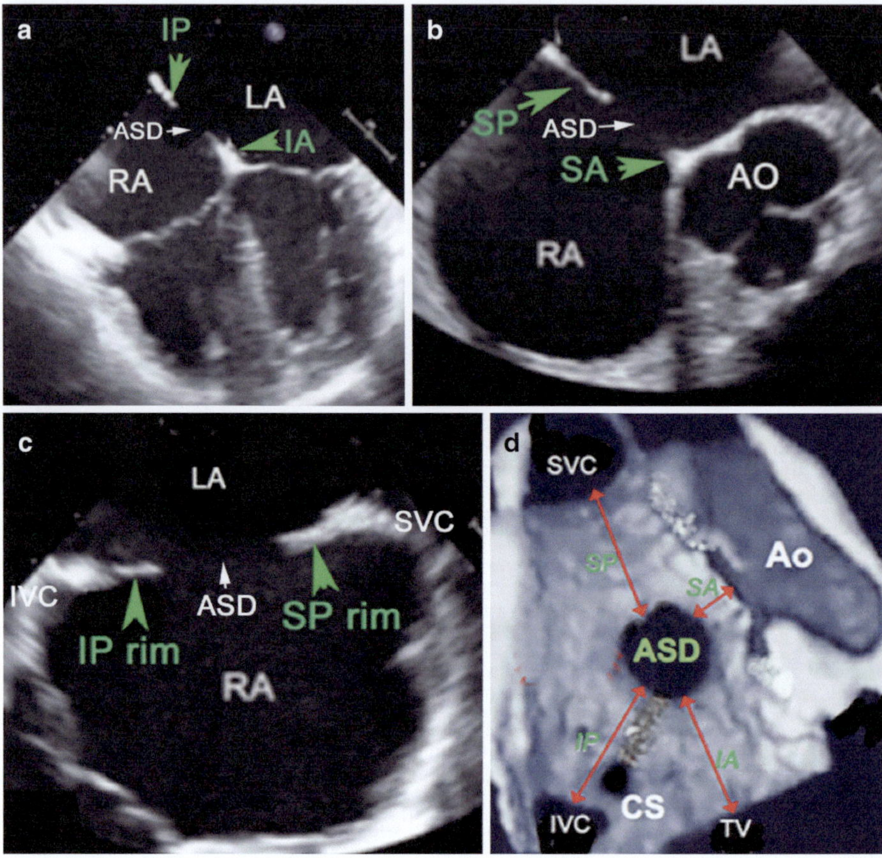

Fig. 8.11 Evaluation of the atrial septal defect (ASD) and associated septal rims through cross-sectional analysis on two-dimensional (2D) and three-dimensional (3D) TEE images. (**a**) ME four-chamber view TEE image demonstrates the inferior anterior (IA) rim and inferior-posterior (IP) rim. (**b**) The ME AV SAX view TEE image demonstrates the anterior-superior (SA) rim and posterior-superior (SP) rim. (**c**) Bicaval view TEE image demonstrates the superior-posterior (SP) and inferior-posterior (IP) rim. (**d**) 3D view provides a clearly the widths of the rims from the ASD to the key anatomies of the aortic locus (AO) in the anterior-superior (SA rim), superior vena cava (SVC) in the posterior-superior (SP rim), inferior vena cava (IVC) in posterior-inferior (IP rim), and tricuspid valve (TV) in anterior-inferior (IA rim), respectively

6. Multiple or Fenestrated ASD.

   Multiple or fenestrated atrial septal defects (ASDs) are characterized by the presence of two or more separate openings in the atrial septum, leading to abnormal blood flow between the atria. Placing multiple occluders in such cases requires precise navigation and positioning within each defect, which can be

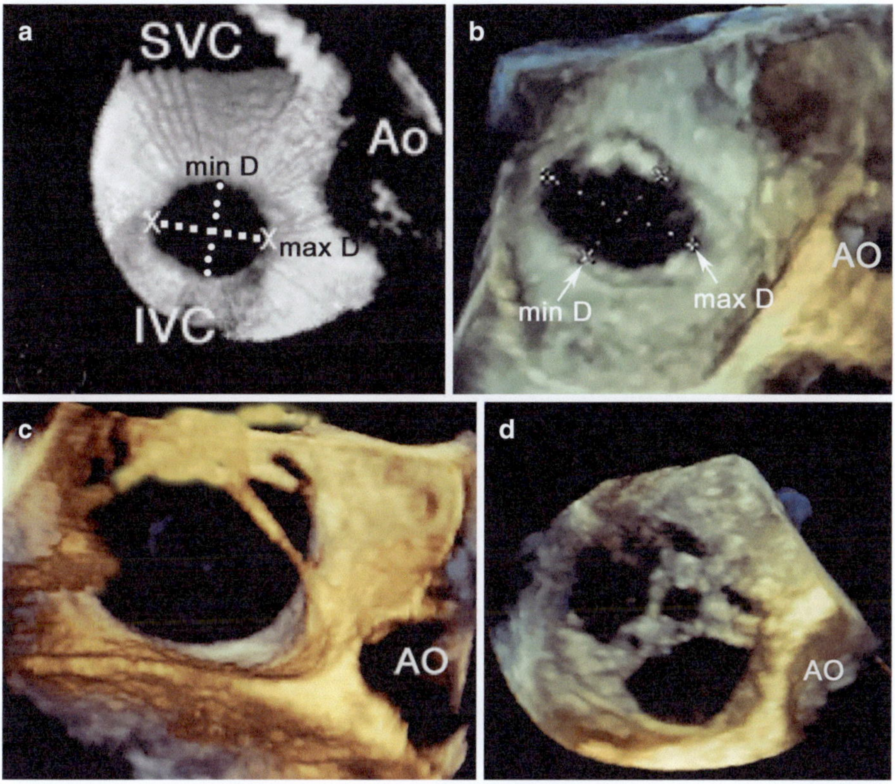

Fig. 8.12 Evaluation of the morphology and diameter of the ASD [maximum (MAX) and minimum (MIN) diameters] on a 3D TEE image. 3D TEE of ASD morphology depicts four common shapes in **a**, **b**, **c**, and **d**. (**a**) Round shape of the ASD as determined by visual analysis or circular Index (MAX D/MIN D) less than 1.3. (**b**) Oval shape of the ASD as determined by visual analysis or circular index (MAX D/MIN D) greater than 1.3. (**c**) An irregular shape of the ASD, characterized by thin and flexible rims. (**d**) An ASD with multiple fenestrations

challenging when the defects are in close proximity or complex in nature. Ensuring proper positioning is crucial to achieve effective sealing without residual shunting, as shown in Fig. 8.17. However, deploying multiple occluders in close proximity carries the risk of device interaction, such as interference, entanglement, or displacement [12–14], as depicted in Fig. 8.18.

However, the cribriform septal occluder is specifically designed to address the management of multiple moderate-sized atrial septal defects (ASDs) with multiple fenestrations. It provides an alternative approach to the conventional single-device closure method, as detailed in Fig. 8.19.

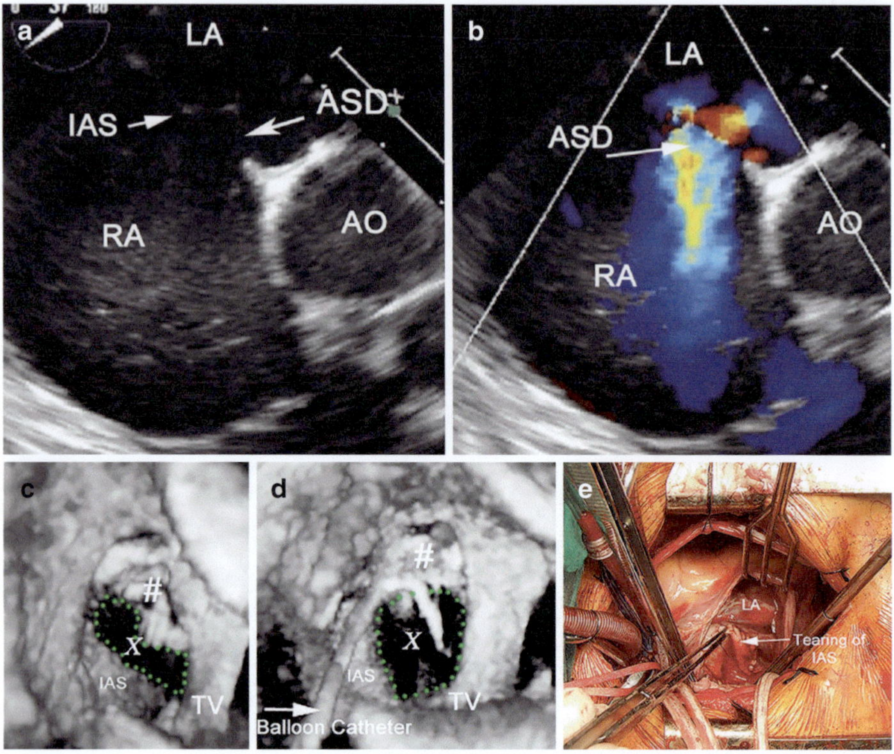

Fig. 8.13 Atrial septal tear due to balloon overstretch during device closure of atrial septal defect (ASD) in a patient with a thin and supple atrial rim. (**a**) Pre-procedural TEE in ME AV SAX reveals dilation of right atrium, an ASD with an attenuated superior-anterior (SA) atrial rim, and an extremely thin and pliable posterior atrial septum. (**b**) Color Doppler TEE displays flow in an ASD, with blood flowing from the left-to-right chambers. (**c**) Enface view of the right atrium using 3D TEE reveals an irregularly shaped ASD (X) with a flexible posterior-inferior rim (#). (**d**) 3D TEE image after balloon sizing reveals an enlarged ASD (X) measuring 40 mm, caused by tearing of the flexible posterior-inferior rim (#) due to the sizing balloon. (**e**) Intraoperative photo depicts tearing of the atrial septum toward the inferior vena cava

7. Isolated Unroofed Coronary Sinus ASD.

   Isolated unroofed coronary sinus ASD (CS-ASD) is a rare type of atrial septal defect where there is a communication between the roof of the coronary sinus and the left atrium. This occurs due to a partial or complete absence of the coronary sinus septum [19, 20]. Surgical closure is currently the preferred treatment option for such defects. Figure 8.20 discusses the successful percutaneous transcatheter closure of an isolated CS-ASD without persistent left superior vena cava using an Amplatzer Septal Occluder in a child.

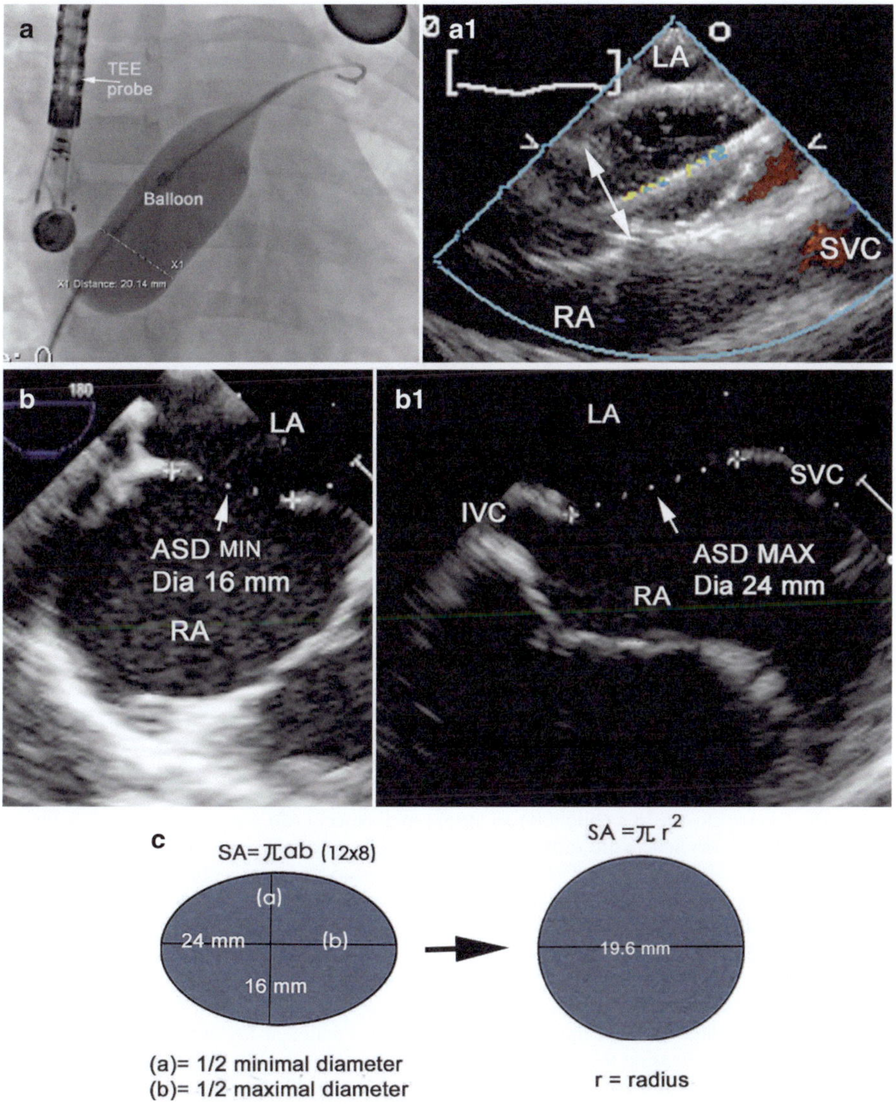

Fig. 8.14 Measurement of ASD diameter without the use of balloon sizing. (**a**) Stretched balloon sizing (BS) is crucial during a transcatheter closure of an ASD and has long been regarded as the gold standard for selecting the appropriate size of the device. (**a**1) A two-dimensional TEE is used to guide the stretched balloon sizing during the catheterization procedure. The view ensures that there is no residual shunt across the septum, while the balloon is fully inflated in the left atrium. By pulling the balloon back against the atrial septum, it helps to prevent over- or under-estimation of the sizing. ASD diameter measurement using 2D TEE multiplanar at different angles in **b** and **b1**. (**b**) In the four-chamber view, the measurement of the minimum diameter (MIN) of the ASD is 16 mm. (**b1**) In the bicaval view, the measurement of the maximum diameter (MAX) of the ASD is 24 mm. (**c**) To accurately size the occluder without the use of balloon sizing. The oval-shaped ASD's size is converted into a circular-shaped occluder using the surface area (SA) equation. The final waist diameter of the occluder is 19.6 mm (2*r*), which is used to select the device size in this case

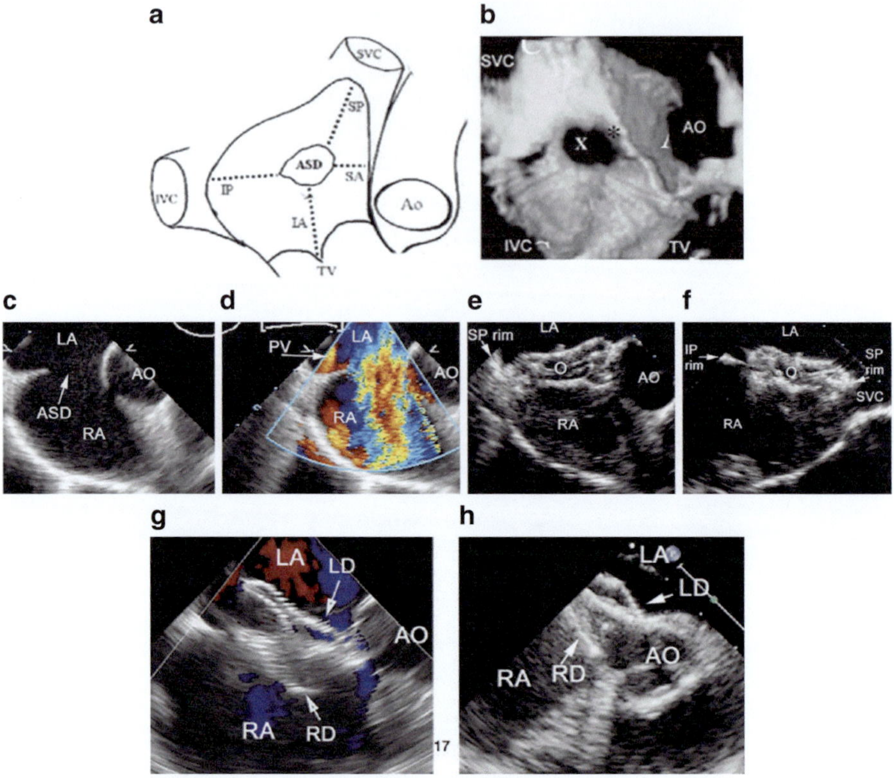

Fig. 8.15 Device closure in a child with an atrial septal defect (ASD) and an attenuated anterior-superior (SA) rim. (**a**) Schematic showing an ASD with four normal septal rims. (**b**) Enface view of the right atrium (RA) using 3D TEE displays an attenuated SA atrial septal rim (*) between the ASD (X) and the aorta (AO). (**c**) Pre-procedural TEE in the ME AV SAX view reveals an atrial defect between the left and right atria with a deficient SA rim. (**d**) Color Doppler TEE in a similar view displays a large left-to-right blood flow. (**e**) After implantation of the Amplatzer septal occluder (O), with both disks of the occluder splayed and secured on the aortic locus. (**f**) Bicaval view displays the occluder (O) in a good position within the defect. Furthermore, acute complications of malpositioned occluder during ASD closure with deficient SA atrial rim, requiring re-implantation before releasing the occluder in **g** and **h**. (**g**) Both the left disk (LD) and right disk (RD) of the occluder are not splayed and are not secured to the aorta. (**h**) Disk edges of the occluder are impacting the aortic locus (arrows) during device closure

8. Large ASD with Pulmonary Hypertension.

   The transcatheter closure of a large atrial septal defect (ASD) can be a complex procedure [15, 16], especially when pulmonary hypertension is present. It is crucial to temporarily occlude the defect with a balloon during balloon sizing to assess the pulmonary artery pressures. This step is essential in determining whether the closure will effectively reduce pulmonary hypertension. In patients with severe pulmonary hypertension, it is feasible to perform transcatheter closure using a homemade fenestrated ASD [17], as depicted in Figs. 8.21 and 8.22.

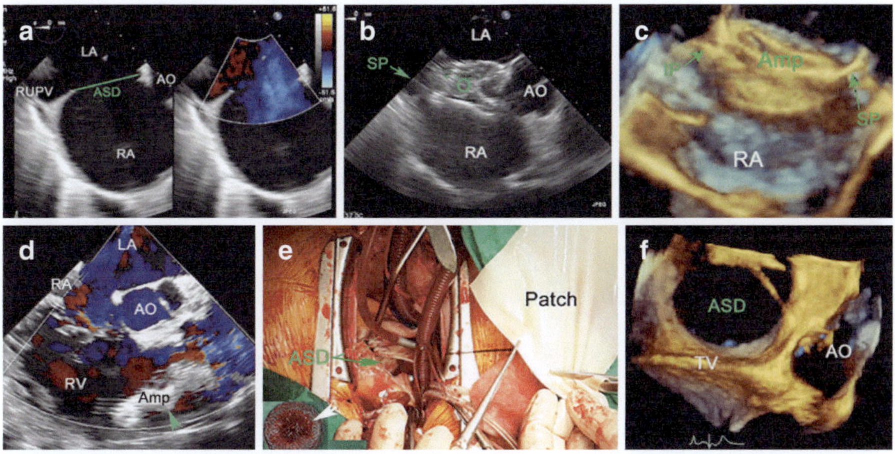

Fig. 8.16 A 14-year-old boy underwent closure of an atrial septal defect (ASD) with a 32-mm Amplatzer device. The device was successfully implanted and embolized to the right ventricular outflow tract the following day. (**a**) During the procedure, TEE in the ME AV SAX view showed a 28-mm diameter secundum ASD with a deficient superior-anterior (SA) rim. A left-to-right shunt was detected using color Doppler in the right diagram. (**b**) Similar plane to **a** after a 32-mm Amplatzer device was successfully deployed. The aortic locus and the superior-posterior (SP) rim were captured and well positioned between by the right and left disks. (**c**) A 3D TEE image in the bicaval view after device implantation showed the device securely in place in both the superior-posterior (SP) rim and inferior-posterior (IP) rim. (**d**) One day after the procedure, the Amplatzer septal occluder (Amp) was embolized in the right ventricular outflow tract (RVOT) as shown on the TEE (indicated by the green arrowhead). (**e**) Intraoperative photograph shows a large atrial septal defect (ASD). The occluder was successfully removed (seen in the left lower small diagram with a white arrow) and repaired surgically using a patch. (**f**) Pre-procedural 3D TEE was reviewed, revealing the presence of a thin and unstable superior-posterior rim, which may result in loosing and dislodge after device implantation

In patients with pulmonary hypertension and a preexisting homemade fenestrated ASD occluder with partial obstruction, a vascular stent was inserted through an Amplatzer™ ASD closure device [18]. This deployment aimed to enable shunt patency, if necessary, as shown in Fig. 8.23.

9. Complications Commonly Associated with Device Closure of ASD [21, 22].

   Common complications associated with ASD device closure include device-related issues such as device embolization (when the device dislodges and moves to a different location within the heart or blood vessels), device malposition, device causing cardiac erosion (rare), and device-related thrombosis. These complications are discussed in Figs. 8.15, 8.16, and 8.24.

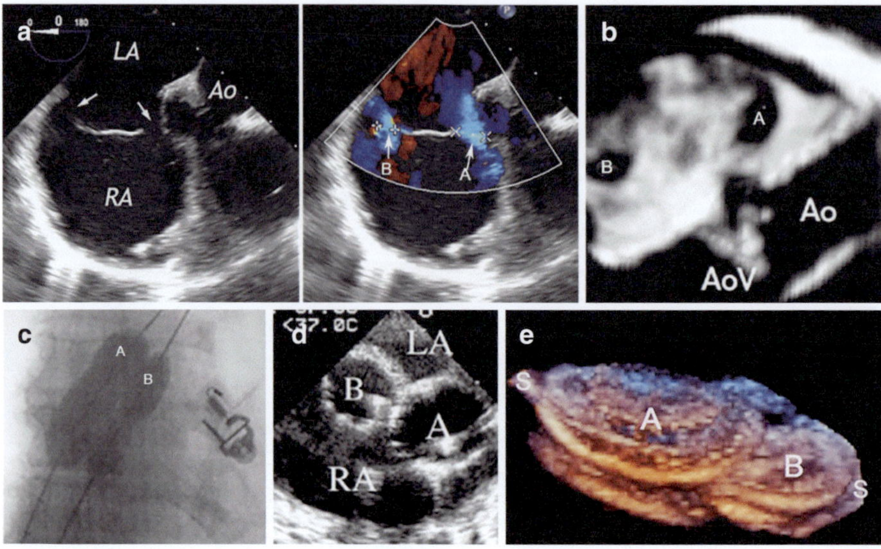

Fig. 8.17 A 6-year-old girl weighing 25 kg underwent closure of multiple atrial septal defects (ASDs) using an Amplatzer device. (**a**) Pre-procedural color Doppler TEE image in the ME AV SUX view displays two ASDs with diameters of 4 mm (B) and 8 mm (A). The distance between the two ASDs is 13 mm. The color Doppler flow image depicts left-to-right shunting flow in the right diagram, indicative of the two ASDs. (**b**) Three-dimensional TEE image in the right atrium (RA) enface view depicts two secundum ASDs, labeled B and A, with diameters of 4 and 8 mm, respectively. (**c**) First defect was occluded using a balloon, which enabled the cannulation of the second defect. Both defects were then simultaneously inflated with balloons. (**d**) TEE guidance was used to size the balloons for the two defects (A and B) to assess any residual flow. The balloon waist was used to determine the appropriate size of the device. (**e**) Three-dimensional TEE image displays two devices (A and B) that have been interleaved after deployment, appearing sandwiched in relation to the septum (S)

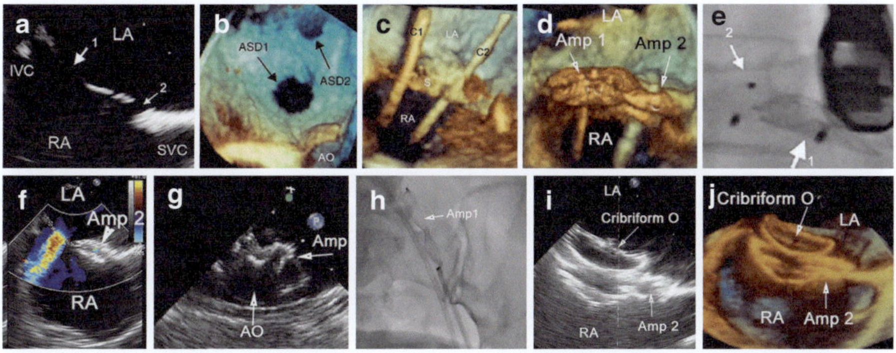

Fig. 8.18 Multiple atrial septal defects (ASDs) were closed using two devices. One of the occluders became embolized and was successfully retrieved percutaneously and re-implanted with another one Amplatzer cribriform occluder. (**a**) Pre-procedural 2D TEE in the bicaval view reveals two secundum ASDs. The first ASD (1) is 8 mm in size and located inferiorly, while the second ASD (2) is 5 mm in size and located superiorly. (**b**) A 3D TEE enface view of the right atrium (RA) shows two ASDs, ASD1 is round and 8 mm in size, and ASD2 is rather ovoid with 5 mm in size. The distance between the two ASDs is 12 mm. (**c**) 3D TEE enface image displays two delivery catheters (C1 and C2) passing through the two separate defects from the RA to the left atrium (LA). (**d**) 3D TEE enface image depicts two ASD occluders (Amp1–12 mm and Amp2–8 mm) deployed successfully and are securely positioned in place. (**e**) Fluoroscopic imaging displays the two occluders in their final proper position, interleaved after being released. (**f**) Upon final check using TEE, the image revealed that the Amp2 occluder remained in place, but Amp1 occluder had disappeared. (**g**) TEE image in the UE DAo LAX view shows that the Amp1 occluder has embolized into the descending aorta (AO). (**h**) Fluoroscopic image demonstrates the retrieval of the device using a 20 mm gooseneck snare with a large sheath at the level of the left iliac artery. The device was successfully caught and brought back into the sheath. (**i**) TEE image after re-implantation of ASD1 shows that it was successfully done using a 25-mm cribriform Amplatzer occluder, which was fully clamped with the Amp2 occluder. (**j**) 3D TEE image displays the final position of the two occluders, appearing sandwiched together after being wiggled and released

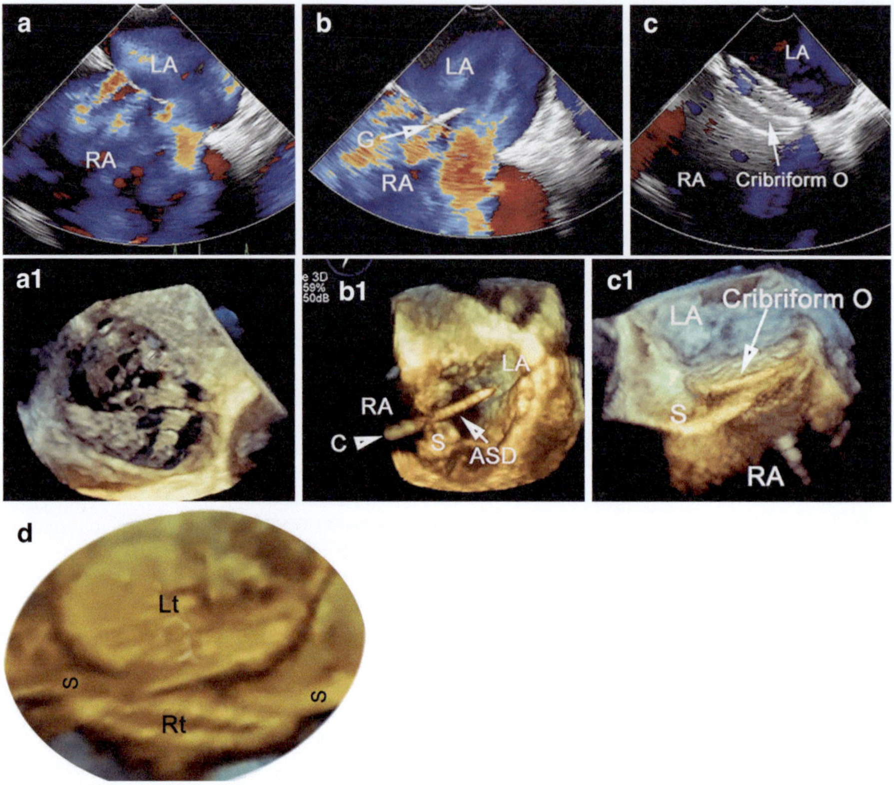

Fig. 8.19 Closure of a fenestrated ASD device in a 16-year-old girl, guided by 2D and corresponding 3D TEE, using a single cribriform occluder. (**a** and **a1**) Pre-procedural TEE with color Doppler in the ME AV SAX view shows a multifenestrated ASD with four openings and dilation of the right atrium (RA) with an aneurysmal atrial septum. (**b** and **b1**) TEE in the same view displays the device catheter (C) crossing the targeted central defect. (**c** and **c1**) A 25-mm cribriform septal occluder (O) was deployed and released successfully. The 2D TEE image shows only a trivial residual leak within the perimeter of the device. (**d**) A 3D TEE imaging model of the Amplatzer cribriform multifenestrated septal occluder shows that it is a non-self-centered device with a small, narrow waist and large atrial disks to cover multiple fenestrations

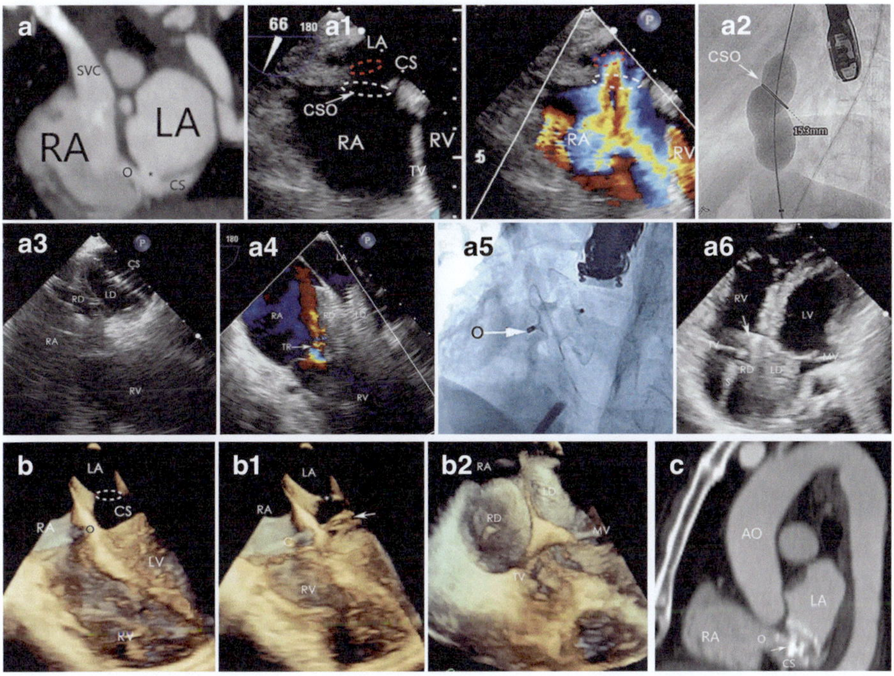

Fig. 8.20 Device closure of an isolated unroofed coronary sinus type atrial septal defect (ASD) in a 1-year-old boy. (**a**) Contrast-enhanced cardiac CT scan in an oblique-coronal image reveals that the coronary sinus (CS) is unroofed only in the terminal portion, measuring 6 mm in diameter (indicated by the asterisk). There is no persistent left superior vena cava. (Note: "O" refers to the ostium of the coronary sinus). (**a1**) A 2D TEE in the ME four-chamber view at 66 degrees shows a dilated right atrium (RA) and right ventricle (RV). Blood is flowing from the left atrium (LA) to the dilated coronary sinus (CS) through a defect in the CS (indicated by the red dotted circle) and then into the RA and RV (on the right diagram). (Note: CSO refers to the ostium of the coronary sinus). (**a2**) Fluoroscopic image shows the balloon sizing of the ostium of the coronary sinus (CSO) with a size of 15.3 mm. (**a3**) 2D TEE in the ME four-chamber view shows the successful deployment and release of the occluder (30 mm Lifetech Scientific CeraFlex ASD occluder) at the CSO. (**a4**) A color Doppler image reveals mild tricuspid regurgitation (TR) after device deployment without evidence of residual hunting. (**a5**) A fluoroscopic image shows the final position of the occluder after release. (**a6**) Post-procedural 2D transthoracic echocardiography in the apical four-chamber view reveals the right disk of the occluder impinges the tricuspid valve (TV) during diastole (indicated by arrow), resulting in mild tricuspid regurgitation (TR) after occluder implantation. (**b**) Pre-procedural 3D TEE image in the four-chamber view displays a defect, represented by the white dotted circle, in the CS region between the LA and the dilated CS. This indicates that the CS has a small unroofed defect. (**b1**) A delivery catheter (C) passed through the CSO from the RA into the CS and began to deploy the left disk of the occluder (arrow), which was clearly viewed on the 3D TEE. (**b2**) Two disks of the Lifetech Scientific CeraFlex ASD occluder (30 mm, LT-ASDf-30) were both deployed and securely positioned at the ostium of the CS, as demonstrated in the 3D TEE image. (**c**) After the procedure, a cardiac CT was performed with an oblique-sagittal view, which revealed that the occluder (arrow) was effectively closing the roof defect located at the terminal CS at the ostium position

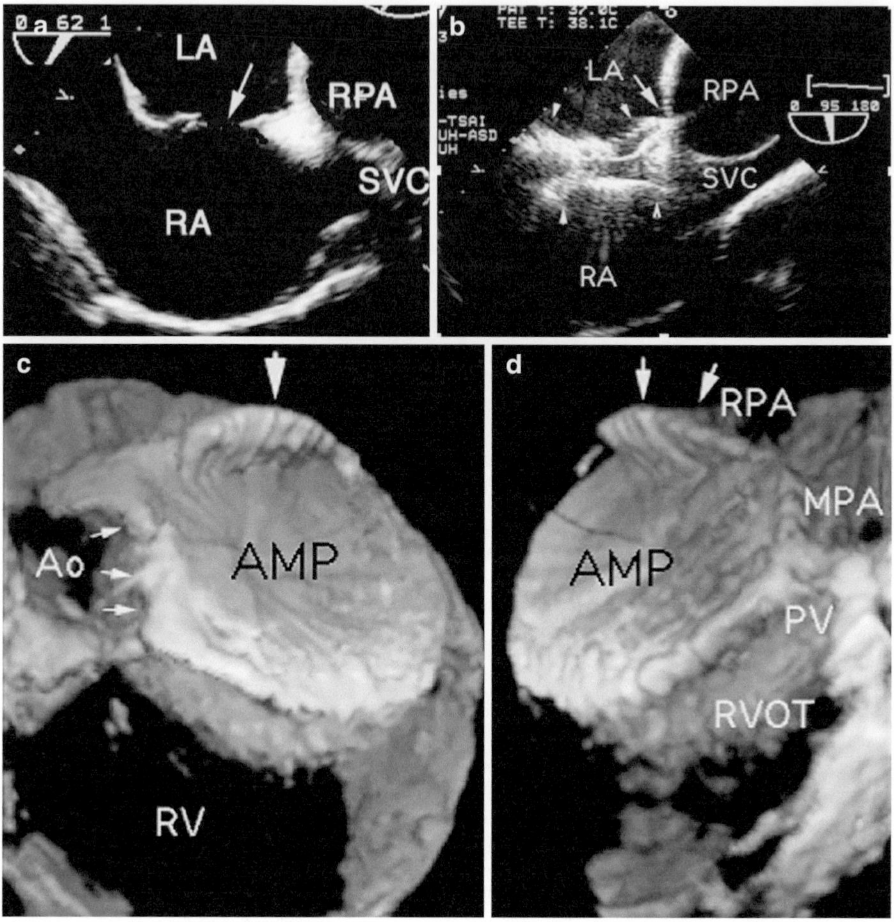

Fig. 8.21 A 17-year-old male patient with an atrial septal defect (ASD) and a right pulmonary artery (RPA) aneurysm who underwent a device closure procedure. (**a**) Pre-procedural 2D TEE image in the bicaval view displays a secundum ASD, indicated by the arrow, with a diameter of 14 mm. This defect is associated with a large RPA aneurysm. (**b**) A 16-mm Amplatzer septal occluder was deployed. The post-procedural 2D TEE image in a similar view shows the occluder in proper position but the left disk impinges against the RPA, as indicated by the arrow. (**c**) 3D TEE image in an enface view of the left atrium (LA) reveals that the left disk of the Amplatzer occluder (AMP) has a partially deformed edge, as indicated by the arrow. (**d**) The 3D TEE in an oblique enface view of the LA displays that the left disk of the AMP has a partially deformed edge, as indicated by the arrow. This is due to compression from the RPA aneurysm, which is demonstrated by the arrows

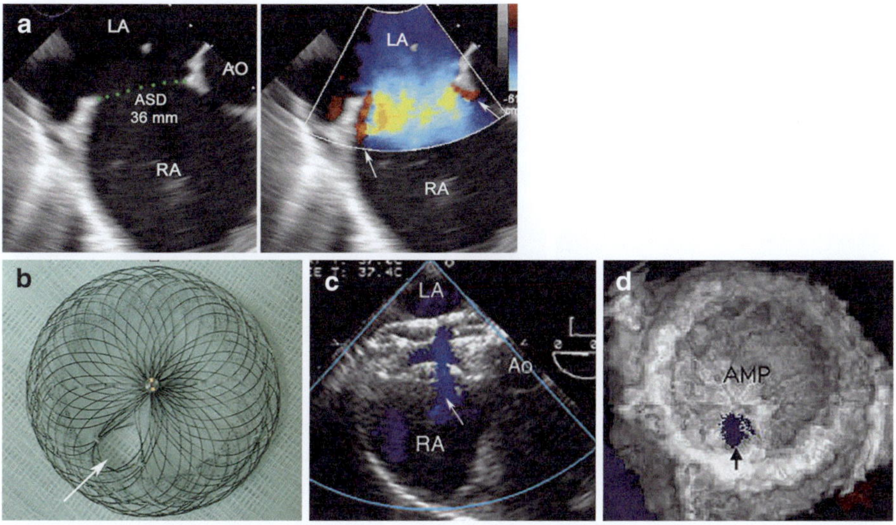

Fig. 8.22 A large atrial septal defect (ASD) with pulmonary hypertension underwent device closure using a homemade, fenestrated septal occluder. (**a**) Pre-procedural 2D TEE with color Doppler in the ME four-chamber view shows a dilated right atrium and a 36 mm diameter secundum ASD with a huge bidirectional shunting (arrows) on the right diagram. (**b**) A photograph shows a 38-mm Amplatzer septal occluder with a 6-mm homemade fenestrated hole (arrow). (**c**) A left-to-right shunting through the homemade fenestrated hole (arrow) is seen on the 2D TEE. (**d**) 3D TEE after device deployment shows complete closure of the ASD with a mild intra-occluder shunting (black arrow) through the homemade fenestrated hole in the peripheral of this occluder

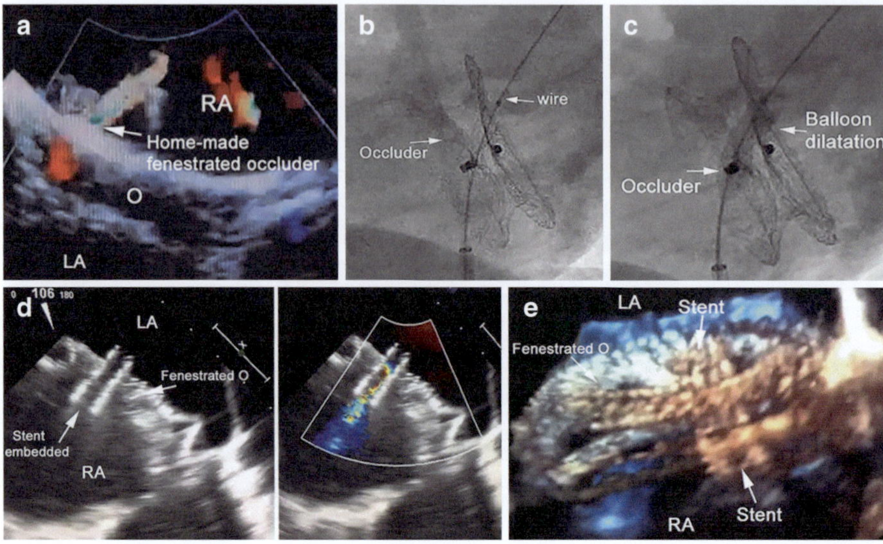

Fig. 8.23 A stent-embedded fenestrated septal occluder used in a child with a persistent pulmonary hypertension. (**a**) A 2D TEE with color Doppler demonstrates narrowing of the fenestration hole in a homemade fenestrated Amplatzer occluder used to treat a preexisting atrial septal defect (ASD) with persistent pulmonary hypertension. (**b**) Fluoroscopic imaging depicts the insertion of a guidewire across the fenestrated hole of the Amplatzer septal occluder. (**c**) Fluoroscopic imaging depicts the use of a balloon to dilate and size the fenestrated hole. (**d**) A 2D TEE in the bicaval view shows a vascular stent deployed across the occluder device via a shuttle sheath. The fenestrated hole was enlarged by an embedded stent, resulting in a left-to-right shunt (on the right diagram). (**e**) 3D TEE with color Doppler shows that the stent-embedded septal occluder is well positioned (Fenestrated O: Fenestrated Occluder)

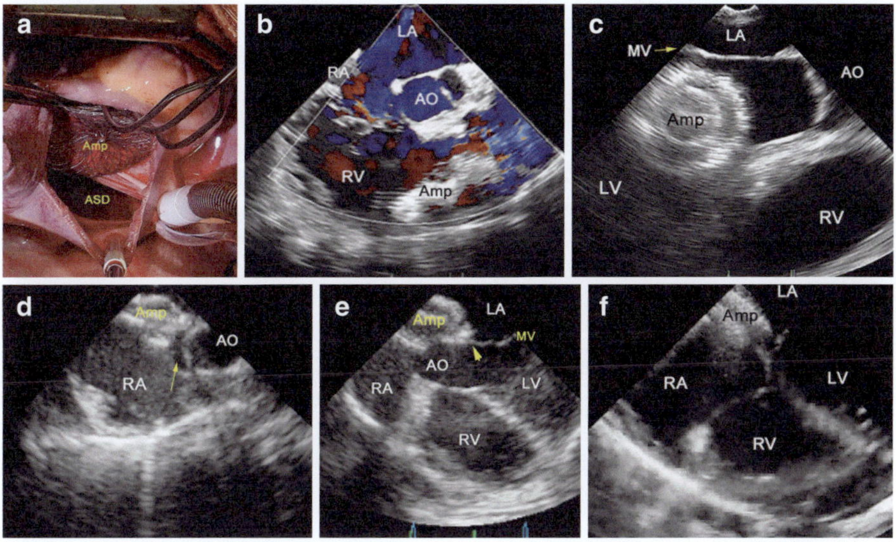

Fig. 8.24 Complications commonly associated with device closure of atrial septal defects (ASD). (**a**) Surgical photograph shows the embolization of the device before the surgical removal and patch repair of the ASD. (**b**) TEE image shows an Amplatzer septal occluder (Amp) that has embolized into the right ventricular outflow tract and protruded into roof of pulmonary valves. (**c**) TEE image depicts an Amplatzer septal occluder (Amp) that has become dislodged and partially embolized in the left ventricular outflow. (**d**) TEE image reveals a periaortic hematoma (thin yellow arrow) following the deployment of the device that tightly impinges on the aortic locus. (**e**) TEE image displays the impingement of the mitral valve (short yellow arrow) after the deployment of the Amplatzer device (Amp). (**f**) TEE image illustrates the Amplatzer device (Amp) resting on the anterior-inferior rim, leading to heart block

References

1. Wang JK, Tsai SK, Wu MH, et al. Short- and intermediate-term results transcatheter closure of atrial septal defect with the Amplatzer Septal Occluder. Am Heart J. 2004;148:511–7.
2. Thomson JDR, Aburawi EN, watterson KG, et al. Surgical and transcatheter (Amplatzer) closure of atrial septal defects: a prospective comparison of results and cost. Heart. 2002;87:466–9.
3. Hayes N, Rosenthal E. Tulip malformation of the left atrial disc in the Lifetech Cera ASD device: a novel complication of percutaneous ASD closure. Catheter Cardiovasc Interv. 2012;79(4):675–7.

4. Butera G, Carminati M, Chessa M, et al. CardioSeal/Starflex versus Amplatzer devices for percutaneous closure of small to moderate (up to 18mm) atrial septal defects. Am Heart J. 2004;148:507–10.
5. Hascoet S, Hadeed K, Marchal P, et al. The relation between atrial defect shape, diameter, and area using three-dimensional transoesophageal echocardiography and balloon sizing during percutaneous closure in children. Eur Heart J Cardiovasc Imaging. 2015;16:747–55.
6. Carlson KM, Justino H, O'Brien RE, et al. Transcatheter atrial septal defect closure: modified balloon sizing technique to avoid overstretching the defect and oversizing the Amplatzer septal occluder. Catheter Cardiovasc Interv. 2005;66:390–6.
7. Hascoet S, Hadeed K, Marchal P, et al. The relation between atrial defect shape, diameter, and area using three-dimensional transesophageal echocardiography and balloon sizing during percutaneous closure in children. Eur Heart J Cardiovasc Imaging. 2015;16:747–55.
8. Wang JK, Tsai SK, Lin SM, et al. Transcatheter closure of atrial septal defect without balloon sizing. Catheter Cardiovasc Interv. 2007;71:214–21.
9. Ackermann S, Quandt D, Hagenbuch N, et al. Transcatheter atrial septal defect closure in children with and without fluoroscopy: a comparison. J Interv Cardiol. 2019:1–9.
10. Lin SM, Tsai SK, Wang JK. Supplementing transesophageal echocardiography with transthoracic echocardiography for monitoring transcatheter closure of atrial septal defects with attenuated anterior rim: a case series. Anesth Analg. 2003;96:1584–8.
11. Huang CF, Fang CY, Ko SF, et al. Transcatheter closure of atrial septal defects with superior-anterior rim deficiency using Amplatzer Septal Occluder. J Formos Med Assoc. 2007;106:986–91.
12. Tillman T, Mulingtapang, R, Sullebarger JT. Approach to percutaneous closure in patients with multiple atrial septal defects. J Invasive Cardiol. 2008;20:E167–E170.
13. Cao Q, Radtke W, Berger F, et al. Transcatheter closure of multiple atrial septal defects. Initial results and value of two- and three-dimensional transesophageal echocardiography. Eur Heart J. 2000;21:941–7.
14. Teoh K, Wilton E, Brecker S, Jahangiri M. Simultaneous removal of an Amplatzer device from an atrial septal defect and the descending aorta. J Thorac Cardiovasc Surg. 2006;131:909–10.
15. Yong G, Khairy P, De Guise P, et al. Pulmonary arterial hypertension in patients with transcatheter closure of secundum atrial septal defects: a longitudinal study. Circ Cardiovasc Interv. 2009;2(5):455–62.
16. Dell'avvocata F, Rigatelli G, Paolo Cardaioli P, et al. Home-made fenestrated Amplatzer occluder for atrial septal defect and pulmonary arterial hypertension. J Geriatr Cardiol 2011;8(2):127–9.
17. Kamali H, Saritas T, Erdem A, et al. Percutaneous closure of large ASD using a home-made fenestrated atrial septal occluder in 18-year-old with pulmonary hypertension. BMC Cardiovasc Disord. 2014;14:74.

18. Yadlapati A, Wax D, Rich S, et al. Novel shunt modification with an adjustable stent-embedded fenestrated septal occluder in a patient with pulmonary hypertension. Catheter Cardiovasc Interv. 2019;93:1382–4.
19. Chungsomprasong P, Durongpisitkul K. Transcatheter closure of coronary sinus atrial septal defect. World J Cardiol. 2014;6:499–503.
20. Panos A, Walsh KP, McGiffin, et al. Transcatheter occlusion of an isolated coronary sinus atrial septal defect. JACC Cardiovasc Interv. 2012;5(9):e19–20.
21. Spence MS, Qureshi. Complications of transcatheter closure of atrial septal defects. Heart. 2005;91:1512–4.
22. Jalal ZJ, Hascoet S, Baruteau AL, et al. Long-term complications after transcatheter atrial septal defect closure: a review of the medical literature. Can J Cardiol. 2016;32:1315e11–e18.

8.4 Transcatheter Closure of Ventricular Septal Defect (VSD)

Ventricular septal defect (VSD) is the most common congenital heart defect and can be categorized as perimembranous, inlet, muscular, and outlet types, according to location of defect within the septum (as depicted in Sect. 3.2). Traditionally, VSDs were closed surgically, which was associated with morbidity and mortality. However, transcatheter closure of VSDs are considered an appropriate treatment option for certain cases. The specific indications for transcatheter VSD closure may vary based on individual patient factors.

Currently, transcatheter techniques have become successful in closing many VSDs, serving as an established alternative to surgical repair [1–4]. The first reported transcatheter closure of VSD took place in 1988, performed by Lock et al. Over time, numerous devices and techniques have been developed, enhancing the potential for routine device closure of VSDs. However, complex VSDs with certain characteristics may not be suitable for transcatheter closure. These characteristics include VSDs that are too large or have complex anatomy, making it challenging to effectively place and secure a transcatheter device. Additionally, VSDs located in specific areas of the heart, such as near the aortic or pulmonary valves, may not be amenable to transcatheter closure due to the risk of interfering with valve function. Furthermore, VSDs accompanied by severe pulmonary hypertension and irreversible pulmonary vascular disease may also preclude transcatheter closure. In such cases, surgical closure remains the preferred treatment option.

8.4.1 Catheterization Procedure

The closure of ventricular septal defects (VSDs) through transcatheter procedures can be performed using two techniques: the antegrade approach and the retrograde approach. The antegrade approach (Fig. 8.25) involves advancing the catheter and device from the right side of the heart to the left ventricle, and it is commonly used

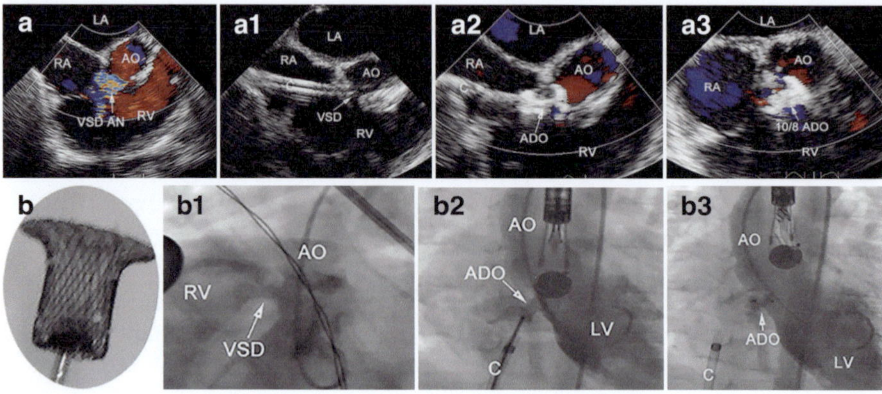

Fig. 8.25 Antegrade percutaneous closure of a perimembranous ventricular septal defect (VSD) using fluoroscopy and transesophageal echocardiography (TEE) imaging together. (**a**) A pre-procedural TEE with color Doppler in the ME AV SAX view reveals a 3 mm perimembranous VSD with left-to-right shunting. In step **a1**, the catheter is seen positioned across the VSD from the right ventricle side. In step **a2**, the left disk of the Amplatzer ductal occluder (ADO 10/8) is shown deploying away from the aortic valve cusp. In step **a3**, the final proper positioning of the device without any residual shunting is displayed. (**b**) A photograph depicts the ADO. In step **b1**, a fluoroscopic image of a left ventricular angiogram shows a VSD indicated by an arrow. In step **b2**, the ADO device is shown deployed. In step **b3**, the final position of the device (ADO) is displayed after it has been released

for perimembranous and muscular VSDs (Fig. 8.25). On the other hand, the retrograde approach (Fig. 8.29) entails advancing the catheter and device from the aorta to the right ventricle, and it is typically employed for subarterial VSDs using ADOII or multifunctional occluder device (MF-Konar).

An arteriovenous (AV) loop is created by passing a guidewire through the VSD and snaring the wire. A long sheath is then advanced to the LV through the AV loop and positioned below the aortic valve. The VSD occluder is deployed through the long sheath with the guidance of fluoroscopy and TEE (Fig. 8.26).

8.4.2 Device Used

Transcatheter closure of a VSD increases additional challenges compared to ASD closure. VSDs are located in close proximity to the heart's valves and conduction. This makes VSD closure technically more challenging. Positioning and stabilizing the device within the ventricular septum can be more challenging than placing a device in the interatrial septum for ASD closure.

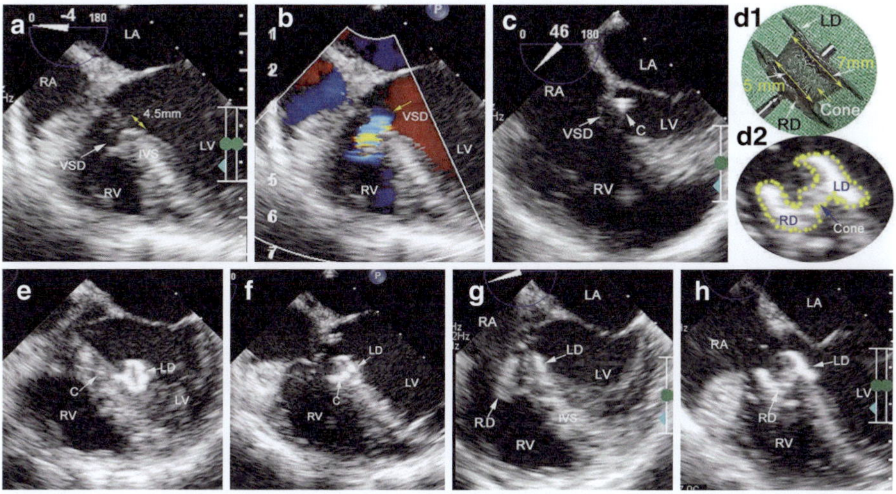

Fig. 8.26 Retrograde percutaneous closure of a perimembrane VSD (pmVSD) in a 5-year-old child using a symmetrical VSD occluder. (**a**) TEE imaging displays a pmVSD with a size of 4.5 mm (LV side) in the four-chamber view. (**b**) Same view with color Doppler displays a left-to-right shunting. (**c**) After creating an AV loop, the four-chamber view shows the delivery sheath (**c**) being introduced into the LV across the defect. (**d1**) Photograph and magnified TEE (**d2**) images of the 5/7 mm Lifetech Konar-MFO symmetrical VSD occluder (a self-expanding double-disk device with a cone-shaped waist). (**e**) LV left disk (LD) of the 5/7-mm Konar-MFO VSD occluder was deployed. (**f**) Left disk (LD) anchoring the ventricular septum is shown in the five-chamber view after pulling back. (**g**) Right disk (RD) is deployed in a good position prior to release. (**h**) Final image in the five-chamber view displays good device positioning

VSD closure devices may have different designs and mechanisms, but they are generally designed to provide a similar function of closing the VSD through a transcatheter approach. The selection of the appropriate device depends on various factors, including the size, location, and anatomy of the VSD.

1. Duct occluders (St, Jude Medical, St. Paul, MN) for pmVSD closure were initially introduced by Hieu in 2002. These devices, including the first-generation Amplatzer™ ductal occluder (ADO) [6, 7] and the second-generation Amplatzer™ ductal occluder (ADO II) [8], are designed to be soft and lack occlusive fabric, facilitating their delivery through small catheters. Both the ADO (Fig. 8.27) and ADO II (Figs. 8.28 and 8.31) are considered safe and attractive options for this procedure. It is recommended to maintain a minimum distance of 3 mm between the defect and the aortic valve when using either the ADO or ADO II, with the device size selected being 1 to 2 mm larger than the defect diameter.
2. Symmetric occluder [9] (Lifetech Scientific, Shenzhen, China; Starway Medical, Beijing, China) (as shown in Fig. 8.26d1, d2) is a new self-expanding double-disk device with a cone-shaped waist and selected device size was 1–2 mm larger than the defect diameter, as shown in Figs. 8.26, 8.29, 8.33, and 8.34.

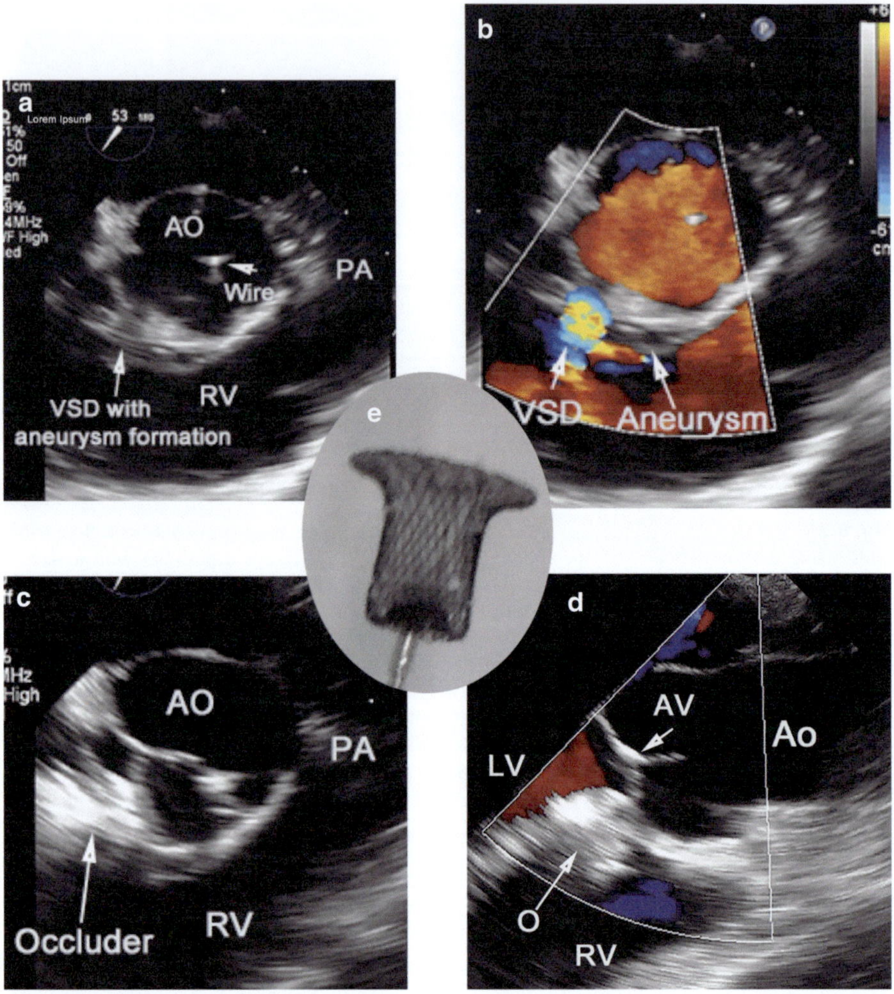

Fig. 8.27 Closure of a perimembranous ventricular septal defect (VSD) in a 6-year-old boy using an Amplatzer duct occluder (ADO) device. (**a**) TEE in the ME AV SAX view displays a VSD with an aneurysm formation measuring 3 mm in diameter on the left ventricular side. (**b**) Color Doppler shows an aneurysm formation with left-to-right shunting. (**c**) In the TEE ME AV SAX view, the deployment of a 5 mm ADO for closure of a VSD is displayed. (**d**) TEE with color Doppler in the ME AV LAX view displays proper deployment of the occluder (O) without any residual shunting. (**e**) Photograph of the ADO

3. The eccentric occluder [10] (Shanghai Shape Memory Alloy, Shanghai, China) features a modified double-disc design. Specifically, the aortic flange of the left disc does not extend beyond the waist, while the opposite flange extends 6 mm beyond the waist (as illustrated in Fig. 8.32b). In this particular case, the distance between the ventricular septal defect and the aortic valve needed to be less than

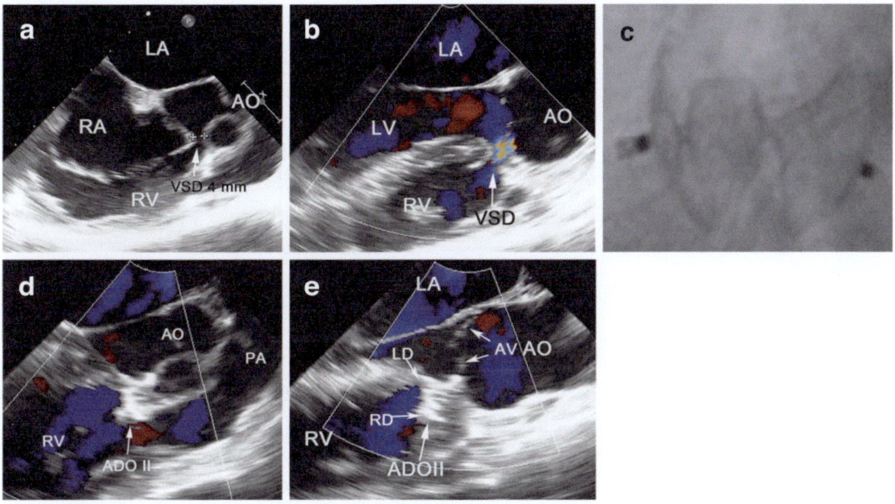

Fig. 8.28 Perimembranous VSD closed in a 16-year-old boy using the Amplatzer ductal occluder II (ADO II). (**a**) Pre-procedural TEE in the ME AV SAX view displays a tiny VSD with a diameter of 4 mm. (**b**) TEE color Doppler in the ME AV LAX view displays a flow across this tiny VSD with a small left-to-right shunting. (**c**) Fluoroscopy image shows the ADO II, a self-expanding nitinol mesh device with two retention disks connected by a waist on either side of the duct. (**d**) TEE in the ME AV SAX view immediately after successful deployment of a 6 × 4 mm ADOII shows the occluder well-seated on the septum without any residual shunting. (**e**) Post-procedural TEE in the ME AV LAX view shows both retention disks aligned with the septum without interfering with the aortic valve (AV). (*LD* left disk, *RD* right disk)

2 mm, and a device size 2–4 mm larger than the defect diameter was selected (as depicted in Fig. 8.32).

4. Amplatzer muscular VSD occluder is a self-expanding, double-disk device made from nitinol wire mesh and designed to facilitate occlusion of muscular VSDs that occur post-myocardial infarction. The 7 mm waist length is designed to accommodate the thickness of the muscular ventricular septal wall as shown in Fig. 8.35.

8.4.3 Transcatheter Closure of Outlet VSD

Perimembranous VSD (pmVSD) accounts for approximately 70% of all VSD cases in asian population. Transcatheter device closure of pmVSD has been widely performed with acceptable mortality and morbidity rates, as depicted in Figs. 8.25, 8.26, 8.27, 8.28, 8.29 and 8.30. On the other hand, outlet VSD can be further classified as muscular outlet VSD and doubly committed (DC) subarterial VSD. Previously, the outlet type of VSD was considered unsuitable for device closure. However, transcatheter closure of outlet VSD in selected children has been proven to be a safe and successful procedure, resulting in good medium- and long-term outcomes [11,

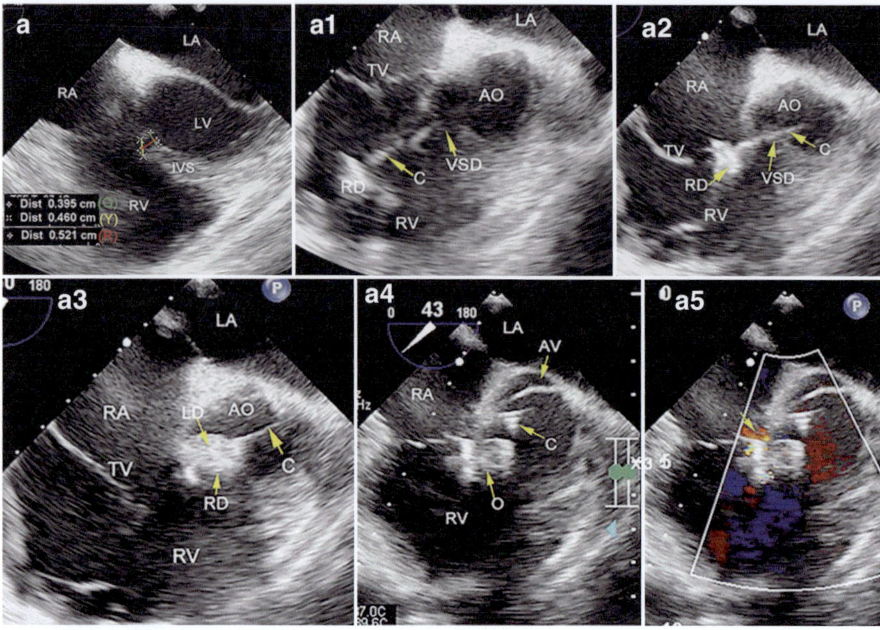

Fig. 8.29 Retrograde percutaneous closure of perimembranous VSD in a child using the Konar-MFO occluder without requiring snaring or exteriorizing a guidewire to form an arteriovenous loop. The closure device was placed directly. TEE shows the procedure steps in the ME AV SAX view (**a**–**a5**) in a 4-year-old boy and ME LAX view (**b**–**b6**) in a 7-year-old girl. (**a**) Appearance of the defect. (**a1**) The catheter is passed through the defect into the RV, and the right disk (RD; 7 × 5 mm Konar-MFO) is deployed. (**a2**) The delivery catheter and RD are pulled back to against on the ventricular septum. (**a3**) The appearance of the left disk (LD) while the RD unfolds. (**a4**, **a5**) The final appearance of the device after release, without residual shunting. (**b**) Defect was measured and (**b1**, **b2**) a wire (yellow arrows) and delivery catheter were passed through the defect into the right ventricle. (**b3**, **b4**) The 7 × 5 mm Konar-MFO occluder's RD was deployed and anchored to the ventricular septum. (**b5**, **b6**) The final image showed the deployed device in a proper position without any residual shunting

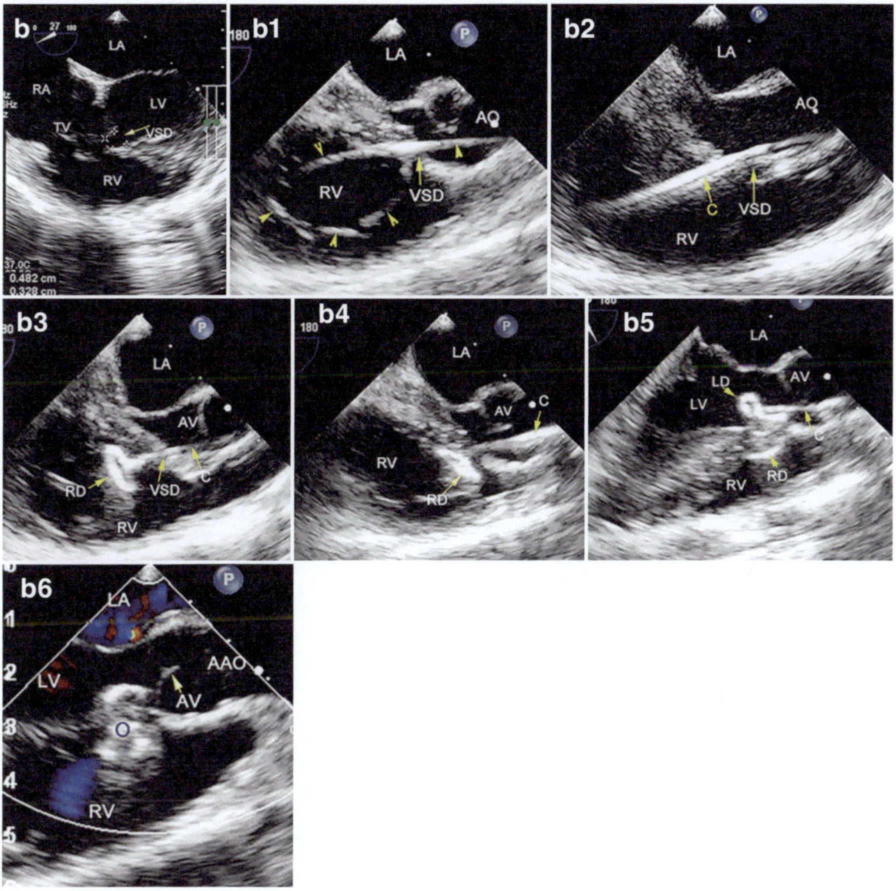

Fig. 8.29 (continued)

12]. The transcatheter approach provides a promising alternative to traditional surgical repair for outlet VSD, as shown in Fig. 8.31, which illustrates the closure of outlet VSD using the ADOII device. Additionally, Fig. 8.32 demonstrates the closure of outlet VSD with an eccentric device, Fig. 8.33 depicts the closure of doubly committed VSD using the Konar-MFO device, and Fig. 8.34 (Videos 8.1, 8.2, 8.3 and 8.4) depicts the closure of doubly committed VSD with aortic valve prolapse using the Konar-MFO device.

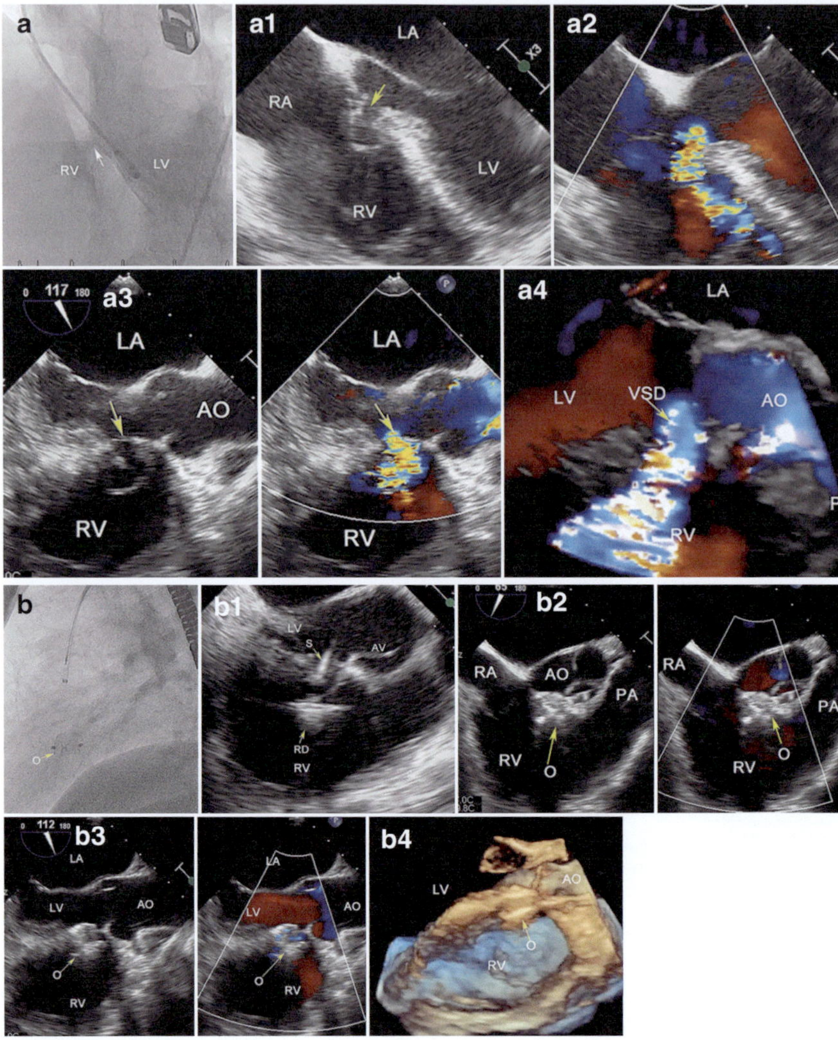

Fig. 8.30 A large perimembranous ventricular septal defect (VSD) with aneurysmal transformation in a child who underwent device closure. (**a**) A pre-procedural left ventriculogram displays a 6.5 mm perimembranous VSD indicated by the arrow. (**a1**) A pre-procedural TEE in the five-chamber view displays the perimembranous VSD with an aneurysm formation (indicated by the arrow). (**a2**) The five-chamber view with color Doppler at the subaortic level displays left-to-right shunting. (**a3**) The ME AV LAX view shows the perimembranous VSD (indicated by the arrow) with aneurysm formation. The color Doppler demonstrates the VSD (indicated by the arrow) with a left-to-right shunting in the right diagram. (**a4**) The pre-procedural 3D TEE color image displays VSD jet flow from the left ventricle to the right ventricle. (**b**) Post-procedural left ventriculography displays the device (Lifetech Scientific KONAR-MF 9-mm VSD occluder, indicated by "O") in proper position after release. (**b1**) The right ventricular disk (RD, indicated by the arrow) was deployed retrogradely from the left ventricle across the defect to the right ventricle. (**b2**) The ME AV SAX view demonstrates that both disks have been released. The color Doppler image displays no residual shunt with trivial aortic regurgitation. (**b3**) The ME AV LAX view displays the device (indicated by "O") well seated with minor residual in the right diagram. (**b4**) The post-procedural 3D TEE reconstruction image shows good positioning and configuration of the device (indicated by "O") after deployment

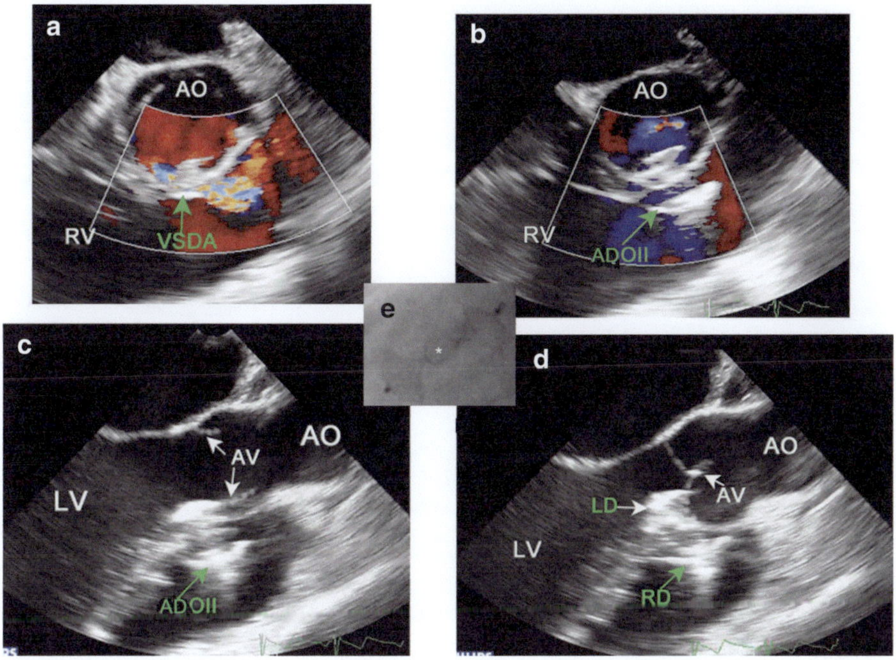

Fig. 8.31 A 12-year-old child who underwent device closure for an outlet ventricular septal defect (VSD) using an Amplatzer duct occluder (ADO) II occluder. (**a**) Pre-procedural "TEE with color Doppler in the ME AV SUX view" depicts an outlet type VSD with an aneurysm (VSDA) and prolapse of the aortic valve. (**b**) After deploying the ADOII occluder, the TEE with color Doppler in ME AV SAX view displays the correct placement of the occluder (ADO II) without any residual shunting. (**c**) TEE in the ME AV LAX view during systole displays the final position of the occluder (ADO II) without any interference with the opening of the aortic valve (AV). (**d**) TEE in the ME AV LAX view during diastole displays the appropriate placement of the occluder (ADO II) without hindering the closure of the aortic valve (AV). (**e**) Fluoroscopy image shows the ADO II occluder, which is a self-expanding nitinol wire with a central lobe (*) and two retention disks on either side of the central lobe

8.4.4 Transcatheter Closure of Muscular VSD

Congenital muscular VSD is characterized by an abnormal opening in the muscular wall (ventricular septum), which can be single or multiple. Acquired muscular VSDs are usually caused by trauma or myocardial infarction. The traditional treatment for muscular VSD is surgical closure, although transcatheter closure is increasingly being undertaken [13–15]. The Amplatzer muscular VSD occluder (AGA Medical Corporation, Golden Valley, Minnesota) has been proven safe and effective for closing muscular VSDs. The transcatheter closure of muscular VSD is depicted in Fig. 8.35, while post-infarction VSD is discussed in Fig. 8.36, and muscular outlet type VSD is discussed in Fig. 8.37.

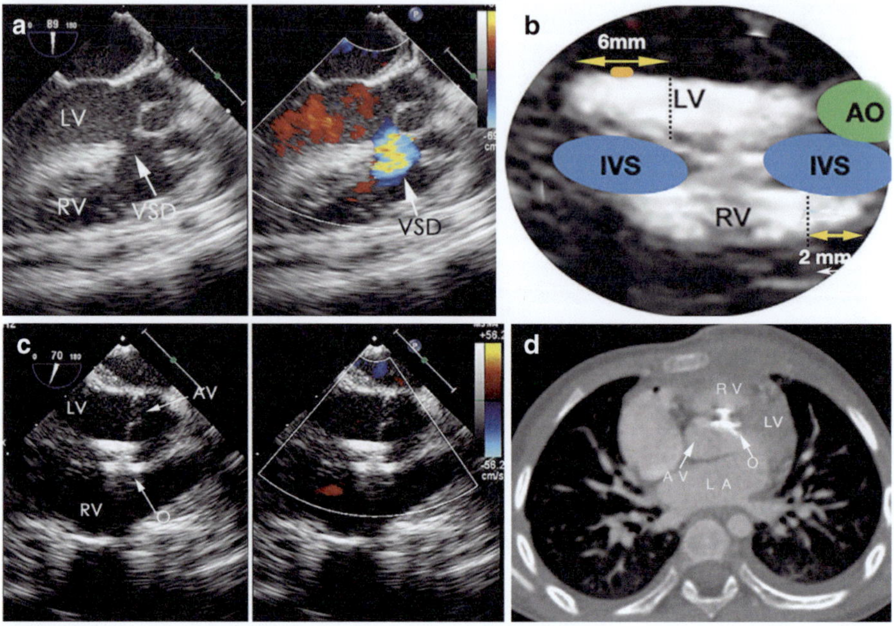

Fig. 8.32 Zero Rim Eccentric ventricular septal defect (VSD) occluder for closure of an outlet VSD in a 3-year-old child. (**a**) Pre-procedural "TEE in the ME AV LAX" displays an outlet VSD with a diameter of 4 mm. There is left-to-right shunting visible in the color flow across the VSD (right diagram). (**b**) Magnified TEE image shows that the Zero Rim Eccentric VSD occluder (Lifetech Scientific in Shenzhen, China) has a modified double-disk design, where the aortic flange of the left disk extends 0 mm beyond the waist, while the opposite flange extends 6 mm beyond the waist. (**c**) After the deployment of the Zero Rim Eccentric VSD occluder (O), the TEE with color Doppler in the ME AV LAX view displays the occluder properly seated and no residual shunting or aortic regurgitation is visible (right diagram). (**d**) Post-procedural chest cardiac CT scans display the eccentric disks properly aligned with the septum and without any interference with the aortic valve (AO) after the deployment. (The statement with permission obtained from Prof. Haibo Song, West China Hospital, Sichuan University)

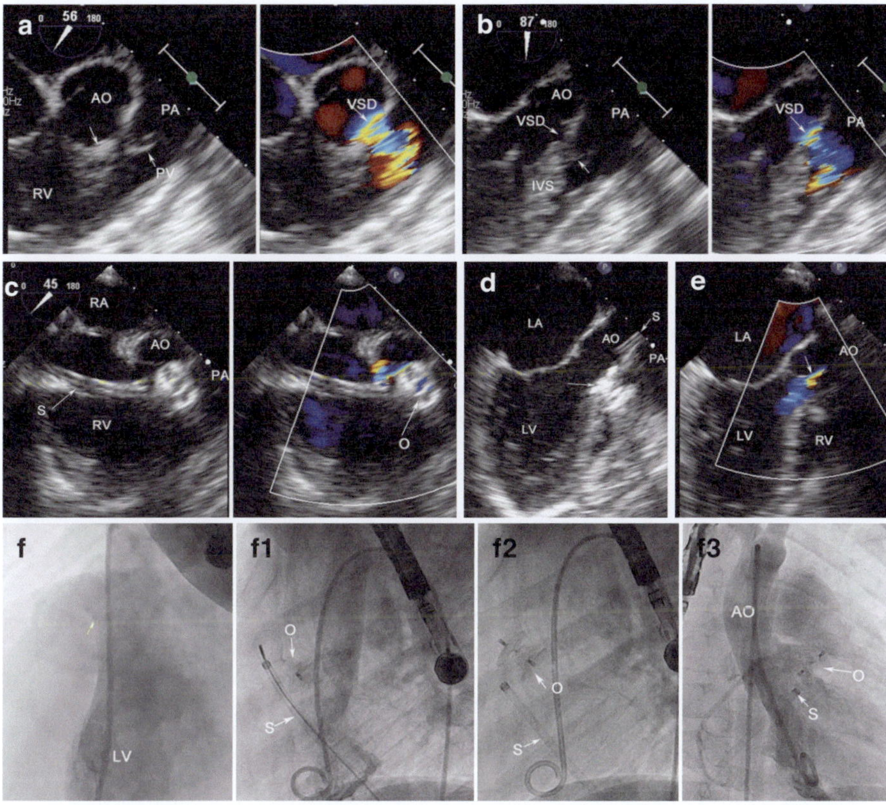

Fig. 8.33 A 3-year-old girl with a doubly committed subarterial ventricular septal defect (dcSA-VSD) that was closed using a device. (**a**, **b**) Pre-procedural transesophageal echocardiogram (TEE) with color Doppler imaging (**a**, **b**) shows a ventricular septal defect (VSD) with prolapse of the aortic valve (arrow). The arterial valves are almost at the same level with fibrous continuity. Right diagram color images show turbulent flow from the aorta to the pulmonary artery (PA). TEE with color Doppler imaging (**c**, **d**) shows the deployment of a Lifetech Scientic KONAR-MF 8-mm occluder (O) via the delivery sheath (S). The trivial aortic regurgitation (arrow) is shown in the ME AV LAX view of the TEE (**e**) after the occluder was deployed. The left ventriculograms during procedure depicts the device closure of the dcSA-VSD are from **f** to **f3**. (**f**) Location of the VSD is indicated by an arrow and measures 5.3 mm in size. (**f1**) Both disks of the occluder have been deployed. (**f2**) The occluder after being released. (**f3**) The final position of the occluder

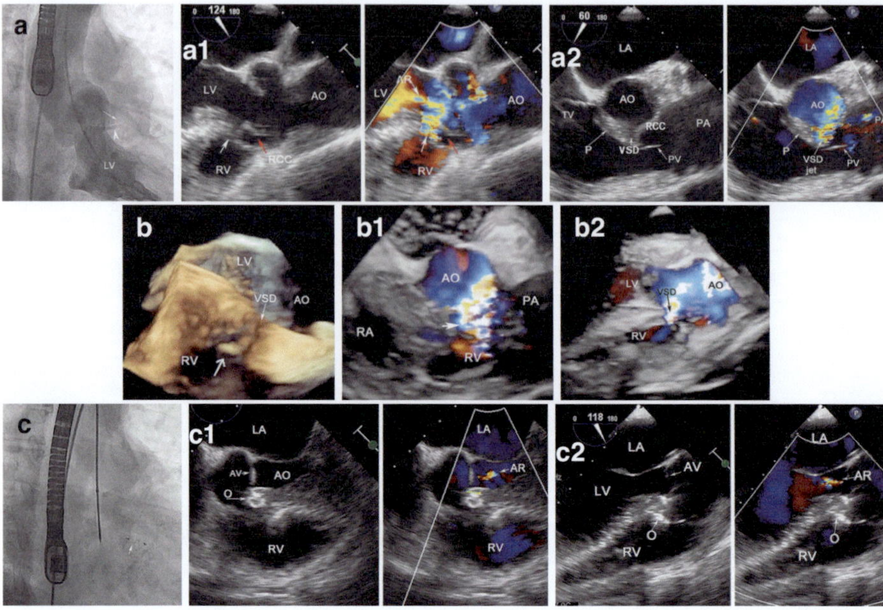

Fig. 8.34 A child diagnosed with a doubly committed subarterial ventricular septal defect (dcSA-VSD) along with aortic valve prolapse and aortic regurgitation, who underwent transcatheter device closure. (**a**) Pre-procedural left ventriculography demonstrates a small ventricular septal defect (VSD) jet (arrowhead) and a severe right coronary cusp prolapse (arrow). (**a1**) Pre-procedural TEE with color Doppler in ME AV LAX shows aortic regurgitation (AR) and right coronary cusp prolapse (red arrow). The native VSD (white arrow) size is 12 mm, and the jet width is 3.5 mm. A VSD jet (white arrow) flows from the left ventricle through the prolapse aortic valve and is directed toward the right ventricular outflow tract (right diagram). (**a2**) ME AV SUX at 60° shows the prolapse (P) of the right coronary cusp and a small VSD channel and an enlarged pulmonary artery (PA). The color Doppler TEE shows a VSD jet flowing from left to right (right diagram). (**b**) Aortic valve prolapse is visible on the enface right ventricular (RV) view of a 3D transesophageal echocardiography (TEE), as indicated by the arrow. The prolapsed aortic valve obstructs the ventricular septal defect (VSD), resulting in only a narrow channel remaining. (**b1**) A 3D TEE image with color Doppler reveals the prolapse of the aortic valve, along with a small VSD jet (indicated by the white arrow) directed toward the pulmonary artery. (**b2**) The long-axis 3D TEE image with color Doppler demonstrates a small VSD jet causing a left-to-right shunt. (**c**) Post-procedural left ventriculography confirms the successful deployment of the Lifetech Scientific Konar-MF 8-mm VSD occluder. (**c1**) The post-procedural color Doppler TEE in ME AV SAX view shows the securely positioned occluder (O) with only a minor degree of aortic regurgitation (AR) following the release of the device. (**c2**) The ME AV LAX view demonstrates a favorable placement and arrangement of the released occluder (O), with only minimal AR observed in the right diagram (a trivial intraprosthetic residual shunt observed on the video clip). Additionally, Video clips of 8.1, 8.2, 8.3, and 8.4 were added

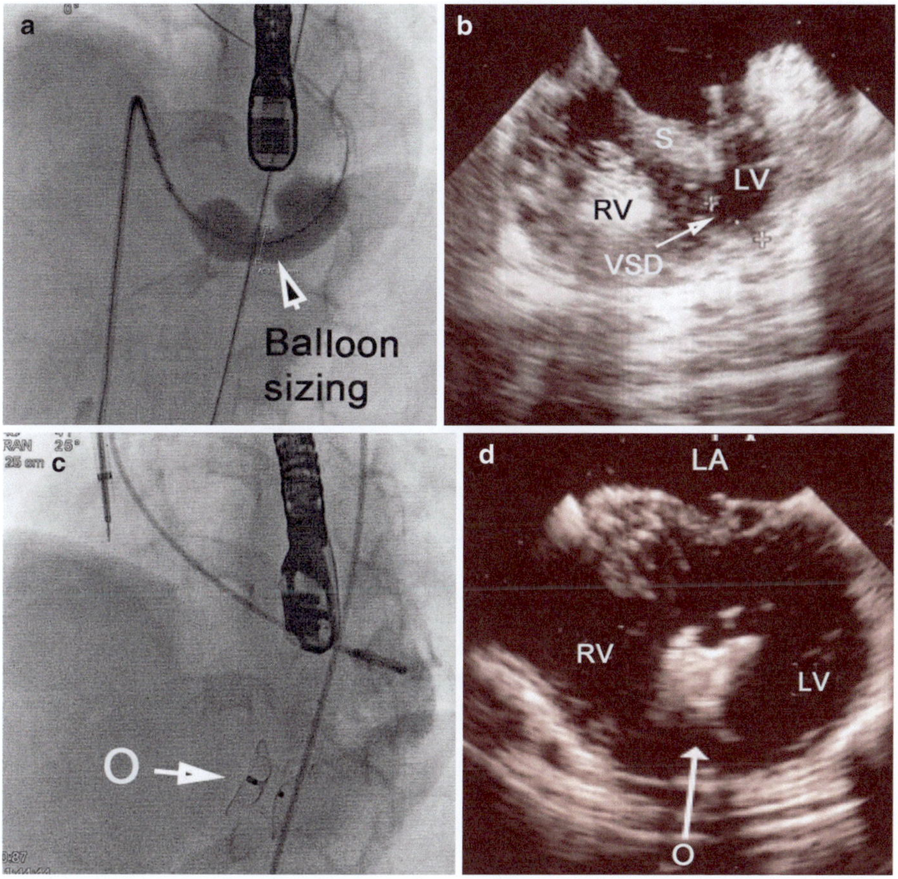

Fig. 8.35 Successful closure of a muscular ventricular septal defect (VSD) in an 8-month-old child using an Amplatzer muscular VSD occluder. (**a**) Pre-procedural fluoroscopic image demonstrates the sizing of the muscular VSD using a balloon, with a diameter of 11 mm. (**b**) Pre-procedural TEE in the ME four-chamber view depicts a muscular VSD with a diameter of 10 mm. (**c**) Post-procedural fluoroscopic image displays the successful deployment of the muscular VSD occluder (O). (**d**) Post-procedural TEE in the ME four-chamber view displays the final location of the occluder (O) in the correct position

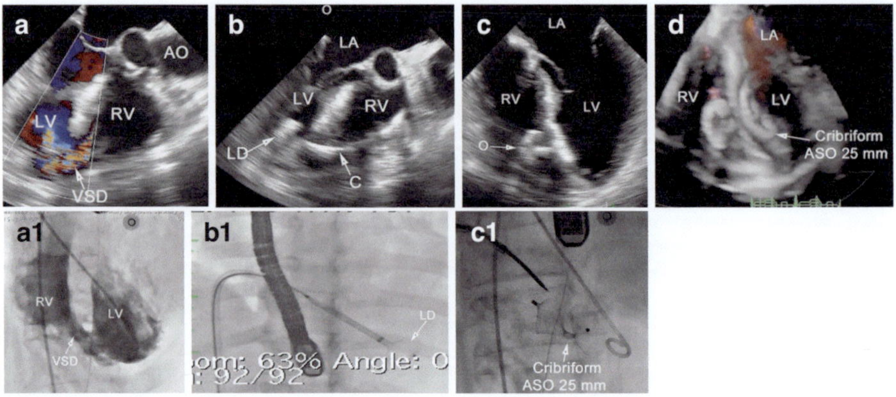

Fig. 8.36 A post-infarction muscular ventricular septal defect (PIVSD) was treated using the Amplatzer cribriform occluder device closure. (**a**) Pre-procedural TEE with color Doppler in the ME AV LAX view revealed a muscular VSD measuring 8 mm in size at the apex region, with a strong turbulent flow crossing from the left ventricle (LV) to the right ventricle (RV). The corresponding fluoroscopic image is shown in **a1**. (**b**) Delivery catheter (C) was passed through the defect from the RV to the LV, and the 25-mm left disk (LD) of the Amplatzer cribriform occluder was deployed. The corresponding fluoroscopic image is shown in **b1**. (**c**) Post-procedural TEE in the ME four-chamber view shows both disks properly anchoring the ventricular septum and in their correct position. The corresponding fluoroscopic image is shown in **c1**. (**d**) Post-procedural 3D TEE with color Doppler imaging demonstrated proper placement of the Amplatzer cribriform occluder with no evidence of residual shunting

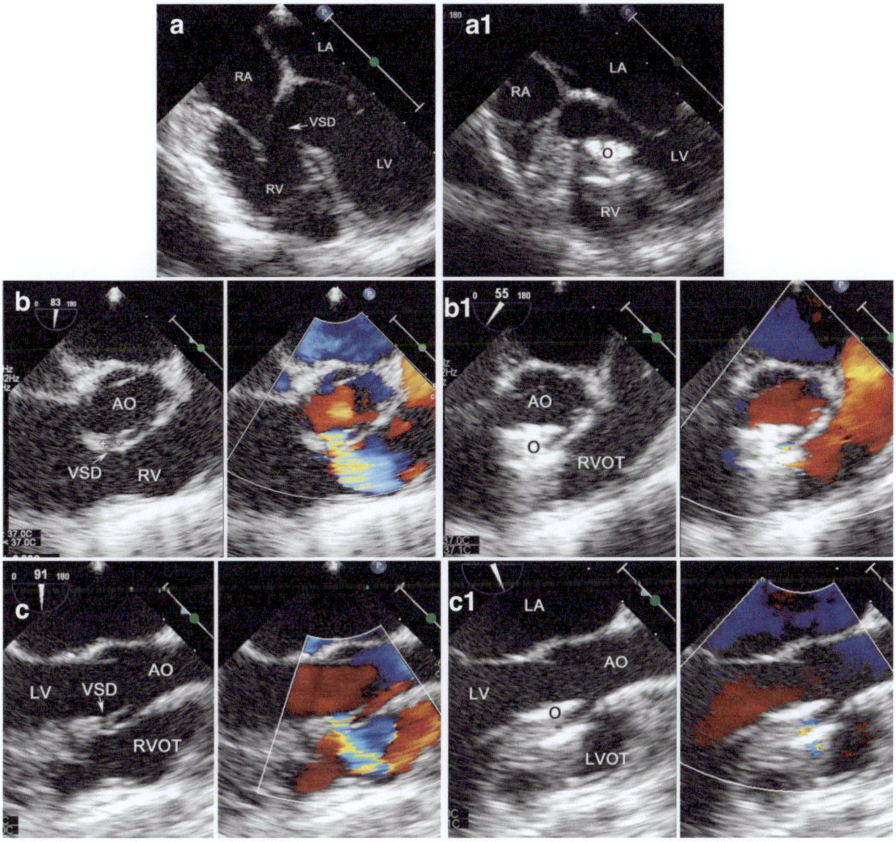

Fig. 8.37 A 5-year-old girl with a ventricular septal defect (VSD) of the muscular outlet type, which was successfully closed using a device. A pre-procedural transesophageal echocardiogram (TEE) with color Doppler imaging was performed. The four-chamber view (**a**) revealed a muscular outlet VSD. The ME AV SAX view (**b**) showed an outlet VSD with a diameter of 4 mm, prolapse of the aortic valve, and a left-to-right shunt. The ME AV LAX view (**c**) also demonstrated an outlet VSD with aortic valve prolapse. A Lifetech Scientific KONAR-MF 4/6-mm occluder (O) was successfully implanted, as confirmed by post-procedural TEE images obtained in views **a1**, **b1**, and **c1**. These images demonstrated complete closure of the ventricular septal defect (VSD) without any residual shunt or aortic regurgitation

8.4.5 Device-Related Complications

1. Embolization of VSD occluder occurring is approximately 0.9% [16]. This condition is discussed in Fig. 8.38.
2. Aortic regurgitation (AR): The rate of AR following VSD device is approximately 3.3% [16]. Surgery was needed to remove the device and close the defect as discussed in Fig. 8.39.

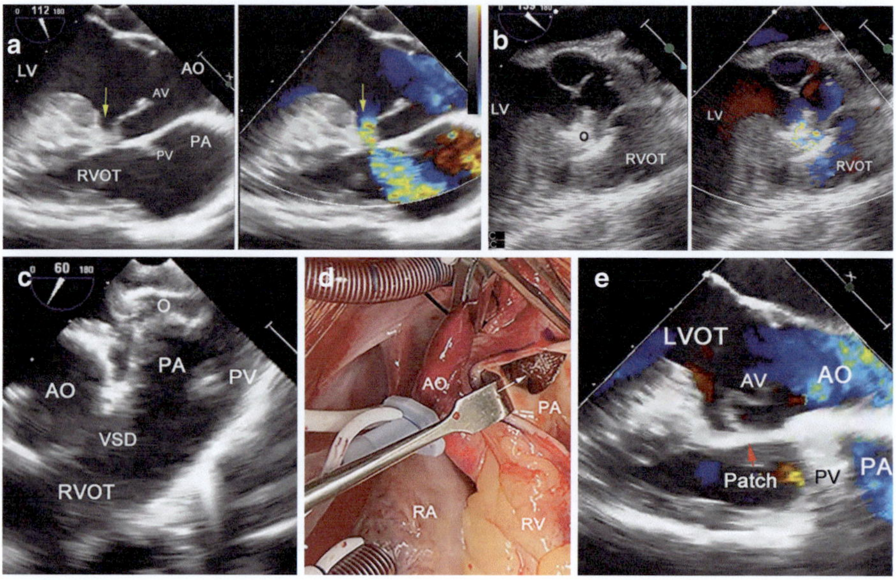

Fig. 8.38 An 8-year-old boy with an outlet VSD and RCC prolapse underwent successful percutaneous device closure. However, the VSD occluder was dislodged the next day and surgical closure of the VSD and removal of the VSD occluder was necessary. The post-operative follow-up was smooth without any complications. (**a**) Pre-procedural TEE with color Doppler, as seen in the ME AV LAX view, displays an outlet VSD with right coronary cusp (RCC) prolapse, indicated by a jet with a width of 5 mm (yellow arrow). (**b**) Post-procedural TEE, viewed from the same perspective, confirms the successful closure of the VSD through the use of the KONAR-MF VSD occluder (O) (LT-MF 8/6 mm), evidenced by minimal residual shunting following deployment. (**c**) On the next day after procedure, TEE imaging shows that the VSD occluder (O) has become dislodged and is situated 1.5 cm above the pulmonary valve (PV). (**d**) The surgical photograph depicts an undamaged VSD occluder (white arrow), seen in close proximity to the pulmonary bifurcation in the main pulmonary artery. (**e**) Post-operative TEE depicts a successful closure of the VSD by a patch after the removal of the dislodged VSD occluder

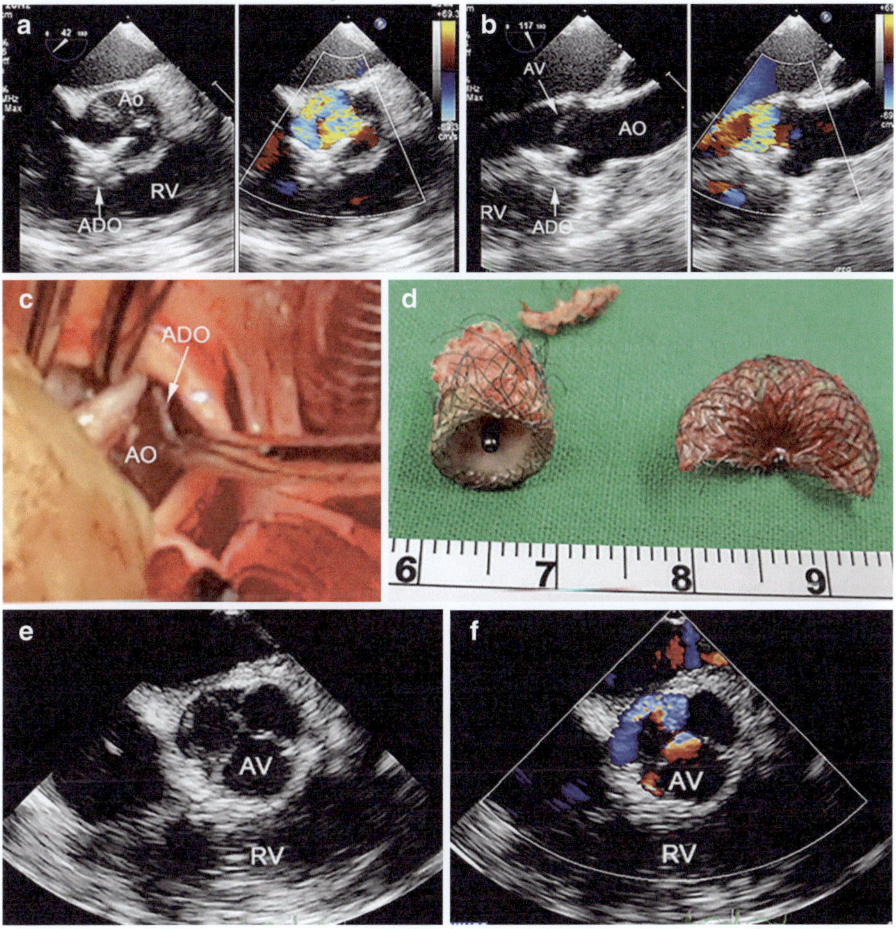

Fig. 8.39 Case of a 6-year-old boy who developed a severe late aortic regurgitation (AR) following a device closure procedure using an Amplatzer ductal occluder (ADO) for perimembranous ventricular septal defect (VSD) at another hospital 10 months prior. He was hospitalized for surgical intervention to remove the device and repair the AR. (**a**) Results of a TEE examination during this admission, showing severe AR following deployment of the ADO occluder (10 × 12 mm). The color Doppler image displays an obvious mosaic flow pattern due to the ADO occluder interferes with the flow through the aortic valve (AO), which creates a prominent turbulence as seen in the ME AV SAX view (right diagram). (**b**) ME AV LAX view demonstrates that the ADO is impinging on the aortic valve, leading to aortic regurgitation as seen in the right diagram. (**c**) Interoperative photograph shows this ADO that is firmly attached to the aortic valve. (**d**) Operative photograph shows the left disk of the occluder being cut off during surgery as it was tightly attached to the LV. (**e**) TEE in the ME AV SAX view depicts the successful surgical repair of the aortic valve. (**f**) Color Doppler TEE in the ME AV SAX view reveals only mild residual AR after surgical repair of the aortic valve (AV)

References

1. Lock JE, Block PC, McKay RG, et al. Transcatheter closure of ventricular septal defects. Circulation. 1988;78:361–8.
2. Butera G, Carminati M, Chessa M, et al. Transcatheter closure of perimembranous ventricular septal defects early and long-term results. J Am Coll Cardiol. 2007;50:1189–95.
3. Carminati M, Butera G, Chessa M. Transcatheter closure of congenital ventricular septal defects: results of the European Registry. Eur Heart J. 2007;28:2361–8.
4. Gu M, You X, Zhao X, et al. Transcatheter device closure of intracristal ventricular septal defects. Am J Cardiol. 2011;107:110–3.
5. Zhou D, Pan W, Guan L, et al. Transcatheter closure of perimembranous and intracristal ventricular septal defects with the SHSMA occluder. Catheter Cardiovasc Interv. 2012;79:666–74.
6. El Said HE, Bratincsak A, Gordon BM, et al. Closure of perimembranous ventricular septal defects with aneurysmal tissue using The Amplatzer Duct Occluder I: Lessons learned and medium term follow up. Catheter Cardiovasc Interv. 2012;80:895–903.
7. Udink Ten Cate FEA, Sobhy R, Kalantre A, et al. Off-label use of duct occluder devices to close hemodynamically significant perimembranous ventricular septal defects: a multicenter experience. Catheter Cardiovasc Interv. 2019;93:82–88.
8. Koneti NR, Sreeram N, Penumatsa RR, et al. Transcatheter retrograde closure of perimembranous ventricular septal defects in children with the Amplatzer Duct Occluder II device. J Am Coll Cardiol. 2012;60:2421–2.
9. Haddad RN, Daou LS, Saliba ZS. Percutaneous closure of restrictive-type perimembranous ventricular septal defect using the new KONAR multifunctional occluder: midterm outcomes of the first middle-eastern experience. Catheter Cardiovasc Interv. 2020;96:E295–E302.
10. Masura J, Gao W, Gavora P, et al. Percutaneous closure of perimembranous ventricular septal defects with the eccentric Amplatzer device: multicenter follow-up study. Pediatr Cardiol. 2005;26(3):216–9.
11. Jiang D, Han B, Zhao L, et al. Transcatheter device closure of perimembranous and intracristal ventricular septal defects in children: medium- and long-term results. J Am Heart Assoc. 2021;10:e02041.
12. Gu M, You X, Zhao X, et al. Transcatheter device closure of intracristal ventricular septal defects. Am J Cardiol. 2011;107:110–3.
13. Thanopoulos BD. Catheter closure of congenital muscular septal defects. Pediatr Cardiol. 2005;26:220–3.
14. Thanopoulos BD, Rigby ML. Outcome of transcatheter closure of muscular ventricular septal defects with the Amplatzer ventricular septal defect occluder. Heart. 2005;91:513–6.
15. Giblett JP, Matetic A, Jenkins D, et al. Post-infarction ventricular septal defect: percutaneous or surgical management in the UK National Registry. Eur Heart J. 2022;43:5020–32.
16. Jortveit J, Leirgul E, Eskedal L, et al. Mortality and complications in 3495 children with isolated ventricular septal defects. Arch Dis Child. 2016;101(9):808–13.

Unusual Shunt and Fistula 9

9.1 Aorta-Right Atrial Tunnel (ARAT)

An aorta-right atrial tunnel, also referred to as an aorto-right atrial fistula, is an abnormal connection between the aorta and the right atrium of the heart. It typically involves an extracardiac vascular channel that starts from one of the sinuses of Valsalva and ends either in the superior vena cava or the right atrium. The tunnel can be classified as anterior or posterior, depending on its position in relation to the ascending aorta. Symptoms of an aorta-right atrial tunnel vary based on its size and orifice, affecting the amount of blood being diverted. Larger tunnels can cause respiratory distress, cyanosis, and congestive heart failure.

Diagnostic tests, such as cardiac catheterization (depicted in Fig. 9.1a) and transesophageal echocardiography (TEE) (depicted in Fig. 9.1b, c), are performed to assess and diagnose an aorta-right atrial tunnel.

The treatment for an aorta-right atrial tunnel typically involves surgical closure or transcatheter closure of the abnormal connection. The details of transcatheter closure are discussed in Fig. 9.1.

Supplementary Information The online version contains supplementary material available at https://doi.org/10.1007/978-981-99-6582-3_9.

S.-K. Tsai et al., *Transesophageal Echocardiography in Pediatric Congenital Cardiac Surgery and Catheter Intervention*, https://doi.org/10.1007/978-981-99-6582-3_9

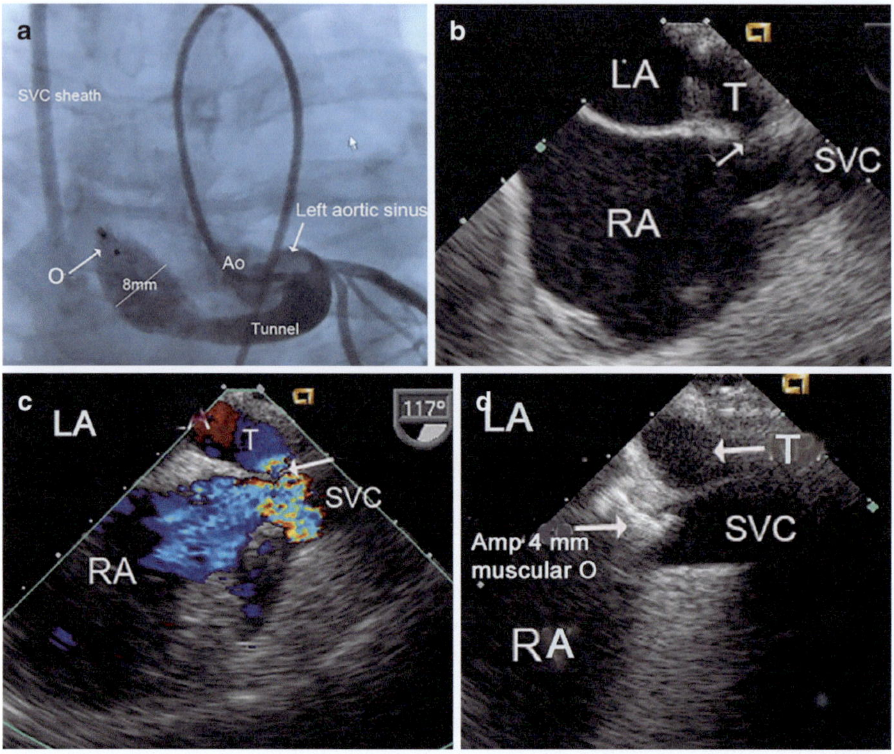

Fig. 9.1 Aorta-right atrial tunnel (A in a 12-year-old child who underwent device closure. (**a**) Cardiac catheterization and angiography revealed a long, tunnel-like structure in the posterior region with an aneurysm. The aneurysm was observed to originate from the left aortic sinus and communicate with the junction between the superior vena cava and the right atrium. A 4-mm Amplatzer muscular ventricular septal defect (VSD) occluder (O) was successfully deployed at the junction of the right atrium (RA) and the superior vena cava (SVC) using a delivery sheath from the SVC. (**b**) Pre-procedural TEE in the bicaval view displaying a posterior tunnel-like structure (T) from the left aortic sinus (not visible in this image) leading into the junction (arrow) between the right atrium (RA) and the superior vena cava (SVC). (**c**) Color image in a similar view demonstrates turbulent flow from the tunnel-like structure (T) into the right atrium (RA) and the superior vena cava (SVC). (**d**) Post-procedural TEE in the bicaval view displays a properly positioned device, the 4-mm Amplatzer muscular occluder, without any residual shunting

References

1. Lee S, Kim SW, Im S II, et al. Aorta-right atrial tunnel is surgical correction mandatory? Circulation. 2016;133:e454–e457.
2. Gajjar T, Voleti C, Matta R, et al. Aorta-right atrial tunnel: clinical presentation, diagnostic criteria, and surgical options. J Thorac Cardiovasc Surg. 2005;130:1287–92.
3. Baykan A, Narin N, Ozyurt A, et al. Aorta-right atrial tunnel closure using the transcatheter technique: a case of a 3-year-old child. Cardiol Young. 2013;23:457–9.

9.2 Ruptured Sinus of Valsalva Aneurysm (RSVA)

The presence of a shunt between the sinus of Valsalva and the cardiac chambers results in a continuous murmur during examination. This left-to-right shunt in the right atrium (RA) is directed toward the center of the tricuspid valve, resembling significant tricuspid regurgitation. The majority of these shunts originate from the right coronary sinus (70% of cases), while the noncoronary sinus accounts for 25% of cases [1, 2]. In cases of rupture, the shunt more commonly develops into the right ventricle (RV) rather than the RA, due to its anatomical proximity to the RV.

Sinus of Valsalva aneurysms can be categorized as congenital or acquired [3]. Acquired aneurysms are linked to causes such as trauma (traumatic sinus of Valsalva [3]), atherosclerosis, and infective endocarditis.

The management of a ruptured sinus of Valsalva aneurysm involves immediate medical intervention, surgical repair, or transcatheter closure. In Fig. 9.2,

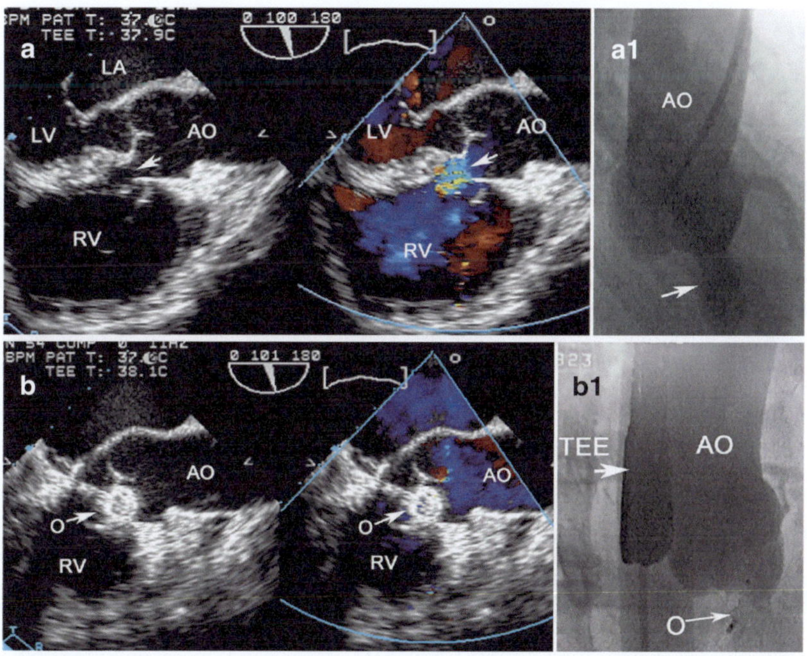

Fig. 9.2 A child underwent device closure with the Amplatzer duct occluder (ADO) for a ruptured sinus of Valsalva aneurysm into the right ventricle (RV). (**a**) A pre-procedural TEE in the ME AV LAX revealed a ruptured aneurysm with an opening of 12 mm in the right coronary sinus. The opening was noted to cause a left-to-right shunt into the right ventricle (RV), as demonstrated by the color Doppler technique. The RV was also noted to be dilated. (**a1**) The aortic root angiogram revealed a ruptured sinus of Valsalva aneurysm, which appeared as a tubular-shaped structure (indicated by the arrow), extending into the right ventricle (RV). (**b**) A transesophageal echocardiogram (TEE) in the ME AV LAX view showed an 18-mm Amplatzer duct occluder (ADO, indicated by the arrow "O") in place across the ruptured sinus of Valsalva. There was no residual shunt or aortic regurgitation observed. (**b1**) An aortic root angiogram displayed the device (indicated by the arrow) positioned across the ruptured sinus of Valsalva

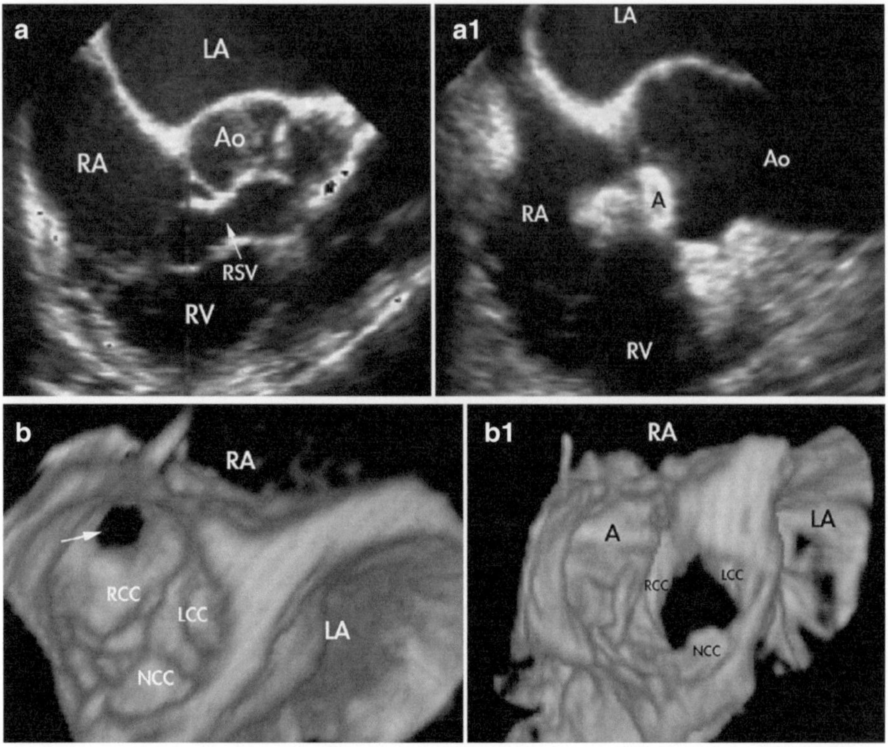

Fig. 9.3 A 12-year-old child underwent device closure for a ruptured sinus of Valsalva aneurysm (RSVA) to the right atrium (RA). (**a**) Pre-procedural 2D TEE in the ME AV SAX view reveals a 7 mm opening of the rupture of the right coronary cusp into the right atrium (RA). (**a1**) "A" labeled a 10-mm Amplatzer ductal occluder (ADO) was successfully implanted without any residual shunting as depicted in **a** with a similar view after device closure. (**b**) 3D TEE image displays a ruptured defect in the right coronary cusp (RCC) indicated by an arrow. (LCC indicating left coronary cusp and NCC indicating noncoronary cusp). (**b1**) 3D TEE image after device closure displays complete occlusion of the defect in the RCC by the ADO labeled as "A."

transcatheter closure using an occluder is shown for the ruptured sinus of Valsalva into the right ventricle (RV), while Fig. 9.3 depicts the ruptured sinus of Valsalva into the right atrium (RA). Additionally, Fig. 9.4 demonstrates the use of three-dimensional (3D) and four-dimensional (4D) transesophageal echocardiography

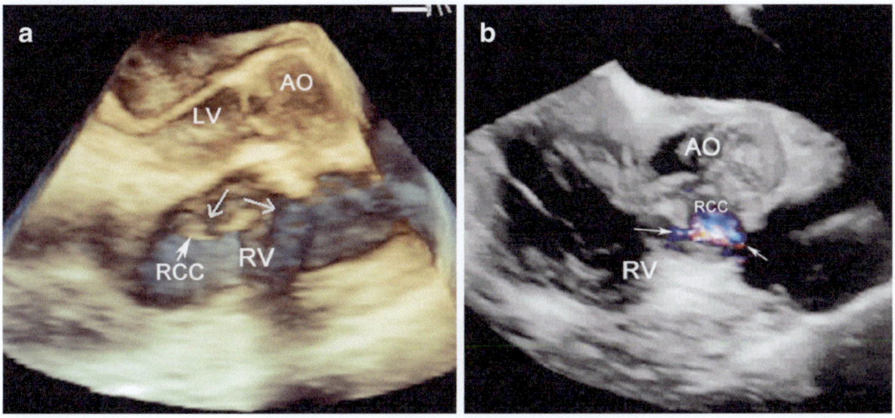

Fig. 9.4 Illustrates the utilization of three-dimensional (3D) and four-dimensional (4D) trans-esophageal echocardiography (TEE) in the planning of transcatheter treatment for a ruptured sinus of Valsalva aneurysm (RSVA) that extends into the right ventricle (RV). (**a**) 3D TEE, taken from an enface right RV view in the modified extended aortic valve long-axis (ME AV LAX) view, clearly shows an RSVA extending into the RV chamber. Additionally, it reveals two exits of the right coronary cusp (RCC) indicated by the presence of two white arrows. (**b**) 4D TEE reveals blood flow draining from the RCC into the RV chamber through two distinct exits, indicated by two arrows. (Online Video 9.1)

(Video clip for Fig. 9.4b) in planning the transcatheter treatment of a sinus of Valsalva aneurysm that extends into the RV. Lastly, Fig. 9.5 addresses intraoperative iatrogenic ruptured of sinus Valsalva during aortic valve surgery.

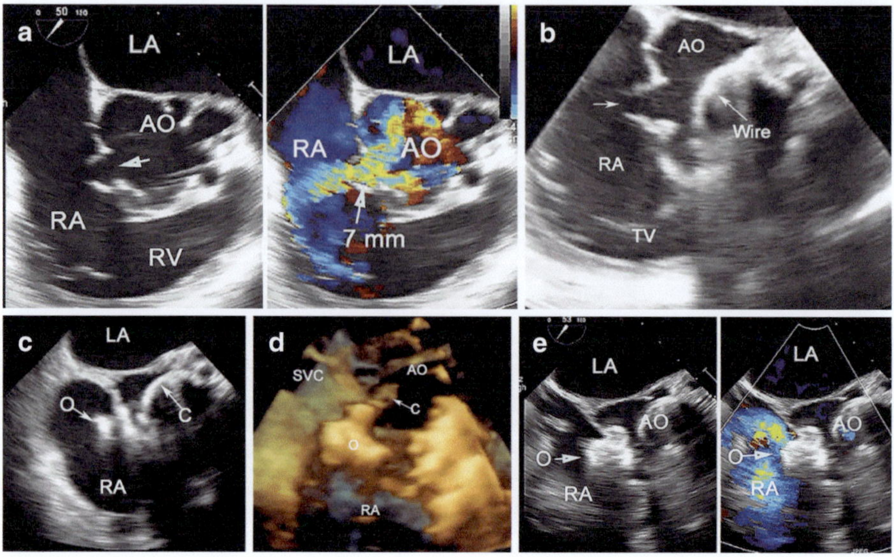

Fig. 9.5 Repair of an iatrogenic ruptured sinus of Valsalva (RSV) during aortic surgery using an intraoperatively deployed Amplatzer ductal occluder (ADO) (**a**) During cardiac surgery, an accidental ruptured sinus of Valsalva occurred, as shown in the intraoperative TEE in the ME AV SAX view. The image reveals a ruptured ostium of the sinus of Valsalva, indicated by an arrow, with an opening of 7 mm and a pronounced left-to-right shunt on the color Doppler (right diagram) between the right coronary sinus and the right atrium (RA). Additionally, mild aortic regurgitation is present. (**b**) An intraoperative, retrograde approach to device closure was performed under TEE monitoring, which depicted difficulty in passing the guide wire (arrow) through the opening of the ruptured ostium of the sinus of Valsalva from the aorta (AO) into the right atrium (RA). (**c**) Successful passage of the wire through the opening of the ruptured ostium of the sinus of Valsalva was achieved by manually manipulating the wire. (**d**) 3D TEE image displays a successful deployment of a Amplatzer ventricular septal defect occluder (O). (**e**) Color Doppler TEE in the ME AV SAX view depicts a properly positioned occluder (O) after release, without any residual shunting or aortic regurgitation

References

1. Takach TJ, Reul GJ, Duncan JM, et al. Sinus of Valsalva aneurysm or fistula: management and outcome. Ann Thorac Surg. 1999;68:1573–7.
2. Moustafa S, Mookadam F, Cooper L, et al. Sinus of Valsalva aneurysms—47 years of a single center experience and systematic overview of published reports. Am J Cardiol. 2007;99:1159–64.
3. Murray EG, Minami K, Kortke H, et al. Traumatic sinus of Valsalva fistula and aortic valve rupture. Ann Thorac Surg. 1993;55:760–1.
4. Kuriakose EM, Bhatla P, McElhinney DB. Comparison of reported outcomes with percutaneous versus surgical closure of ruptured sinus of Valsalva aneurysm. Am J Cardiol. 2015;115(3):392–8.

9.3 Aorto-Left Ventricular Tunnel (ALVT)

Aorto-left ventricular tunnel (ALVT) is a congenital extracardiac channel that connects the ascending aorta, located above the sinotubular junction, to either the left or right ventricular cavity. It was initially described by Levy et al in 1963 [1]. The severity of symptoms associated with ALVT depends on the size and location of the tunnel, as well as the degree of aortic regurgitation [2, 3] (as depicted in Fig. 9.6). In the context of aneurysmal ALVT, an aneurysm refers to the development of dilation specifically within the tunnel connecting the aorta and the left ventricle. ALVT accompanied by a sinus of Valsalva aneurysm (SVA) [4] can lead to difficulties in diagnosis and repair.

The treatment of choice for ALVT with severe regurgitation is surgical management. Transcatheter tunnel closure is reserved for cases where the tunnel is located away from the coronary ostia, and there is no distortion of the aortic valvular cusp or significant valvular aortic regurgitation. The details of the transcatheter repair are discussed in Fig. 9.6. Additionally, the management of ALVT with a large SVA is discussed in Figs. 9.7 and 9.8.

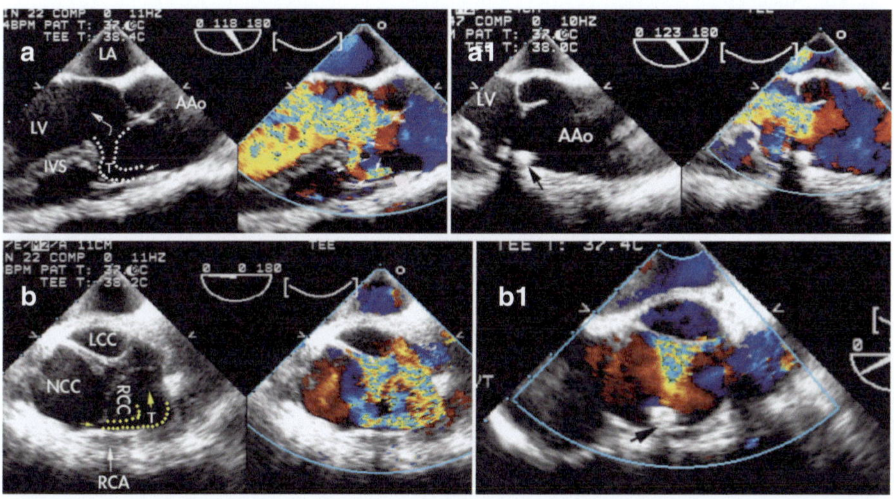

Fig. 9.6 Device closure of aorto-left ventricular tunnel (ALVT) in a10-year-old boy. (**a**) Pre-procedural transesophageal echocardiography (TEE) with color Doppler in the ME AV LAX view displays the 4-mm-sized aorto-left ventricular tunnel (ALVT) (white dotted line) originating from the aorta. The color Doppler image highlights the severe diastolic aortic regurgitation via the tunnel. (**a1**) Following device closure, the post-procedural color Doppler TEE in the ME AV LAX view depicts a 7-mm Amplatzer duct occluder (ADO) (indicated by the black arrow) effectively sealing the ALVT, with mild-to-moderate aortic regurgitation (AR) present at the valve. (**b**) Pre-procedural TEE with color Doppler in the ME AV SAX view displays a significant diastolic aortic regurgitation (AR) jet originating from the aorta and flowing through the aorto-left ventricular tunnel (ALVT, indicated by yellow dotted line). (**b1**) TEE in the ME AV SAX view depicts the Amplatzer occluder (O) (indicated by a black arrow) completely occluding the aorto-left ventricular tunnel (ALVT) and still displaying mild-to-moderate aortic egurgitation from the aortic valve

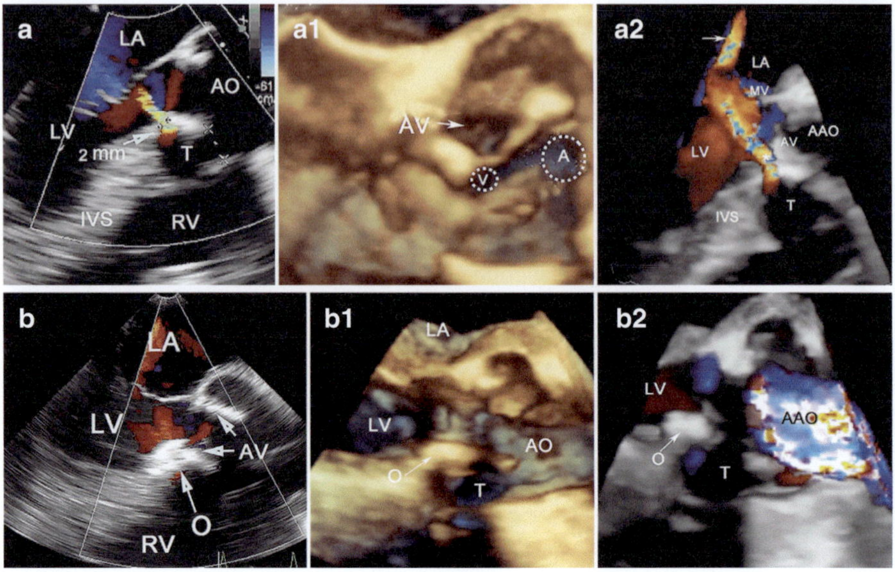

Fig. 9.7 Aneurysmal aorto-left ventricular tunnel (ALVT) undergoing device closure. (**a**) Before the procedure, a 2D TEE with color Doppler in the ME AV SAX view reveals a tunnel-like structure (T) communicating between the ascending aorta and left ventricle (LV). This structure has a pouch-like appearance anterior to the aorta and measures 2 mm in diameter at the LV opening and 4 mm at the aortic orifice. There is no evidence of aortic regurgitation. (**a1**) 3D TEE image of the aortic valve view showing the aortic opening "A" of the tunnel, which measures 4 mm and is positioned anterior to the aortic valve. The ventricular opening of the tunnel is indicated by "V." (**a2**) 3D TEE with color image showing a significant color jet running from the ventricular orifice (asterisk) of the tunnel to the LV and hitting the MV causing mitral regurgitation (arrow). (**b**) Post-procedural 2D TEE image in the ME AV LAX view showing a 4-mm ADO occluder (O) successfully implanted, completely occluding the ALVT and without any residual shunting. (**b1**) Post-procedural 3D TEE image shows complete occlusion of the tunnel by the occluder (O). (**b2**) 3D color TEE image showing complete occlusion of the tunnel without any residual shunting and without any evidence of mitral regurgitation

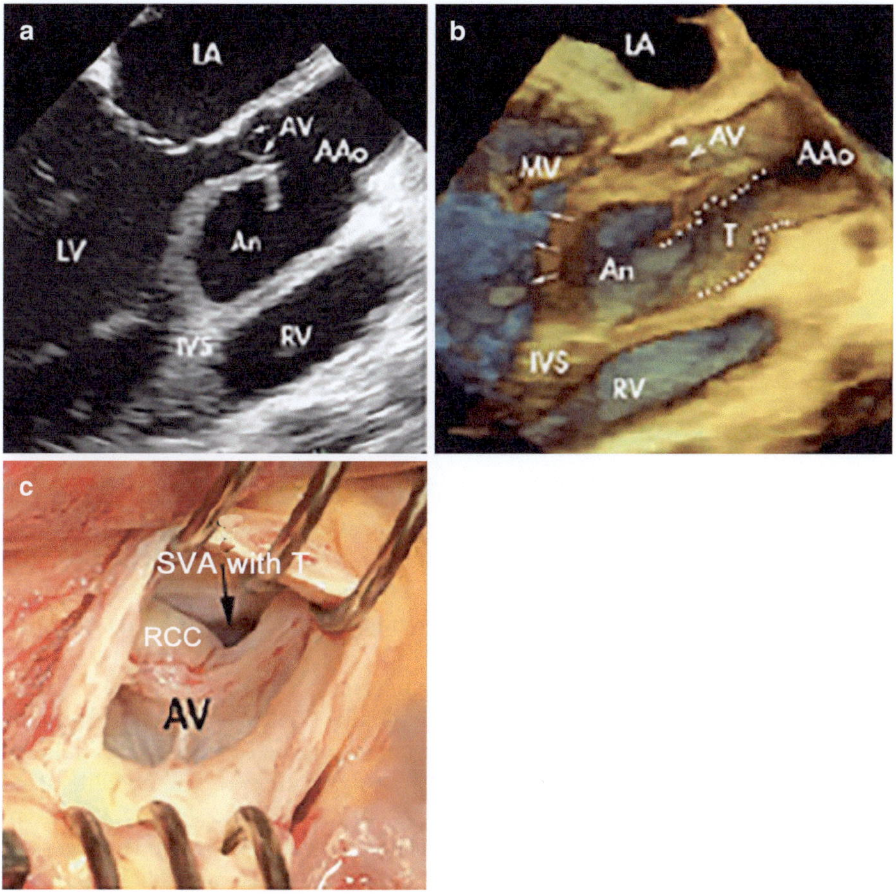

Fig. 9.8 Closure of aneurysmal aorto-left ventricular tunnel (ALVT). (**a**) Two-dimensional TEE showing the dilated ascending aorta and its connection to an interventricular aneurysm in the ME AV LAX view. (**b**) Three-dimensional TEE Illustrates a significant tunnel starting from the ascending aorta (AAo) and entering the left ventricle (LV) through an aneurysm (An) of the tunnel (white dotted line). The aneurysm causes displacement of the interventricular septum and results in partially blocked left ventricular outflow. Surgical repair is required as device closure is not feasible. (**c**) Surgeon's view of the orifice of the aorta into the tunnel (T), with the aortic orifice of the tunnel measuring 1.5 × 1 cm in diameter, consistent with TEE findings

References

1. Levy MJ, Lillehei CW, Anderson RC, et al. Aortico-left ventricular tunnel. Circulation. 1963;27:841.
2. Okoroma EO, Perry LW, Scott LP, McClenathan JE. Aortico-left ventricular tunnel: clinical profile, diagnostic features and surgical considerations. J Thorac Cardiovasc Surg. 1976;71:238–44.
3. Kathare P, Subramanyam RG, Dash TK. Diagnosis and management of aorto-left ventricular tunnel. Ann Pediatr Cardiol. 2015;8:103–7.
4. Spooner EW, Dunn JM, Behrendt DM, et al. Aortico-left ventricular tunnel and sinus of Valsalva aneurysm case report with operative repair. J Thorac Cardiovasc Surg. 1978;75:232–6.

9.4 Aortic Injury During Electrophysiological Studies (EPSs)

Complications of cardiac electrophysiological studies (EPS) may include arterial injury (0.4%), thrombophlebitis (0.6%), systemic arterial embolism (0.1%), pulmonary embolism (0.3%), and cardiac perforation (0.2%) [1]. Inadvertent aortic injury can occur during EPS when catheters are inserted and manipulated, particularly in patients with anatomical variations. Acute traumatic aortic injury (ATAI) is associated with significant morbidity and mortality [2].

Rapid detection is crucial for diagnosing inadvertent aortic injury and planning the management. Transesophageal echocardiography (TEE) is particularly valuable in the acute setting as it can be performed quickly at the bedside and offers detailed information about the location, extent, and severity of the aortic injury (illustrated in Fig. 9.9). The appropriate treatment strategy depends on the severity and extent of the injury. Surgical repair may be necessary in certain cases, while successful intraprocedural transcatheter closure with an occluder is also an additional option and will be discussed in Fig. 9.9.

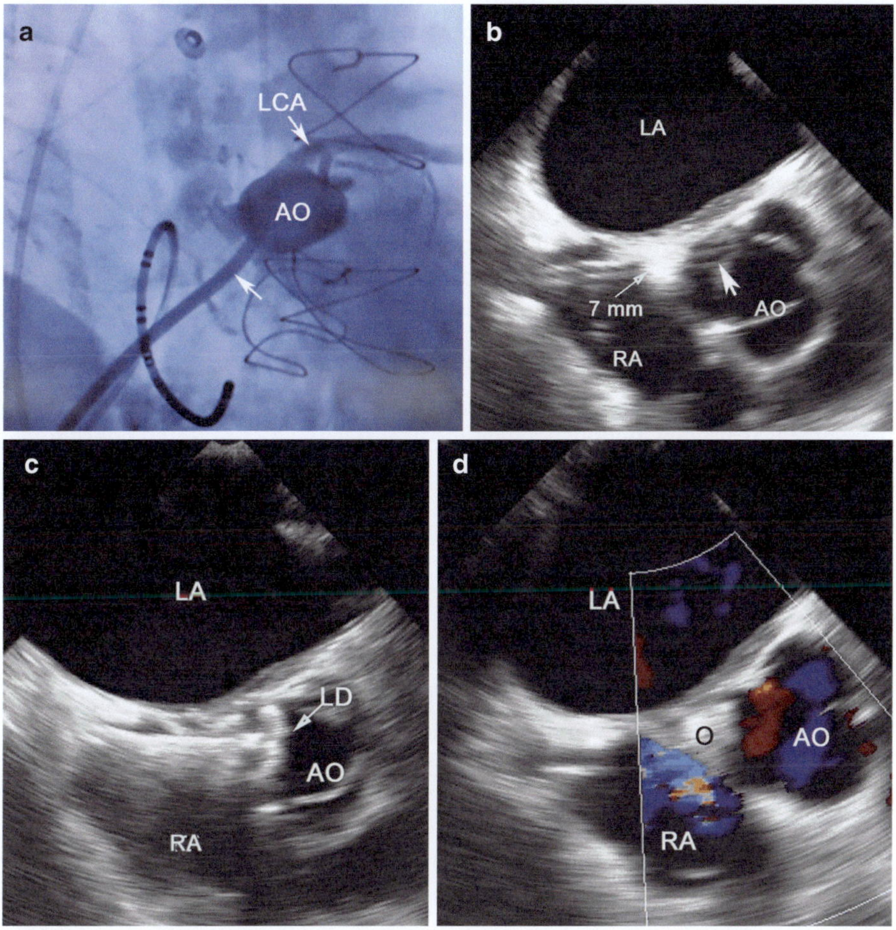

Fig. 9.9 Inadvertent aortic penetration injury during electrophysiology study (EPS) procedure. (**a**) Left anterior oblique (LAO) fluoroscopic image reveals the aortic root and left coronary artery (LCA) following a test injection of contrast medium using a Mullins sheath (indicated by arrow), signifying an accidental penetration injury to the aorta. (**b**) Transesophageal echocardiogram in ME AV SAX view showing the penetration of the Mullins sheath (arrow) from the right atrium into the aorta with a 7 mm opening in the aortic wall. (**c**) Guided wire and delivery sheath were introduced into the aorta through the Mullins sheath, and a 7-mm Amplatzer ASD occluder was deployed. TEE image shows the left disk (LD) in the aorta. (**d**) Final position of the device (O) is securely seated at the perforation site, as shown by color Doppler TEE with mild residual shunt. The recovery was uneventful

References

1. Horowitz LN, Kay HR, Kutalek SP. Risks and complications of clinical cardiac electrophysiologic studies: a prospective analysis of 1,000 consecutive patients. J Am Coll Cardiol. 1987;9:1261–8.
2. Brown SR, Still SA, Eudailey KW. Acute traumatic injury of the aorta: presentation, diagnosis, and treatment. Ann Transl Med. 2021;9:1193.

9.5 Patent Ductus Arteriosus (PDA)

After birth, the ductus arteriosus usually closes within 48 h shortly, enabling proper blood flow from the pulmonary artery to the lungs for oxygenation. However, in cases of patent ductus arteriosus (PDA), the ductus arteriosus remains open (patent), resulting in abnormal blood flow between the aorta and the pulmonary artery. If untreated, a large PDA can lead to complications including heart failure, pulmonary hypertension, infective endocarditis, and an elevated risk of respiratory infections.

PDA is typically diagnosed using diagnostic tests like echocardiography (transthoracic or transesophageal, as shown in Fig. 9.10c) or cardiac catheterization (as shown in Fig. 9.10a).

The treatment for PDA varies based on the size of the ductus arteriosus and the presence of symptoms. Small PDAs may close without intervention, but in preemies if treatment is needed, options include medical treatment prescribing nonsteroidal anti-inflammatory drugs (NSAIDs) like indomethacin or ibuprofen to promote closure of the ductus arteriosus, or in severe cases or when other treatments are not

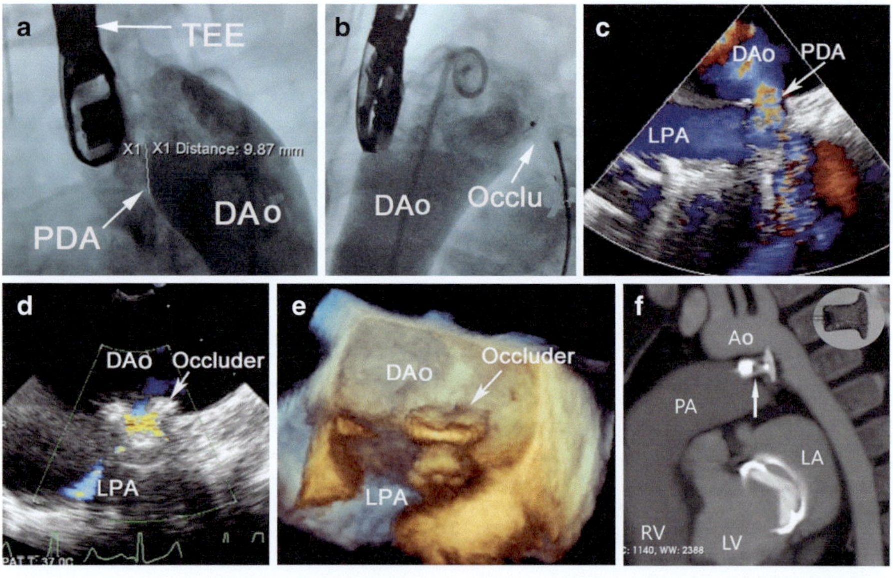

Fig. 9.10 TEE and angiogram images demonstrating device closure of PDA. (**a**) Pre-procedural aortic root angiogram showing a patent ductus arteriosus (PDA) with a diameter of 9.87 mm. (**b**) Post-procedural aortic root angiogram showing the deployment of a 12-mm PDA occluder (Occlu, ADO) in the duct. (**c**) Pre-procedural TEE image in the UE DAO SAX view displaying a large PDA with left-to-right shunting into the left pulmonary artery (LPA). (**d**) Post-procedural TEE image displaying an Amplatzer ductal occluder (ADO) positioned within the duct with a minimal residual shunt. (**e**) 3D TEE image displaying the occluder positioned within the duct in the correct location. (**f**) Contrast-enhanced CT with oblique maximal intensity projection (MIP) reconstruction reveals the Amplatzer ductal occluder (arrow) in a good position. Furthermore, the circle diagram on the upper right shows an Amplatzer duct occluder (ADO)

feasible, open-thoracic surgery or transcatheter closure may be performed to close the PDA, as mentioned in Sect. 5.2.6.

Transcatheter closure of PDA in infants is a viable alternative to surgical ligation [1, 2] (as depicted in Fig. 5.1). It is particularly considered when an infant with extremely low birth weight (ELBW) continues to experience heart failure despite receiving appropriate medical treatment and positive pressure ventilation [3, 4]. This alternative approach is discussed in Fig. 9.11.

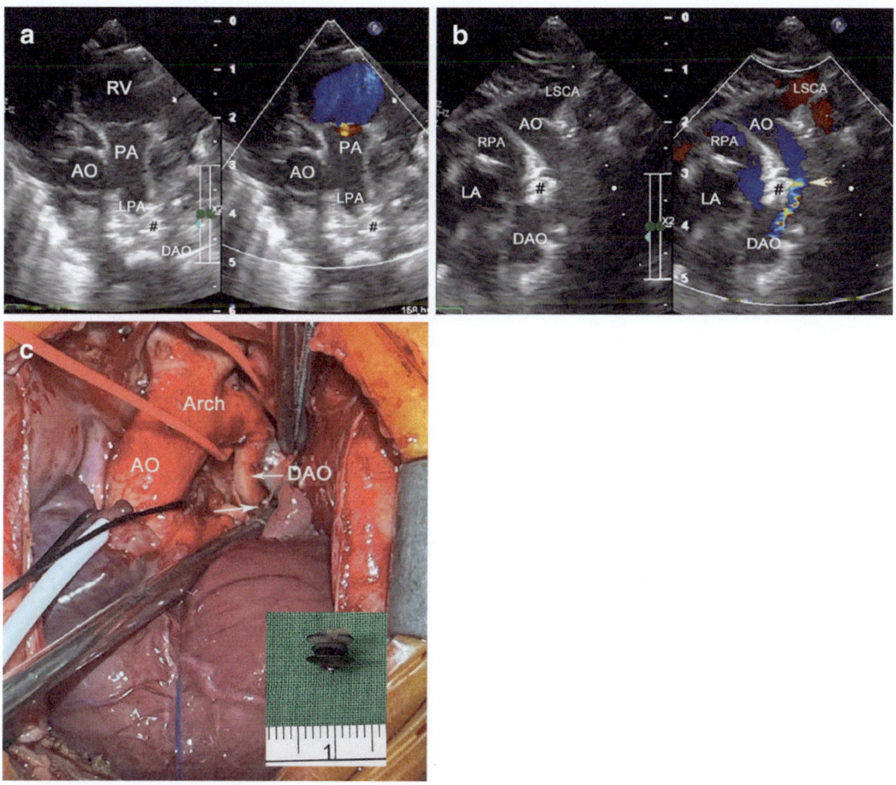

Fig. 9.11 A 6-week-old premature baby weighing 2 kg, who had undergone patent ductus arteriosus device closure at 16 days of age in another hospital. The device had migrated to the aorta, causing severe obstruction and requiring surgical intervention. The baby was admitted for this procedure. (**a**) On admission, a 2D view from the suprasternal notch in the short-axis view (right plane with color image) shows a patent ductus arteriosus (PDA) status post-transcatheter closure with an Abbott Amplatzer Piccolo Occluder (5/2 mm #) without any residual shunt. (**b**) In the right plane color image, it can be seen that the Piccolo PDA Occluder (#) has migrated to the descending aorta, causing severe obstruction (indicated by the arrow) with a pressure gradient of 27 mmHg. (**c**) This intraoperative photograph shows the successful surgical removal of the Piccolo PDA Occluder (bottom right), which had migrated and caused aortic obstruction (indicated by the arrow) at the junction of the left pulmonary artery and descending aorta. (Please note that no trans-esophageal echocardiogram (TEE) was available for this sick patient)

Device-related complications [5, 6] of transcatheter PDA closure include device embolization (when the device becomes dislodged and travels to another part of the blood vessels), device malposition, and migration (improper positioning of the device to close the PDA). The management of device migration, particularly when it causes obstruction of the descending aorta in a premature baby, is discussed in Fig. 9.11.

References

1. Azhar AS, Abd El-Azim AA, Habib HS. Transcatheter occlusion of PDA is safe and effective alternative to surgery. Ann Pediatr Cardiol. 2009;2:36–40.
2. Butera G, De Rosa G, Chessa M, et al. Transcatheter closure of persistent ductus arteriosus with the Amplatzer duct occluder in very young symptomatic children. Heart. 2004;90:1467–70.
3. Muacevic A, Adler JR. Transcatheter closure of a Patent Ductus Arteriosus Occluder using a Piccolo Ductu occluder. Cureus. 2022;14:e28226.
4. Malekzadeh-Milani S, Akhavi A, Douchin S, et al. Percutaneous closure of patent ductus arteriosus in premature infants: a French National Survey. Catheter Cardiovasc Interv. 2020;95:71–7.
5. Chien YH, Wang HH, Lin MT, et al. Device deformation and left pulmonary artery obstruction after transcatheter patent ductus arteriosus closure in preterm infants. Int J Cardiol. 2020;312:50–5.
6. Tomasulo CE, Gillespie MJ, Munson D, et al. Incidence and fate of device-related left pulmonary artery stenosis and aortic coarctation in small infants undergoing transcatheter patent ductus arteriosus closure. Catheter Cardiovasc Interv. 2020;96:889–97.

Postoperative Residual Defect

10

Catheter-based interventions can be an alternative to additional surgery when there is a remaining shunt or defect following certain congenital heart surgeries. Reoperating on these residual defects or shunts carries increased risks and mortality rates. Unlike typical defects or shunts, postoperative residual defects or shunts often exhibits morphological irregularities. These irregularities can make it challenging to determine the diameter of the remaining defects or shunts and difficult in selecting the appropriate devices for transcatheter procedures.

Indications for transcatheter intervention for residual shunt includes:

S.-K. Tsai et al., *Transesophageal Echocardiography in Pediatric Congenital Cardiac Surgery and Catheter Intervention*, https://doi.org/10.1007/978-981-99-6582-3_10

10.1 Residual ASD

When there is a residual defect such as ASD [1, 2] (as shown in Fig. 10.1) after surgery.

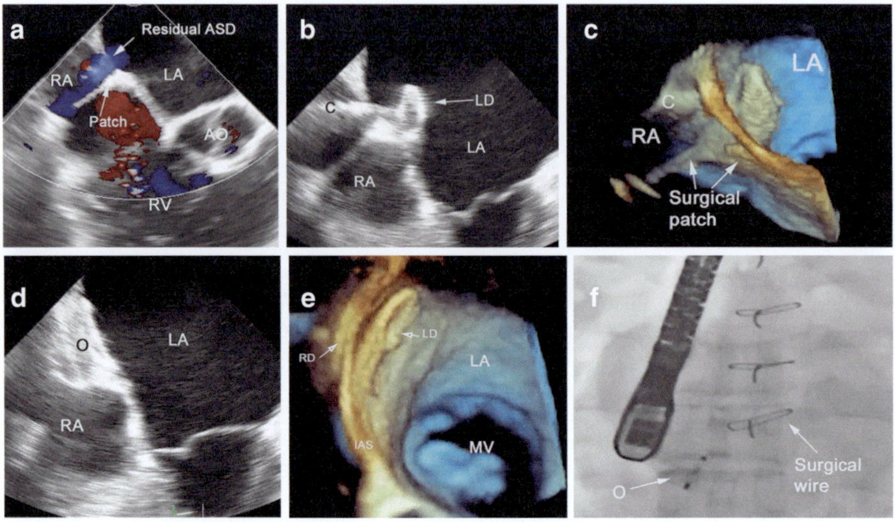

Fig. 10.1 A 10-year-old boy with exertional dyspnea underwent a device closure to address a residual atrial septal defect (ASD). (**a**) A 2D TEE image depicts a residual 8-mm ASD due to a detached surgical patch (indicated by an arrow) as seen in a ME AV SAX view. (**b**) A 2D TEE in the four-chamber view depicts the deployment of the left disk (LD) of a 10-mm Amplatzer septal occluder. (**c**) A 3D TEE image in a similar view displays a detached surgical patch and the deployment of the left disk of the occluder in the left atrium (LA). (**d**) A 2D TEE image displays the successful deployment of the occluder in the four-chamber view. (**e**) A 3D TEE image in a similar view displays the final position of the occluder (RD indicating right disk, MV indicating mitral valve, and IAS indicating interatrial septum). (**f**) A post-procedural chest fluoroscopy image displays the surgical wire and the final position of the deployed occluder (O)

10.2 Residual VSD

Postoperative residual VSD [3, 4] (as shown in Fig. 10.2).

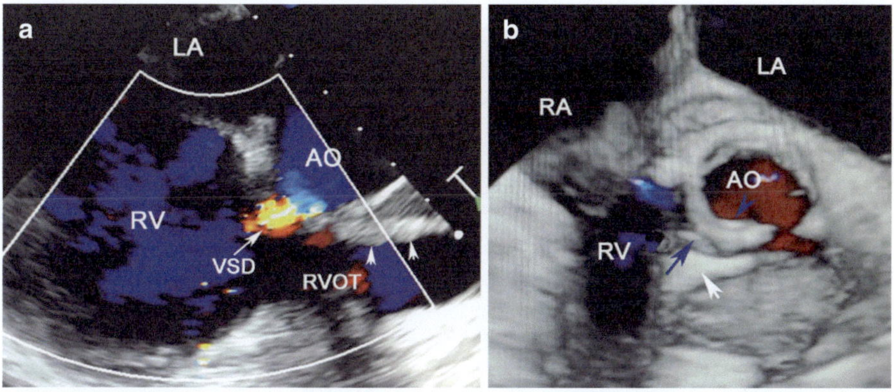

Fig. 10.2 A 12-year-old boy with exertional dyspnea underwent a device closure to address a residual ventricular septal defect (VSD). (**a**) A 2D color TEE image depicts a residual 6-mm VSD due to a detached surgical patch (indicated by white arrowheads) as seen in a ME AV SAX view. (**b**) A 3D color Doppler TEE image in the ME AV SAX view displays a detached surgical patch (indicated by a white arrow) and successful deployment of a Lifetech Scientific KONAR-MF 10/8 mm VSD occluder in a good position (indicated by a blue arrow for the right disk and a blue arrowhead for the left disk) without any residual shunt

10.3 Recurrent PDA

Catheter intervention can be used for recurrent PDA closure [5, 6] (as shown in Fig. 10.3).

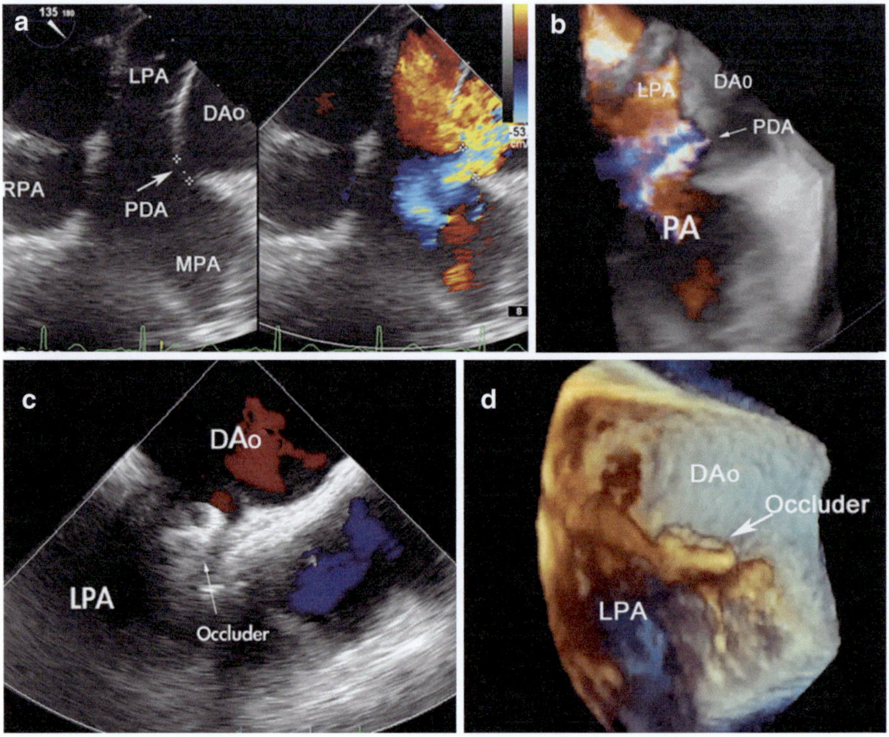

Fig. 10.3 Device closure for a recurrent patent ductus arteriosus (PDA) after a loosened PDA surgical ligation during infancy. (**a**) A 2D TEE image depicts a 7mm diameter patent ductus arteriosus (PDA) seen from an upper esophageal descending aortic view, with accompanying color Doppler image (right plane) showing left-to-right shunting through the ductus. (**b**) A 3D TEE image with color Doppler, in a similar view, depicts flow from the patent ductus arteriosus (PDA) to the junction of the pulmonary arteries. (**c**) 2D TEE image of a 10 mm ADO (Amplatzer ductal occluder) deployed, as seen from a UE DAo view. (**d**) A 3D TEE image in a similar view displays the ADO occluder securely positioned in the ductus without any remaining shunting

10.4 Fenestration Closure

Catheter-based intervention for closure of penetration holes after TCPC (as shown in Fig. 10.4) is safe and effective, with high success rates and low complication rates.

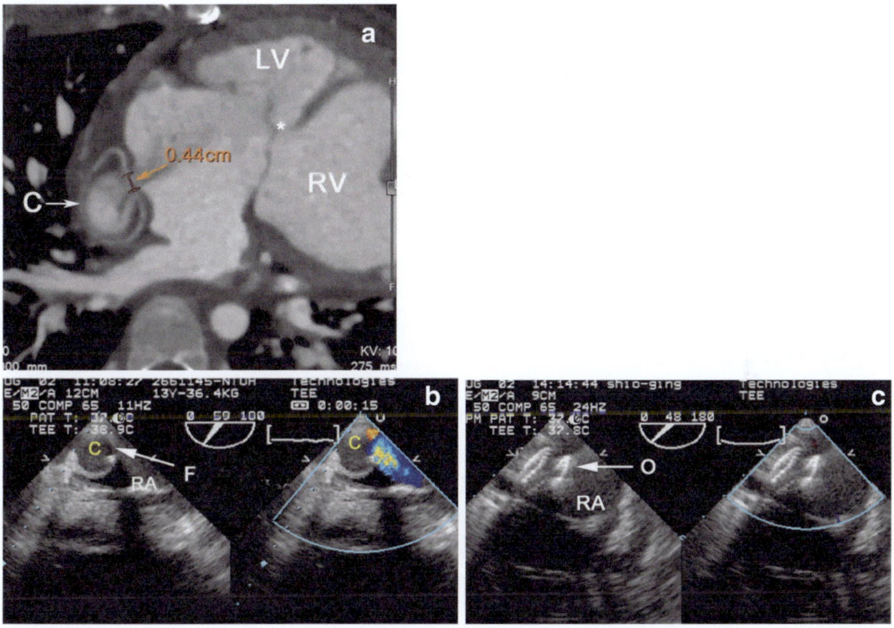

Fig. 10.4 Closure of a fenestration with an Amplatzer septal occluder in a 13-year-old patient with ccTGA/TA/PS/ASD/VSD following total cavo-pulmonary connection (TCPC). (**a**) A cardiac CT study depicts a fenestration with a diameter of 0.44 cm between the extracardiac conduit (C) of the TCPC and the common atrium. (* indicates VSD). (**b**) A 2D TEE image of a fenestration (F) as seen from a ME four-chamber view, along with a color Doppler image in the right diagram, displays shunting through the fenestration (F) between the RA and the conduit (C). (**c**) A 2D TEE image with color Doppler in a similar view after the implantation of an occluder displays a 5-mm Amplatzer septal occluder (O) securely positioned in the fenestration hole without any residual shunting

Catheter interventions for residual defects or shunts after some CHD surgeries have advantages over reoperation because they are:

1. Less Invasive: They are minimally invasive and do not require a large incision in the chest, resulting in faster recovery time, less pain, and scarring.
2. Lower Risk: They have a lower risk of complications like bleeding, infection, and damage to surrounding structures compared to reoperation.
3. Quicker Recovery: Patients may be able to return to their normal activities sooner with catheter interventions.
4. Cost-Effective: They are typically less expensive than reoperation due to shorter hospital stays and lower complication rates.
5. Better Cosmetic Outcome: They result in minimal scarring, which is important for patients concerned about their outlooking after surgery.

References

1. Krasuski RA. Catheter-based interventions versus repeat surgical procedures for patients with residual septal defects. J Invasive Cardiol. 2006;18(7):305–10.
2. Butera G, Carminati M, Chessa M, et al. Transcatheter closure of residual shunts after surgical closure of atrial septal defects: early and midterm results. J Thorac Cardiovasc Surg. 2005;129(3):497–501.
3. Momenah TS, Ebeid MR, Al-Fayyadh MM, et al. Percutaneous device closure of residual shunts following surgical repair of atrial septal defects: a systematic review and meta-analysis. Heart Lung Circ. 2020;29(2):250–5.
4. Forbes TJ, Kim DW, Du W, et al. Comparison of surgical, stent, and transcatheter closure of ventricular septal defects: a multicenter prospective study. JACC Cardiovasc Interv. 2018;11(23):2459–65.
5. Bass JL, Lucas VW, Brauner R, et al. Amplatzer duct occluder to treat recurrent patent ductus arteriosus after surgical ligation. JACC Cardiovasc Interv. 2008;1(1):84–6.
6. Jayaram N, Beekman R, Benson L, et al. Recurrent ductal patency after surgical ligation and transcatheter closure: a comparative study. Heart. 2011;97(24):2034–9.
7. Nguyen HT, Kim DW, Nguyen T, et al. Transcatheter closure of residual fenestrations after Fontan operation. JACC Cardiovasc Interv. 2015;8(8):1142–8.

Hybrid Procedure for Congenital Heart Diseases (CHDs)

11

11.1 Perventricular Device Closure of VSDs

The transcatheter closure of VSD using various devices has shown positive outcomes for over two decades, as reported in studies [1]. However, the perventricular technique for VSD device closure is a hybrid procedure that accesses the heart through a small chest wall incision under general anesthesia. Transesophageal echocardiography (TEE) is used to locate the VSD. A guided wire is then inserted through the incision and carefully directed across the VSD from the right ventricle to the left ventricle, guided by TEE. Once the delivery sheath is correctly positioned, the occluder device is deployed and released to seal the defects. The procedure involves a minimally invasive technique, enabling easy passage through the defects and precise device placements [2].

Transcatheter closure of muscular VSDs in infants [3–5] is challenging and poses a high risk of complications due to the disparity between the sheath size and the vascular access in the patient. Figure 11.1 addresses the minimally invasive perventricular device closure technique for muscular VSDs.

Additionally, in children with an outlet VSD, the spiraling path of the ventricular septum adds complexity to percutaneous transcatheter closure procedures. However, the perventricular approach allows for easier passage of a short sheath directly through the defect and precise device positioning [6]. This technique is detailed in Fig. 11.2.

S.-K. Tsai et al., *Transesophageal Echocardiography in Pediatric Congenital Cardiac Surgery and Catheter Intervention*, https://doi.org/10.1007/978-981-99-6582-3_11

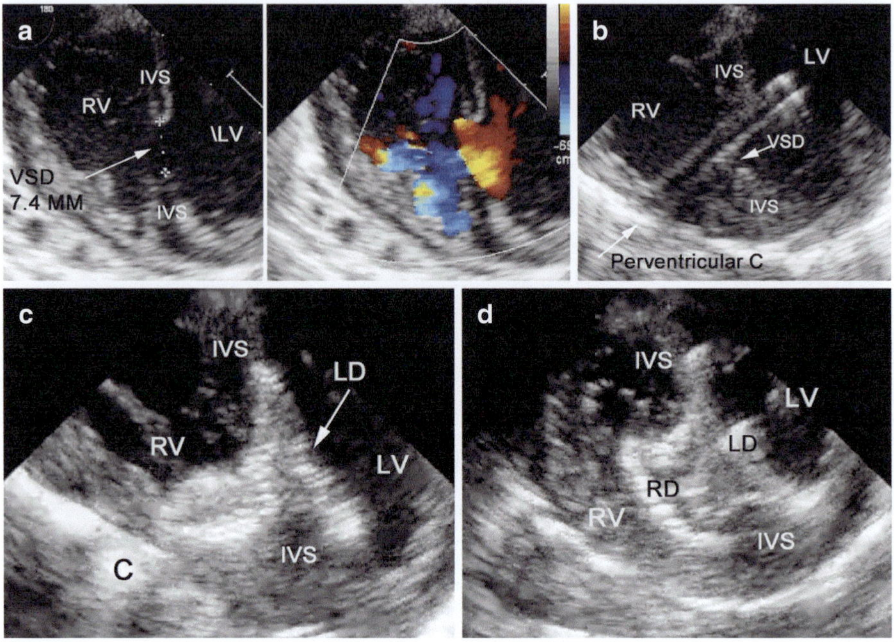

Fig. 11.1 A one-month-old infant with a muscular ventricular septal defect underwent a hybrid procedure for device closure. (**a**) A 2D TEE image of a muscular ventricular septal defect measuring 7.4 mm is shown in a four-chamber view, with a color Doppler image that displays left-to-right shunting through the defect. (**b**) A 2D TEE image in the modified four-chamber view reveals a perventricular catheter passing through the right ventricular wall to the left ventricle via the muscular ventricular septal defect, as guided by TEE. (**c**) A 2D TEE image in the modified four-chamber view shows the deployment of the left disk in the left ventricle. (**d**) A similar view of TEE displays the final position of a 10-mm muscular occluder

References

1. Carminati M, Butera G, Chessa M, et al. Transcatheter closure of congenital ventricular septal defects: results of the European Registry. Eur Heart J. 2007;28:2361–8.
2. .Xing Q, Pan S, An Q, et al. Minimally invasive perventricular device closure of perimembranous ventricular septal defect without cardiopulmonary bypass: multicenter experience and mid-term follow-up. J Thorac Cardiovasc Surg. 2010;139:1409–15.
3. Holzer R, Balzer D, Cao QL, et al. Device closure of muscular ventricular septal defects using the Amplatzer muscular ventricular septal defect occluder: immediate and mid-term results of a U.S. registry. J Am Coll Cardiol. 2004;43:1257–63.
4 Bacha EA, Cao QL, Galantowicz ME et al. Multicenter experience with perventricular device closure of muscular ventricular septal defects. Pediatr Cardiol. 2005;26:169–175.
5. Bacha EA, Cao QL, Galantowicz ME. Multicenter experience with perventricular device closure of muscular ventricular septal defects. Pediatr Cardiol 2005;26:169–75.

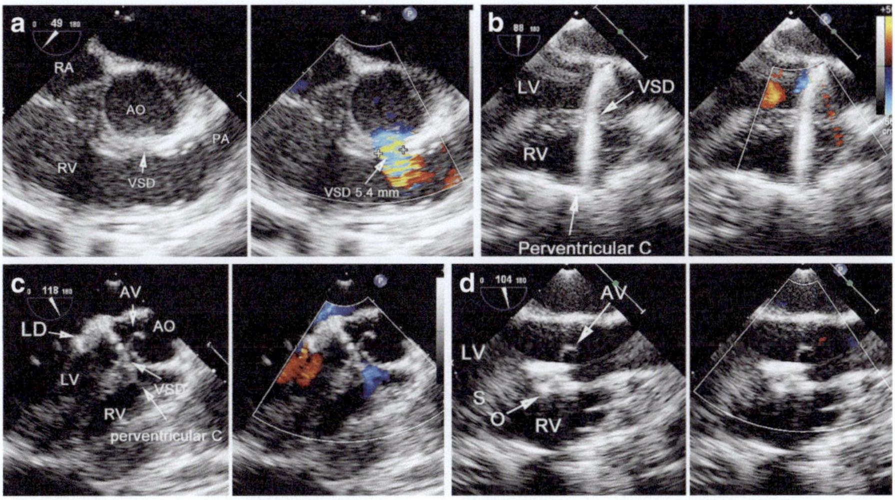

Fig. 11.2 A four-month-old infant with an outlet ventricular septal defect underwent perventricular closure of the defect. (**a**) A 2D TEE image of an outlet ventricular septal defect measuring 5.4 mm is shown in a ME AV SAX view, and a color Doppler image displays left-to-right shunting through the defect. (**b**) A TEE-guided ME AV LAX view under TEE guidance shows a perventricular catheter passing through the right ventricular wall to the left ventricle via the ventricular septal defect. (**c**) A 2D TEE in a ME AV LAX axis view displays the deployment of the left disk (LD) in the left ventricle. (**d**) A ME AV LAX axis view shows the successful release of the asymmetrical ventricular septal defect occluder without shunting. "Permission obtained from Professor Haibo Song MD, at West China Hospital, Sichuan University, China"

6. Zhu D, Lin K, Tang ML, et al. Midterm results of hybrid perventricular closure of doubly committed subarterial ventricular septal defects in pediatric patients. J Card Surg. 2014;29:546–53.

11.2 Hybrid Procedure for Newborn Baby with Complex CHDs

11.2.1 Hybrid Procedure of Surgical Bilateral Pulmonary Artery Banding and Percutaneous Patent Ductus Arteriosus (PDA) Stenting in a Newborn with Hypoplastic Left Heart Syndrome (HLHS)

The purpose of the hybrid procedure for a newborn with hypoplastic left heart syndrome (HLHS) [1–3] is to serve as a bridge to subsequent surgical stages and to stabilize the patient's condition that provides time for further growth and development before more definitive surgical interventions for Norwood procedure (as mentioned in Sect. 4.3).

The hybrid procedure includes a surgical pulmonary artery banding to restrict blood flow to the lungs, thereby balancing the blood flow between the systemic and pulmonary circulation. Additionally, a percutaneous transcatheter PDA stent is

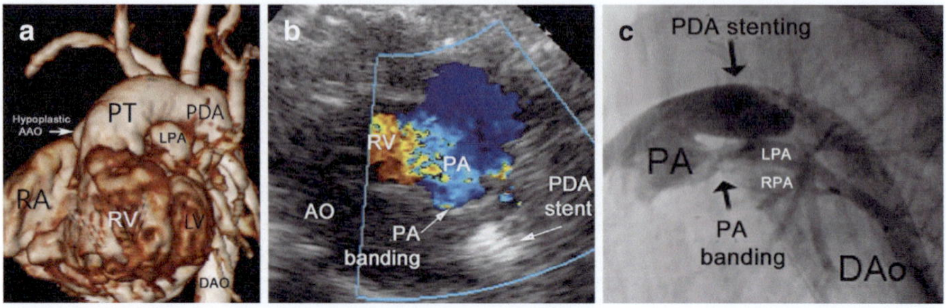

Fig. 11.3 A newborn with a hypoplastic left heart syndrome underwent a hybrid procedure that involved stenting of the patent ductus arteriosus and banding of the pulmonary artery. (**a**) A 3D volume cardiac image of the hypoplastic left heart syndrome displays a very hypoplastic ascending aorta, a large pulmonary trunk (PT), and a patent ductus arteriosus (PDA). (**b**) A transthoracic parasternal short-axis view after median sternotomy shows banding of the pulmonary artery (PA) and transcatheter stenting of the patent ductus arteriosus. (Note: The newborn is too weak to undergo transesophageal echocardiography). (**c**) Pulmonary angiography displays the stented patent ductus arteriosus and banding of the pulmonary artery (Permission obtained from Professor FU YC MD, at Taichung Veterans General Hospital, Taichung, Taiwan)

combined used to maintain blood flow to the body. Figure 11.3 addresses the hybrid procedure for HLHS in a newborn.

References

1. Galantowicz M, Cheatham JP, Phillips A, et al. Hybrid approach for hypoplastic left heart syndrome: intermediate results after the learning curve. Ann Thorac Surg. 2000;69(3):893–7.
2. Murphy MO, Bellsham-Revell H, Morgan GJ. Hybrid procedure for neonates with hypoplastic left heart syndrome at high-risk for Norwood: midterm outcomes. Eur J Cardiothorac Surg. 2014;46:14–9.
3. Laranjo S, Costa G, Freitas I. The hybrid approach for palliation of hypoplastic left heart syndrome: immediate results of a single center experience. Rev Port Cardiol. 2015;34:347–55.

11.2.2 A Hybrid Procedure of Trans-Right Ventricular Outflow Tract (Trans-RVOT) Pulmonary Valvuloplasty in a Newborn with Critical Pulmonary Stenosis

Critical pulmonary valve stenosis can be life-threatening in newborns, causing cyanosis. Percutaneous balloon pulmonary valvuloplasty (BPV) is the preferred treatment, usually performed through the femoral venous approach. However, if a newborn has critical pulmonary stenosis and inferior vena cava interruption, the traditional femoral venous approach is not possible. In such cases, alternative trans-pulmonary approaches, like the trans-RVOT (trans right ventricular outflow tract) approach for BPV, can be used. A balloon catheter is inserted through a small

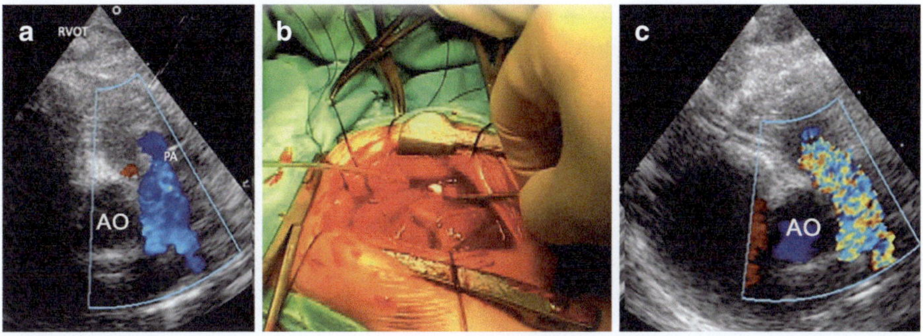

Fig. 11.4 A premature baby with a critical pulmonary stenosis underwent a hybrid procedure for balloon pulmonary valvuloplasty (BPV) due to inferior vena cava interruption. (**a**) A transthoracic echocardiogram (TTE) in the parasternal short-axis view displays the critical pulmonary stenosis. (**b**) After median sternotomy, a delivery catheter for balloon pulmonary valvuloplasty was directly inserted from the right ventricular outflow tract. (**c**) Transthoracic echocardiogram demonstrates an adequate pulmonary flow after BPV procedure (Permission obtained from Professor FU YC MD, at Taichung Veterans General Hospital, Taichung, Taiwan)

surgical incision, crossing the narrowed pulmonary valves, and guided to the pulmonary valves using direct visualization. Balloon dilation can be repeated under fluoroscopic guidance to achieve the desired outcome. Figure 11.4 provides additional information on this approach.

References

1. Kan JS, White RI Jr, Mitchell SE, et al. Percutaneous balloon valvuloplasty: a new method for treating congenital pulmonary-valve stenosis. N Engl J Med. 1982;30:540–2.
2. Rao PS. Percutaneous balloon pulmonary valvuloplasty: state of the art. Catheter Cardiovac Interv. 2007:69:747–63.

11.2.3 A Hybrid Procedure of Blade Atrioseptostomy in an Infant with Mitral Atresia and Severely Restrictive Atrial Septal Defect (ASD)

Infants with mitral atresia and hypoplastic left heart syndrome (HLHS) or transposition of the great arteries (TGA) often require immediate catheter-based septostomy to establish interatrial communication before surgical palliation. The standard approach is percutaneous transcatheter balloon atrial septostomy (BAS) for critical cyanotic congenital heart diseases in neonates. However, traditional percutaneous BAS may be challenging or unsuccessful in infants with intact or highly restrictive atrial septum. To address this, a hybrid procedure involving blade atrial septostomy is performed, guided by transesophageal echocardiography (TEE). This procedure entails incising the right atrium (RA) and using a specialized transeptal puncture blade or dilator to cross the interatrial septum from the right atrium to the left atrium, creating an adequate opening under TEE guidance. The objective is to facilitate improved blood flow and mixing between the atria. Once the desired septal opening size is achieved, the blade is retracted and removed. For more details, refer to Fig. 11.5, which discusses the novel method of perforating the interatrial septum using the hybrid procedure with blade atrial septostomy.

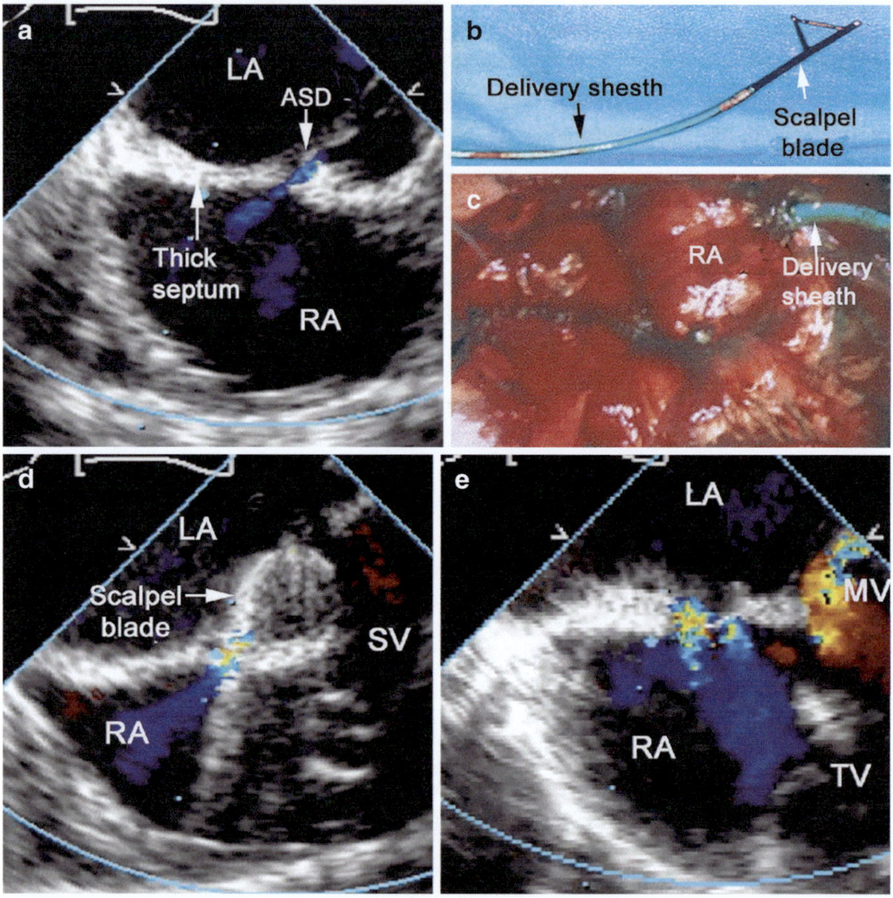

Fig. 11.5 A 1-month-old infant with severe cyanosis was diagnosed with mitral atresia and severely restrictive atrial septal defect (ASD). Standard balloon atrial septostomy was attempted but failed due to a thick interatrial septum. A hybrid procedure with an off-pump blade atrial septostomy was performed to improve the severe cyanosis. (**a**) A TEE image in the modified four-chamber view demonstrates a severely restricted ASD and a thickened interatrial septum. (**b**) This photograph displays a self-expanding triangular scalpel fully extended beyond its delivery sheath. This instrument is used within the left atrium after passing through a restrictive ASD to create a large ASD by retracting it back. (**c**) After median sternotomy, a delivery catheter with a closed scalpel blade was inserted from the right atrium (RA). (**d**) Under TEE guidance, this catheter was advanced through the restrictive ASD and into the left atrium (LA), and then, a triangular scalpel blade was opened before it was pulled back to create an atrial septostomy. (**e**) TEE image of the same patient shown in fig. (**d**) demonstrates successful enlargement of the ASD with adequate interatrial shunting

References

1. Rashkind WJ, Miller WW. Transposition of the great arteries: results of palliation by balloon atrioseptostomy in thirty-one infants. Circulation 1968;38:453–62.
2. Vlahos AP, Lock JE, McElhinney DB. Hypoplastic left heart syndrome with intact or highly restrictive atrial septum: outcome after neonatal transcatheter atrial septostomy. Circulation 2004;109:2326–30.
3. Rychik J, Rome JJ, Collins MH, et al. The hypoplastic left heart syndrome with intact atrial septum: atrial morphology, pulmonary vascular histopathology and outcome. J Am Coll Cardiol. 1999;34:554–60.
4. Gordon BM, Levi DS, Shannon. Electrosurgical energy in combination with a transseptal needle: a novel method for the creation of an atrial communication in hypoplastic left heart syndrome with intact atrial septum. Catheter Cardiovasc Interv. 2009;73(1):113–6.

Valvular Abnormalities

12

12.1 Percutaneous Trans-Septal Mitral Valvuloplasty Used for Treating Congenital Mitral Stenosis in Infants and Children

12.1.1 Congenital Mitral Stenosis (MS)

Congenital MS is a heart condition present from birth, characterized by a narrow or stiff mitral valve that obstructs blood flow from the left atrium to the left ventricle. This leads to congestive symptoms and potential complications, with varying severity depending on the degree of narrowing.

Diagnosis of congenital mitral stenosis usually involves a comprehensive assessment, including medical history, physical examination, and diagnostic imaging tests such as cardiac CT (Fig. 12.1a) and transesophageal echocardiography (TEE, Fig. 12.1b, c).

Surgical repair or replacement of the mitral valve in infants and young children is rarely performed due to higher mortality rates and poor long-term outcomes. However, percutaneous balloon mitral valve valvuloplasty (PBMV) offers a minimally invasive alternative to surgery. This procedure involves guiding a balloon catheter through the atrial septal defect into the left atrium and then inserting it across the narrowed mitral valve. The balloon is inflated to widen the valve opening, resulting in improved blood flow. PBMV is a safer alternative to surgery for congenital mitral stenosis, even in infants. Further details are discussed in Fig. 12.1

Supplementary Information The online version contains supplementary material available at https://doi.org/10.1007/978-981-99-6582-3_12.

S.-K. Tsai et al., *Transesophageal Echocardiography in Pediatric Congenital Cardiac Surgery and Catheter Intervention*, https://doi.org/10.1007/978-981-99-6582-3_12

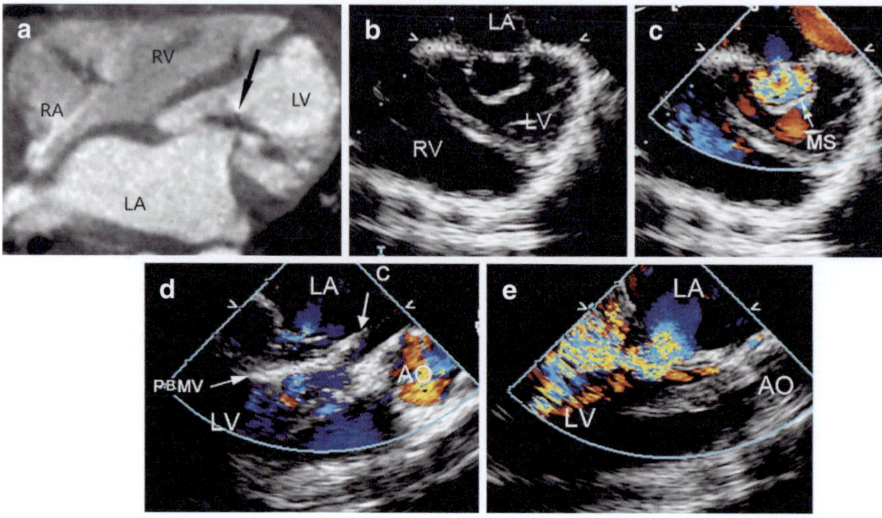

Fig. 12.1 A 6-month-old child who presented with congestive heart failure and was diagnosed with congenital mitral stenosis. The patient underwent a percutaneous transseptal balloon mitral valvuloplasty (PBMV) procedure. (**a**) Four-chamber view of contrast-enhanced cardiac CT reveals an irregular, nodular pattern affecting the mitral valves, resulting in limited opening during the ventricular diastolic phase. Additionally, the LA appears dilated, causing the interatrial septum to bow toward the RA. (**b**) A typical TEE image of a stenotic mitral valve in the ME four-chamber view shows thickened chordae and nearly nonexistent orifices in the chordal apparatus, resulting in severe mitral stenosis. (**c**) Color Doppler in a similar view shows a dilated left atrium, small left ventricle, and dispersed jets of mitral inflow through the small orifices. (**d**) TEE image in the MEAV LAX view shows a balloon catheter passing through the stenotic mitral valve into the LV. (**e**) After PBMV, the obstruction to ventricular inflow is relieved, as seen in the similar view as shown in fig. (**c**)

References

1. Gunther T, Mazzitelli D, Schreiber C, et al. Mitral-valve replacement in children under 6 years of age. Eur J Cardiothorac Surg. 2000;17:426–30.
2. Caldarone CA, Raghuveer G, Hills CB, et al. Long-term survival after mitral valve replacement in children aged <5 years: a multi-institutional study. Circulation. 2001;104(1):I143–7.
3. Kojori F, Chen R, Caldarone CA, et al. Outcomes of mitral valve replacement in children: a competing-risks analysis. J Thorac Cardiovasc Surg. 2004;128:703–9.
4. Vohra HA, Laker S, Stumper O, et al. Predicting the performance of mitral prostheses implanted in children under 5 years of age. Eur J Cardiothorac Surg. 2006;29:688–92.
4. Alday LE, Juaneda E. Percutaneous balloon dilatation in congenital mitral stenosis. Br Heart J 1987;57:479–82.
5. Kveselis DA, Rocchini AP, Beekman R, et al. Balloon angioplasty for congenital and rheumatic mitral stenosis. Am J Cardiol. 1986;57(4):348–350.

12.1.2 Mitral Stenosis in a 6-Year-Old Children

Mitral stenosis (MS) is more prevalent among adults, but it can also occur in children, although it is relatively uncommon in pediatric populations. In children, mitral stenosis is frequently linked to rheumatic heart disease [1]. Mild cases may exhibit no symptoms or minimal symptoms, while severe cases can severely compromise heart function.

MS is typically diagnosed through a thorough evaluation that encompasses physical examination and a range of diagnostic imaging tests. These tests may include transesophageal echocardiography (TEE), as depicted in Fig. 12.2a, b.

Percutaneous balloon mitral valve valvuloplasty (PBMV) [2–4] offers a minimally invasive alternative.

PBMV can be a life-saving intervention in this pediatric group, as discussed in Fig. 12.2. However, it carries the potential complication of mitral valve regurgitation [5], which may occur if the procedure causes damage to the mitral valve leaflets.

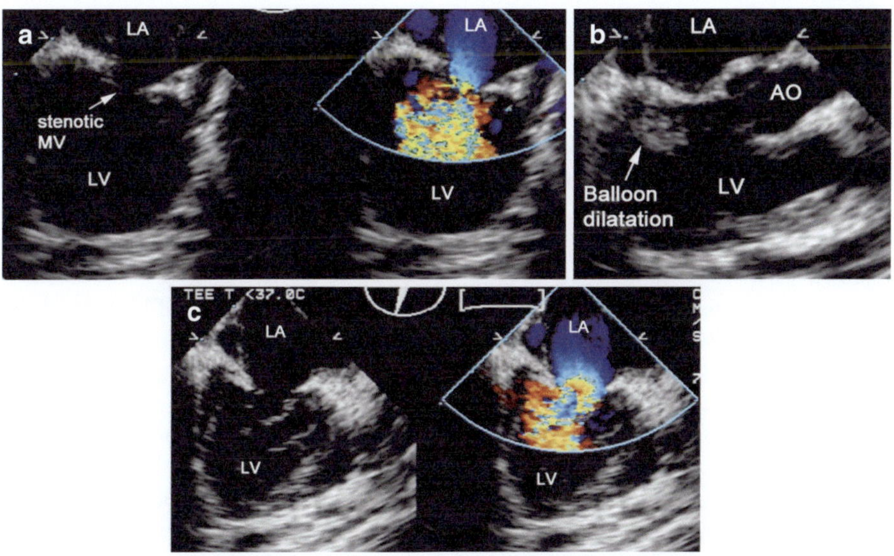

Fig. 12.2 A 6-year-old girl who presented with exertional dyspnea and was diagnosed with mitral stenosis. She underwent percutaneous transseptal balloon mitral valvuloplasty (PBMV). (**a**) 2D TEE image displays mitral stenosis with the bileaflet thickening and reduced opening. The color Doppler image (right diagram) shows a turbulent mosaic flow passing through the mitral valve. (**b**) TEE-guided balloon catheter is passed through the MV into the LV and the balloon is inflated, as seen in the ME AV LAX view. (**c**) After the PBMV intervention, there is a larger mitral valve opening and increased blood flow to the LV as seen in the color image of the bi-commissural view

References
1. Reale A, Colella C, Bruno AM. Mitral stenosis in childhood: clinical and therapeutic aspects. Am Heart J. 1963;66:15–28.
2. Sarkar A, Patil S, Ahmed I. Balloon mitral valvotomy in youngest documented rheumatic mitral stenosis patient. Catheter Cardiovasc Interv. 2015;86(5):E213–6.
3. Kveselis DA, Rocchini AP, Beekman R, et al. Balloon angioplasty for congenital and rheumatic mitral stenosis. Am J Cardiol. 1986;57:348–50.
4. Kveselis DA, Rocchini AP, Beekman R, et al. Balloon angioplasty for congenital and rheumatic mitral stenosis. Am J Cardiol. 1986;57(4):348–50.
5. Nair M, Agarwala R, Kalra GS. Can mitral regurgitation after balloon dilatation of the mitral valve be predicted? Br Heart J 1992;67:442–4.

12.2 Transcatheter Pulmonary Valve Implantation (TPVI) in Patients with Right Ventricular Outflow Tract Dysfunction After Surgical Correction of Tetralogy of Fallot

Transcatheter pulmonary valve implantation (TPVI) is a minimally invasive procedure used to treat valvular dysfunction in the right ventricular outflow prosthetic conduit. It is especially beneficial for patients who have previously undergone corrective surgery for tetralogy of Fallot (TOF) [1–3]. Traditional TOF repair surgery aims to correct defects, including widening the narrowed right ventricular outflow tract. However, in some cases, the pulmonary valve conduit may narrow again over time after surgery, resulting in recurrent pulmonary stenosis and pulmonary insufficiency.

TPVI involves delivering a new artificial valve, typically made of biological tissue, to the narrowed pulmonary valve site using a catheter. This procedure eliminates the need for repeated cardiac surgery and has demonstrated positive outcomes [4]. However, in cases where branch pulmonary artery stenosis is also present, additional interventions such as peripheral pulmonary dilation and stenting may be required.

Complications during the TPVI procedure may include the dislodgement of the stent/valve apparatus and pulmonary artery (PA) perforation. However, these complications can be carefully avoided with advances in technique and effectively managed using catheter techniques [1].

The assessment of prosthetic conduit and right ventricular dysfunction is discussed in Fig. 12.3. Transesophageal echocardiography (TEE) guidance during the TPVI procedure is discussed in Fig. 12.4. Illustrations of 3D and color Doppler images for the procedure are provided in Figs. 12.5 and 12.6 (Video 12.1).

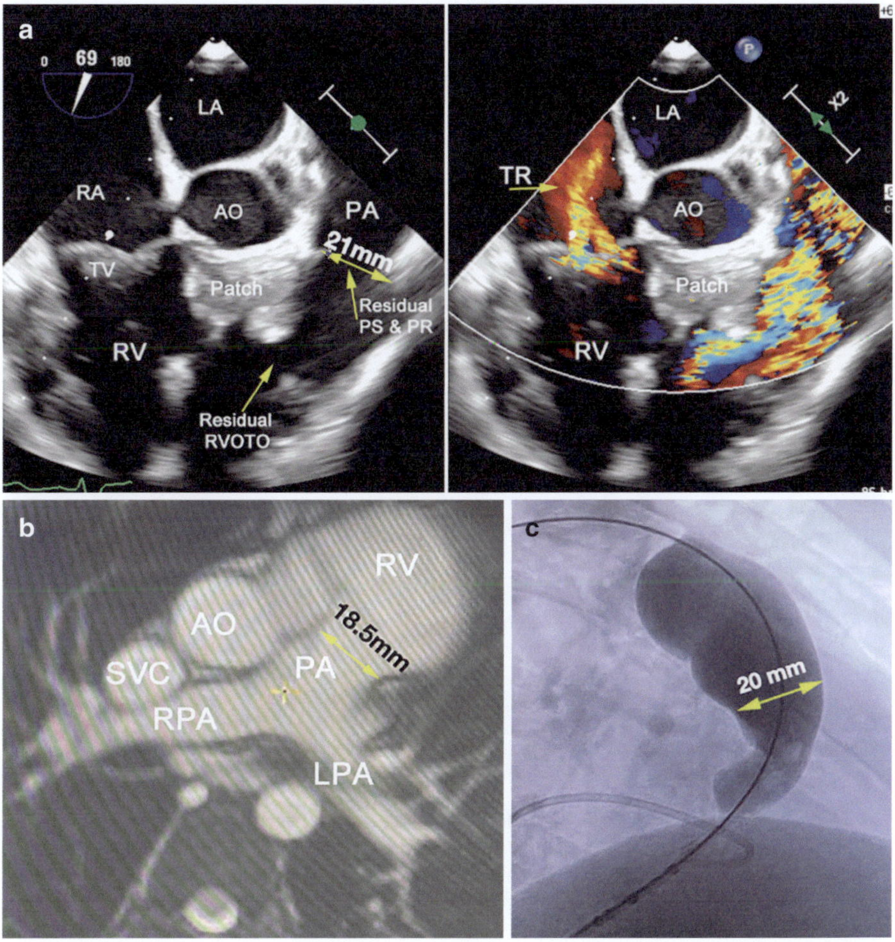

Fig. 12.3 TPVI (transcatheter pulmonary valve implantation) performed on a 17-year-old patient with severe pulmonary conduit regurgitation caused by TOF (tetralogy of Fallot). The patient had previously undergone total correction and Rastelli conduit replacement at the age of 2. (**a**) 2D TEE image displays typical residual pulmonary stenosis (PS) and pulmonary regurgitation (PR) after total correction of TOF with Rastelli PA conduit replacement. The pulmonary valve (PV) diameter measures 21 mm. The color image (right plane) shows moderate tricuspid regurgitation (TR), PS, and PR. (**b**) CT scan image reveals a PV diameter of 18.5 mm. (**c**) Balloon PA angiography shows a PV diameter of 20 mm

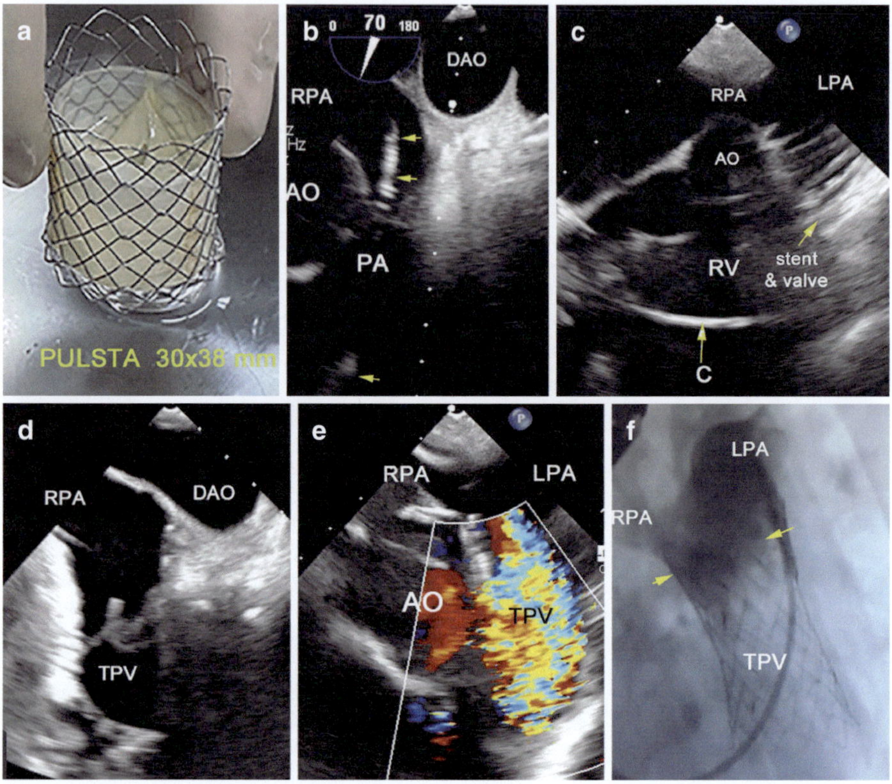

Fig. 12.4 Same patient Fig 12.3 who underwent the TPVI procedure. (**a**) Photograph depicts the implantation of a self-expandable transcatheter pulmonary valve (30 × 38 mm Pulsta valve) using a knitted nitinol wire backbone and a trileaflet a-Gal-free porcine pericardial valve. (**b**) 2D TEE in the UE PA SAX view shows the delivery catheter (indicated by yellow arrows) passing the pulmonary annulus. In (**c**), the deployment of the transcatheter Pulsta valve (TPV) at the pulmonary artery (PA) can be seen. The release of the transcatheter Pulsta valve is depicted in (**d**). The color Doppler TEE image in (**e**) shows a mosaic turbulent flow at the TPV. (**f**) A post-procedural PA angiograph displays the transcatheter Pulsta valve (indicated by yellow arrows) positioned in the PA below the PA bifurcation

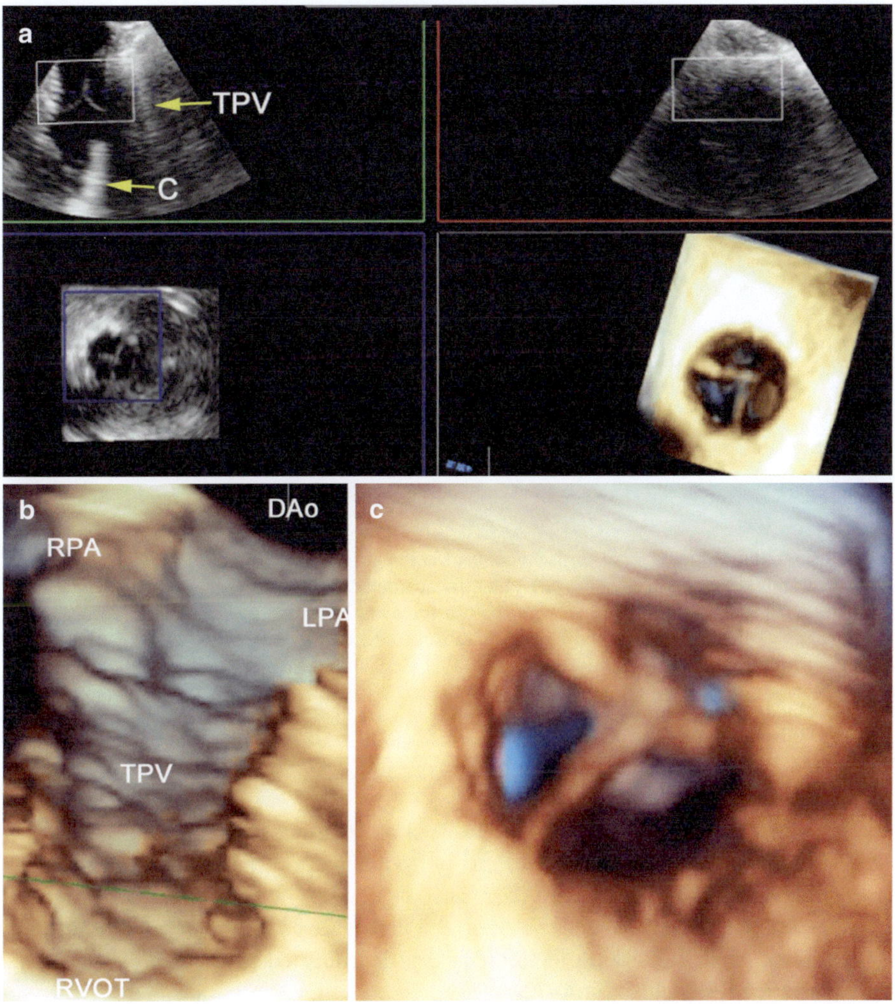

Fig. 12.5 Three-dimensional TEE was performed for transcatheter pulmonary valve implantation with Pulsta bioprosthetic valve in the same patient. (**a**) 3D TEE and MPR were conducted on the pulmonary valve after successful implantation of the Pulsta bioprosthetic valve. The plane in green bounding box provides an en profile view of the transcatheter Pulsta valve (TPV), and the plane in blue bounding box displays an enface view. The 3D planimetry of the TPV in mid-systole is depicted in the plane in yellow bounding box. (**b**) In the 3D TEE mode, the LAX view showcases the perspective of the pulmonary artery (PA) and right ventricular outflow tract (RVOT). The Pulsta bioprosthetic valve was implanted at the pulmonary trunk between the RVOT and the bifurcation of the PA. (*RPA* right pulmonary artery, *LPA* left pulmonary artery, *DAo* descending aorta). (**c**) 3D TEE mode shows an enface view from the perspective of the pulmonary valve. The number of leaflets and coaptation can be observed

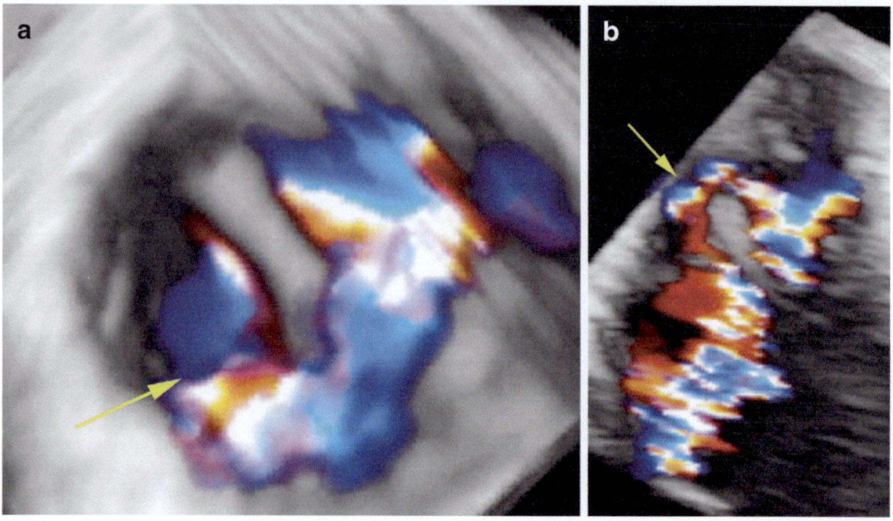

Fig. 12.6 A three-dimensional transesophageal echocardiography (3D TEE) image with color Doppler of the same patient who underwent a transcatheter pulmonary valve implantation (TPVI) procedure. (**a**) En face horizontal view of the transcatheter Pulsta valve (TPV) in a 3D TEE color Doppler image displays mild valvular regurgitation (indicated by an arrow (Video 12.1). (**b**) 3D TEE en profile longitudinal pulmonary artery (PA) view shows that one leaflet of the TPV is not fully expanding, causing mild regurgitation (indicated by an arrow), which suggests that the TPV is oversized (Video 12.2)

References

1. Bonhoeffer P, Boudjemline Y, Saliba Z, et al. Percutaneous replacement of pulmonary valve in a right-ventricle to pulmonary-artery prosthetic conduit with valve dysfunction. Lancet. 2000;356:1403–5.
2. Lurz P, Coats L, Khambadkone S, et al. Percutaneous pulmonary valve implantation: impact of evolving technology and learning curve on clinical outcome. Circulation. 2008;117:1964–72.
3. Chatterjee A, Bajaj NS, McMahon WS, et al. Transcatheter pulmonary valve implantation: a comprehensive systematic review and meta-analyses of observational studies. J Am Heart Assoc 2017;6:e006432.
4. Muller J, Engelhardt A, Fratz S, et al. Improved exercise performance and quality of life after percutaneous pulmonary valve implantation. Int J Cardiol. 2014;173:388–92.

MIX
Papier aus verantwortungsvollen Quellen
Paper from responsible sources
FSC® C105338

If you have any concerns about our products,
you can contact us on
ProductSafety@springernature.com

In case Publisher is established outside the EU,
the EU authorized representative is:
Springer Nature Customer Service Center GmbH
Europaplatz 3, 69115 Heidelberg, Germany

Printed by Libri Plureos GmbH
in Hamburg, Germany